Principles and Techniques for the Beauty Specialist

Also published by Stanley Thornes (Publishers) Ltd:

Ann Gallant	*Body Treatments and Dietetics for the Beauty Therapist*
Ann Gallant	*Principles and Techniques for the Electrologist*
W E Arnould-Taylor	*The Principles and Practice of Physical Therapy (2nd Edition)*
W E Arnould-Taylor	*A Textbook of Anatomy and Physiology*
Joyce Allsworth	*Skin Camouflage: A Guide to Remedial Techniques*
Ann Gallant	*Beauty Guides:*
	Muscle Contraction Treatment
	Figure Treatment
	Galvanic Treatment
	Epilation Treatment

Principles and Techniques for the Beauty Specialist

2nd Edition

Ann Gallant

.S.H.B.Th., Int.B.Th.Dip., DRE.(Tutor),
Teachers Certificate in Further Education

Formerly Lecturer Responsible
for Beauty Therapy at
Chichester College of Technology, and
Gloucestershire College of Art and Technology, England

Stanley Thornes (Publishers) Ltd

First edition published in 1975 by

Stanley Thornes (Publishers) Ltd.,
Old Station Drive,
Leckhampton,
CHELTENHAM
England GL53 0DN

Second edition completely reset and with new material added 1980
Reprinted 1982
Reprinted 1983
Reprinted 1984 with minor amendments
Reprinted 1985 with minor amendments, especially in the section on galvanism.
Reprinted 1986
Reprinted 1987

British Library Cataloguing in Publication Data

Gallant, Ann
    Principles and techniques for the beauty
    specialist.—2nd ed.
    1. Beauty culture
    I. Title
    646.7'2   TT957

ISBN 0 85950 444 1
ISBN 0 85950 449 2 Pbk

Set in 10/11 VIP Bembo by
Martins of Berwick
Printed and bound in Great Britain at
The Bath Press, Avon

Foreword to First Edition

A textbook on the theory behind the technical aspects of the many skills of beauty therapy has been needed for a considerable time and I therefore welcome this excellent and comprehensive book written so concisely by Ann Gallant. She states the standard required for correct skills to be acquired during a course of beauty therapy training.

It is not always understood by the general public that such a great deal of theory has to be assimilated, and a very high level of physical endeavour expended in beauty therapy training if correct methods are to be used and the proper standard of expertise achieved. Wherever the body is handled, the beauty therapist requires to work with the highest standard of ethics and care, and unless the student can learn to diagnose what she can and cannot do, which way the therapy should be done, how much is needed, and in what way she should use apparatus involved, she cannot be confident.

This book will give that confidence. It is being published at a time when courses are being re-structured and newly established in many Schools and Colleges, and recognition in the form of certificates from national sources agreed. It should receive approval. It also makes some useful suggestions for employment after training in the many choices of career available for the student qualified in the various fields within the whole subject.

Ann Gallant has given great care to writing her book, and the wealth of detail coupled with her illustrations reflect her very extensive experience. It should succeed in its aims.

Mrs J. R. Gordon. B.Sc. FHCIMA. FAHE.
Head of Department,
Department of Food, Health, Fashion and Art,
Chichester College of Technology
1975

Preface to Second Edition

I am indebted to Stanley Thornes (Publishers) Ltd. for providing the opportunity to produce a new edition of *Principles and Techniques for the Beauty Specialist*, for it makes it possible to keep the guide up to date on techniques, which are always changing and developing.

This edition includes new information on the latest procedures, both electrical and cosmetic, that have been developed recently (such as cool wax and sun beds). Manual techniques have been completely reillustrated and expanded to aid comprehension, and the makeup chapter expanded to include makeup for the dark skin.

Many suggestions for additional material, received from students and practitioners, have been incorporated, and further suggestions will be included in future books on camouflage and electrology and in teachers' guides. For all these suggestions I am grateful.

I hope that this edition will help beauty specialists all around the world to raise their standards even higher.

Ann Gallant

Acknowledgements

The author is especially indebted for much invaluable advice to Mrs J R Gordon, former Head of Department of Food, Health, Fashion and Art at the Chichester College of Further Education. To Mr John Puntis BSc for his advice on certain aspects of the scientific background to the textual matter. The author and Stanley Thornes (Publishers) Ltd wish to thank Messrs. Oxford Illustrators and Mrs Angela Lumley for their work in illustrating the book.

Contents

Chapter 1

Reception and Client Preparation

CLIENT RECEPTION

A client seeking treatment and guidance for skin improvement may have been prompted into action by a critical self-appraisal, and have already accepted the need for professional help. National or local press coverage of available skin treatments may have stimulated the interest, or a personal recommendation of satisfactory results obtained from the salon. Whatever the reason for the inquiry, the result should be client satisfaction, and confirmation of an individually designed treatment programme. The importance of the client to the salon should be evident in the reception approach and interest shown in her individual problem.

The initial impression the client receives of the beauty salon will be based on a visual appreciation of her surroundings, and the manner in which she is received at the reception. A professional atmosphere should be created, where solutions to the problems posed can be discussed without embarrassment, and adapted to suit individual requirements.

Calm efficiency and business organization should be apparent to the client from her first contact with the salon, and will instil confidence in the professional skills offered. Experienced reception technique is vital to a successful business, and an interested and knowledgeable response to an inquiry increases the possibility of the client undertaking a course of therapy from which she can gain maximum benefit. Understanding the effects and purpose of the various treatments will increase the therapist's advisory ability, and will indicate circumstances where only a personal consultation will determine the client's exact condition and its remedy.

The personal nature of the facial specialist's work will mean that a large majority of the treatments booked will follow a preliminary consultation, where the ideal opportunity exists to promote the professional services available. Much of the therapy promotion of a small clinic is undertaken by the beauty staff, as the specialized nature of the work needs to be handled proficiently to sustain treatment programmes, promote cosmetic sales, and introduce new ideas to existing clients.

A tentative inquiry, dealt with patiently, can be converted into a confirmed booking, by offering constructive advice as to the most advantageous method of treatment, and giving guidance as to the cost and time commitment required. Client satisfaction should result from fulfilling individual wishes, rather than high pressure salesmanship.

Interest in the client's minor problems will build a professional relationship within which more important areas for treatment will be revealed, which would otherwise have been hidden.

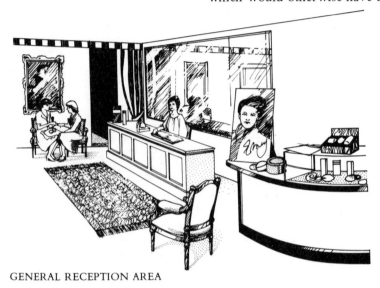

GENERAL RECEPTION AREA

PROFESSIONAL ETHICS

Development of this client relationship will depend on trust and confidence in the standard of expertise, acquired through training and experience. An evident interest in the work increases respect for the operator's personal standards and knowledge, and improves the status of facial specialists in whatever aspect of therapy they are involved. A thorough training will prepare the therapist for any situation, and enable her to adapt her knowledge and presentation to the differing demands of practical therapy, sales promotion, or demonstration techniques.

Personal appearance must be immaculate, and indicate the nature of the work. It will be a continual advertisement and example to clients. The operator's appearance and manner form the immediate visual impression which inspires or reduces client confidence, and can decide the success of the business. Disinterest in the work is quickly evident in the lowering of standards, and subsequent loss of trade due to client dissatisfaction and is both unprofessional and dishonest.

MAINTENANCE OF SALON RECORDS

To promote efficiency, salon treatment cards should contain not only the home address, telephone number, and medical background of the client, but also form a record of treatments completed and results achieved. Skin diagnosis information (Chapter 2), existing abnormalities, sensitivity, and previous allergic reactions should give guidance as to suitable treatment. Observation of changes occurring during a course of therapy must be noted, as improvement and progress may depend on a reappraisal and possible change of treatment being indicated. Both standard and supplementary treatments should be recorded, i.e. facial therapy and eye lash tinting, to determine general progress and the lasting properties of additional items. Records of depilatory treatment can also show changes in hair growth pattern needing further investigation and a more remedial approach.

HEALTH & BEAUTY CLINIC

Name	Address	Tel.
Mrs. P. Smith	21 Bantland Rd., Felixport FX1 2GB	9674

Skin diagnosis Dehydrated skin. Tendency to dilated capillaries. Sensitive to lanolin. Loss of skin tone in neck area.

Date	Treatment record	Special care & cosmetic sales
19·9·79	Continental facial. Lip wax	HOME CARE ADVISED - cleansing preparations
26·9·79	Continental facial. Eye brow shape	- toner (tissue firmer)
3.10·79	Warm oil mask therapy	- night cream
10·10·79	" " "	- under makeup nutrient base
24.10·79	Continental facial / Indirect H/F	
31·10·79	" " Lash + brow tint	MAKEUP PREPARATIONS - tinted foundations
	Makeup	- powder/cream eye shadows
12·11·79	Facial with muscle toning. Lip wax	- non-allergic lipstick; tawny pink
		- mascara; dark brown

SALON RECORD CARD

Maintained salon record cards give the therapist a complete résumé of treatments applied, progress achieved and problems encountered, and help her to decide the client's future needs. In difficult skin conditions, where medical approval is required, the record card shows both the successful and regressive aspects of the therapy, and can indicate future direction. Electrical treatments which are progressive, i.e. sun tanning, or muscle contraction, are of particular importance to record, to ensure safe levels of application. In times of illness or staff changes, the client's records form a valuable guide to possible treatment, and give cautionary suggestions as to method and client tolerance.

BOOKING AN APPOINTMENT

Telephone or personal inquiries should be dealt with clearly, and the exact nature of the treatment, and the time required, determined prior to booking. Client satisfaction will result if suggestions regarding the treatments and sequence can be agreed before the appointment is made. Additions to basic therapy, i.e. eyebrow shape, or manicure, must be booked, and a time allowance allocated, both for preparation purposes, and as a reminder when preparing the account.

Salon price lists and explanatory leaflets can instigate inquiries, and should be attractively presented, with details of the treatments available. Telephone inquiries may sometimes be best resolved by sending a treatment leaflet, and price guide, particularly on specialized routines requiring detailed information. Potential clients may then avail themselves of the consultation service offered, to determine exact needs.

A selection of treatments should be displayed both in price lists and show cards, giving a cost indication to the client. Listing all available treatments is unnecessary and confusing.

THE INITIAL TREATMENT

The first treatment should be basic in its application and allow time for discussion to determine the skin diagnosis and suitable home care. Previous skin behaviour, problems encountered, and history of allergic reaction will add background to the skin condition observed during treatment. Therapy and cosmetic advice may be discussed at appropriate times during the facial sequence, and product application demonstrated. Confirmation of a course of facial therapy depends both on the client's confidence in the operator's abilities, and the sales approach to further treatment and cosmetic care.

COSMETIC SALES

Cosmetic and makeup advice should be entered on the client's personal skin chart for home purchases, and maintenance of skin care between professional visits. A salon record of the sale gives information regarding periods of usage, and is useful for stock control purposes. To ensure successful

Beauty Clinic

£   p

Facial cleanse and makeup
Facial treatment

Specialized facial treatments for
dry, greasy or dehydrated skin
conditions by consultation from

Mature skin treatment

Treatment to include muscle
toning and electrical stimulation

Manicure

Pedicure

Eyebrow shaping from

Eyelash tinting

Shaping & tinting brows & lashes

Lip bleach

Course of eight or more treatments at a
special price.

Beauty Perfection

Beauty is so many things—well groomed
hair, clear and glowing complexion and a
youthful figure.

YOUR HAIR
Should be your crowning glory. Let us
help you to achieve this by expert cutting,
styling and conditioning treatments.

YOUR SKIN
This should be youthful and glowing
with firm contours. We can help you
achieve this image with expert beauty
therapy treatments.

YOUR FIGURE
Almost every woman has a potentially
graceful and attractive figure. We can help
you to attain this with our continental electrical treatments and manual massage
therapy.

For the convenience of our business
clients, the Hair Salon will remain open
until 7.30 p.m. on Friday evening.

A free consultation is advised prior to all
therapy treatments to decide the most
advantageous method of treating the skin
or body condition.

Epilation

(Removal of unwanted hair)

£   p

Lip and chin
15 mins
20 mins
Legs and Bikini
½ hr
1 hr

Waxing

(Depilatory for hair removal)

Lip
Chin
Lip and chin
Leg (to knee) from
Full Leg from
Under Arm
Bikini

SALON PRICE LIST

cosmetic sales, details of the purpose and application of the preparations advised must be concluded prior to the actual purchase from the reception or sales area.

skin care		makeup	
General Advice		Moisture Base _____	
_____		Tinted Foundation _____	
_____		Cheek Blusher _____	
Day Care	**Night Care**	Contours _____	
_____	_____	Lip Colour _____	
_____	_____	Eye Makeup _____	
Special Treatment		Additional Items _____	
_____		Skin Preparations etc._____	
_____		_____	
_____		_____	

COSMETIC AND SKIN CARE CHART

Attractive display positions will promote treatment and cosmetic sales, and must be supported by adequate stock reserves. The success of enthusiastic sales methods depends on product availability, and client disappointment can result in a loss of both treatment and cosmetic business.

PROFIT FACTORS

Salon profitability relies on the therapist's efficiency and skilful appointment planning to build trade. Punctuality and preparation for the treatment should ensure adequate time allowance for successful results and client satisfaction. Sufficient time allowance for completion of all items booked should prevent clients ever being kept waiting and avoid irritation.

A time-to-profit ratio can be used to decide which areas of therapy are self supporting, and those which require revising or recosting. Short duration items, such as lip wax or manicure, should ideally be combined with longer treatments to form a more profitable service. Even as introductory treatments they must be planned into the day's programme to fill time gaps between more profitable areas. Skilful reception techniques can ensure client satisfaction, with an efficient service achieved with maximum profit and staff utilization.

CLINIC LAYOUT

Creating a quiet and pleasant atmosphere, conducive to relaxation, is of prime importance in successful facial therapy. A balance should be set between the clinical and luxurious aspects of therapy so that all areas of treatment fit easily into the working situation. Modern multi-purpose chairs permit a large range of treatment applications, and the furnishings of the cubicles should reflect this flexibility, whilst not losing the intimacy or comfort expected.

The clinical appearance of modern apparatus can be softened by richness of colour and texture in the complementary cubicle décor. Over-elaborate or austere surroundings restrict relaxation and limit successful results. A harmonious theme of colour in salon design, furnishings, and client robes, promotes a feeling of continuity and avoids discordant elements.

Cubicle layout should provide for maximum treatment use and client comfort, whilst retaining an air of spaciousness and efficiency. Natural daylight provides colour blending accuracy in makeup applications, and reduces operator strain in detailed treatments demanding meticulous results. Use of illuminated magnifiers during treatment increases skin information and improves the standard of work possible. A flexible facial couch, providing comfortable support for differing body postures, permits application of various treatments with minimum client disturbance. Vanitory units combining washing facilities with storage space can ease floor use restrictions and give a streamlined appearance. Large equipment, either floor-based or wall-mounted, must be neatly and safely positioned to prevent accidents and avoid undue wear and tear. Small apparatus, planned into a trolley layout, with commodities and makeup requisites, must be placed for operator ease and safety in application.

General salon hygiene to prevent cross-infection, can be maintained by a regular system of cold sterilization for small implements, and use of an antiseptic cleansing agent for general work surfaces. A high standard of personal and treatment hygiene guards against the risk of infection, an essential for maintaining client confidence.

CLIENT PREPARATION

Client satisfaction can be assured by forethought in preparation and prompt attention to individual requirements. A smooth client flow will increase efficiency and salon use, and enable maximum time to be spent in personal contact and conversation. Knowledge of the day's work sequence permits preparation of record cards and treatment area for the necessary range of applications.

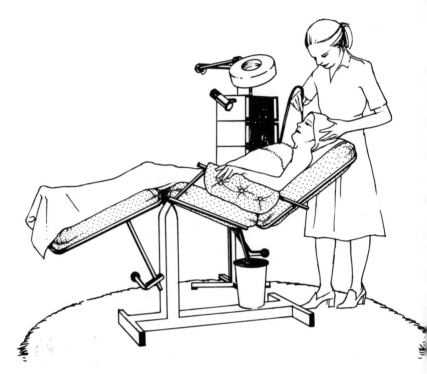

GENERAL FACIAL TREATMENT POSITION

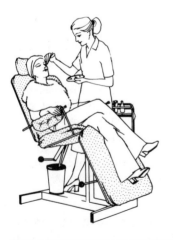

SEMI-UPRIGHT CHAIR POSITION

Equipment and stock maintenance completed in readiness for use avoids unnecessary movement or noise during facial therapy. A professional approach to the client, evident by attitude and method of work, will permit formation of a personal relationship based on trust and confidence in the operator's skill. Personal contact and guidance gives a feeling of security throughout the facial sequence, and increases client relaxation and enjoyment. To avoid uncertainty and confusion, instructions should indicate clearly the treatment sequence and participation required.

The nature of the facial therapy chosen will dictate both the method of client robing, and the situation best equipped to achieve satisfactory results. Couch positions may be adjusted to individual tastes, but should hold the body in a semi-reclining posture, whilst giving support to the spine and shoulder areas.

Complete therapy routines require a robing procedure which frees the face and shoulder areas for treatment, whilst maintaining client modesty and comfort over the extended period. Adequate chair and clothing protection prevents staining or damage and reduces cleaning costs.

Cosmetic facial applications and short duration treatments, planned to a shorter time allocation, require less preparation and client disrobing. A more upright chair position is suitable, and use of disposable materials reduces costs whilst maintaining hygiene and comfort.

Treatments involving client participation, such as makeup instruction, require a mirror reflection, adequate lighting, and the client in a natural position in order to gain a true impression of facial contours and individual personality.

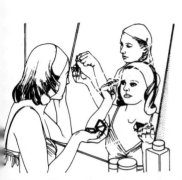

MAKEUP POSITION

RELAXATION AND CLIENT CONVERSATION

To ensure full benefit is gained from the treatment routine, relaxation should be encouraged by skilful client handling and use of conversation if desired. Client awareness will give guidance as to the amount of conversation necessary to achieve relaxation. Once a rapport has been established between the therapist and her client, very little verbal communication is required and relaxation becomes automatic. Even a client determined to chat, who gains enjoyment from the personal contact involved, can be encouraged to lose her nervous tensions under the persuasive hands and calm personality of a skilled therapist.

Topics of conversation should be neutral, avoiding controversial areas, such as politics or religion. Many clients enjoy relating personal incidents to increase self-esteem or release tensions, and this aspect of the therapist's rôle is one that must be accepted and treated with integrity. With experience little impression is retained of client's personal problems, as it is important to realize that the therapist is someone who will only listen, not give advice.

Wherever possible avoid instigating topics of conversation, and keep to professional matters relating to treatment or home care whilst the client is adjusting to the salon atmosphere.

The ability to relax does not happen automatically, it has to be developed, and the therapist's success in this area depends largely on her own personality and calmness of attitude.

Chapter 2

Skin Cleansing: the Basis of Skin Perfection

The many factors which contribute to the well being and appearance of the skin are complex and depend entirely on the client's physical and emotional elements being in balance. In normal health the skin is taken for granted, and often the problems which arise stem from ignorance of how skin functions, and how easily its balance is in fact altered. Caring for the skin of the client is one of the most important responsibilities the therapist must undertake. The basis of perfection is undoubtedly skin cleansing, through both its professional application within the salon and advice to the client for home care.

With the sophistication of products and apparatus available it is possible to deep cleanse skin extremely thoroughly, without over stimulation of surface capillaries or disturbing the delicate balance of the skin's pH (acid/alkaline balance). The usual facial routine practised in many salons does not seem to attach enough importance to the cleansing of the skin, often encouraging the addition of products to the skin rather than the freeing from its surface of adhesions and waste products, thus allowing it to function more efficiently and improve its capacity to naturally regulate its own hydrous and oil balance. This method of treatment has the additional benefit of accelerating the regeneration process, both for young and mature skins.

Diagnosis of the skin is the basis of the therapist's choice when planning a treatment routine, and whilst proceeding through the facial sequence, she must give attention to changes occurring, so that the effectiveness of the treatment can be assessed. Most skins change fairly frequently, due to internal and external factors as well as the emotional condition of the client at the time of the treatment. To diagnose a skin correctly requires a very sound knowledge of how the body functions, and a comprehension of the many different conditions which may be present at the same time on the skin of the subject. The professional therapist must decide what results she hopes to achieve with her applications, and as she has a vast range of cosmetic preparations and different electrical techniques at her disposal she should be able to blend manual and electrical treatment to produce the desired effect

Knowledge of the cosmetic chemistry function of the products used, is essential if the correct result is to be achieved. The skin should be left clean and neither stripped of its natural protective barrier, nor overstimulated, which may cause dilated blood vessels or other imperfections. Choice of the cleansing preparation is important, and consideration should be given to the task it has to fulfil, of removing makeup preparations normally worn, as well as its suitability for the individual skin texture. Extremely active cleansing products should be used with caution, as it is possible to create irritation or even an allergic reaction.

Electrical methods of skin cleansing, including brush massage, are becoming increasingly popular, and if well applied, provide a fast, professional method of deftly and thoroughly cleansing the skin. They do lack the personal touch aspects of manual methods, are not as relaxing, and do not give the therapist as much diagnosis information because the hands are not in direct contact. However, electrical cleansing is becoming more widely used, and is liked by many of the younger clients, where it normally precedes an electrically biased facial treatment, designed to accomplish a task rather than relax the client.

Use of the correct movements during the manual cleansing routine adds greatly to the effectiveness of this section of the treatment and avoids overstimulation of the skin. Skilful massage technique is important as, apart from preparing the skin's surface for further applications, it sets the mood for the entire sequence, enabling the client to become accustomed to the feel of the therapist's hands and to her personality. The client's age and temperament need to be considered carefully, and any treatment which is effective but traumatic is out of place when dealing with the more mature individuals. In their case the improvement in appearance comes as much from the rest and tranquillity of spirit they have gained, as from the actual routine of cleansing, stimulation and toning used in the treatment. With clients of different temperaments it is important to consider how best the skin's respiration can be increased through salon treatment, without upsetting the client's confidence in her therapist or spoiling the relaxation normally enjoyed. Manual methods should always be employed whilst building this rapport with the older client, and in this way the therapist can make an accurate assessment of the client's personality and willingness to cooperate with the home care guidance that is necessary.

MANUAL SKIN CLEANSING

Method of Work   When the client is correctly prepared, hair and underclothing adequately protected and a relaxed posture achieved, the cleansing procedure may be completed as a preparation to further facial treatment. The routine of cleansing strokes deeply cleanses the surface layers of the skin, and the continuous sweeping strokes of the sequence accustom the client to the feel of the therapist's hands, whilst with quiet conversation she can ensure relaxation and increased benefit from the latter sections of the facial treatment. With flowing effleurage massage movements, performed with even pressure, and in a rhythmical fashion, the cleansing preparation can be applied to all areas of the throat and face, the

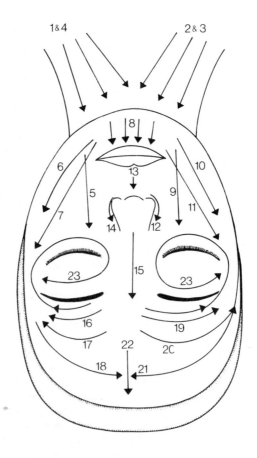

ROUTINE OF CLEANSING STROKES

hands covering the area in a superficial manner in order to distribute the cleansing cream or milk. The routine is then repeated with careful rollpatting strokes, attention being given in varying degrees to all areas depending on the amount of makeup worn and the distribution of the sebaceous (oil) glands in any area. The centre of the forehead, the nose and chin all require more repetitions of the cleansing strokes, due to the greater number of sebaceous glands in these areas, and the subsequent skin blockage which frequently results from over secretion of this sebaceous matter.

A successful cleansing routine must release all the tinted preparations from the superficial layers of the skin, remove surface adhesions such as cellular matter, and should gently stimulate the venous network of the superficial layers of the skin, causing coloration of the surface and a rise in local skin temperature.

Routine of Work

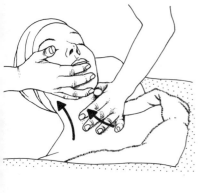

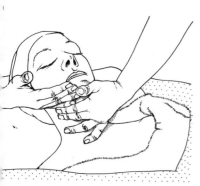

ROLLPATTING ON THE NECK

The entire palmar surface of the hand should be in contact with the skin, where the surface area allows, and adjustments can be made according to the position of the supporting bony prominences of the skull. For sensitive areas such as the upper cheeks, eyes, and trachea (wind-pipe) where heavy pressure would be uncomfortable, the speed, repetition and pressure of the strokes can be altered.

The amount of the hand or fingers used for the strokes depends on the size of the therapist's hands and the area under treatment.

The hands first mould around the neck, fitting its contours, lifting the platysma muscle from the base of the neck to the mandible (lower jaw bone), avoiding heavy pressure over the trachea. The movements work across the neck and chest area, from left to right, returning to the left side. The movement repeats more deeply and then the hands move onto the face from the left side with contouring jawline strokes. Movements on the superficial cheek muscles follow the direction of the muscle fibres, and care must be taken to avoid distorting the mouth or touching the nose. Movements should be more specific and controlled in the cheek area, with less fingers used if necessary. The position and tension present in the cheek muscles gives guidance as to suitable pressure and repetition of the effleurage strokes.

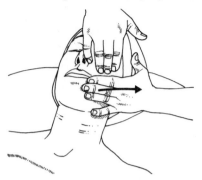
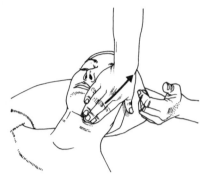

ROLLPATTING ON THE CHEEK

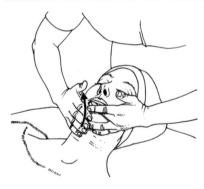

Changing direction, the hands work deeply into the chin fold and the cheek movements are repeated on the right side. Treatment of the nose follows, with detailed attention to the removal of makeup preparations in this area. The hands progress to the forehead, the movements become lighter and the speed slows to a relaxing, restful pace. Treatment on any bony area of the face should be slower, and with less pressure than is used on the rest of the face.

CROSSING THE CHIN TO THE OTHER CHEEK

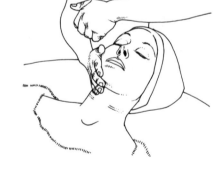

DETAILED WORK ON THE NOSE

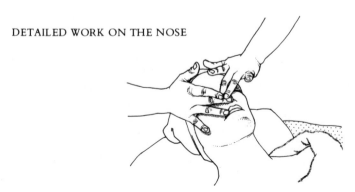

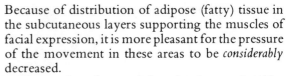

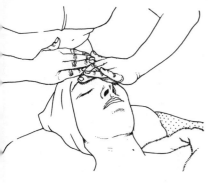

Because of distribution of adipose (fatty) tissue in the subcutaneous layers supporting the muscles of facial expression, it is more pleasant for the pressure of the movement in these areas to be *considerably* decreased.

The routine of manual cleansing is completed by gentle circles around the eye area, releasing the tinted eye makeup and mascara, whilst endeavouring not to spread them onto the facial areas. The sequence is concluded with gentle, even, upward pressure on the temples.

FOREHEAD ROLLPATTING

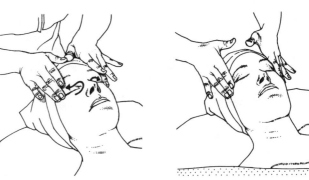

SLOW CAREFUL STROKES AROUND THE EYES

CLEANSING REMOVAL SEQUENCE

The effect of the cleansing sequence should be evident at once, in that the client appears relaxed, with less tension in her facial expression due to the reflex response of the sensory nerve endings in the superficial layers of the skin. This relaxed attitude must be maintained throughout the entire facial routine, and harsh or sudden movements avoided. It is important that the cleansing preparation is thoroughly removed from the face and throat, and this is accomplished with damp cotton-wool tissues, previously prepared. The eye and lip makeup is always removed first if present in order to avoid spreading the tinted, extremely fine textured cosmetics to other parts of the face. It is essential to remove the eye makeup very gently due to the fine textured skin around the eyes and the danger of irritation to the eye itself. Small triangular cotton-wool tissues are used, folded to achieve a flat point, and the skin of the upper lid can be supported by one hand, whilst the other hand removes the cleansing cream and eye makeup.

Eye Makeup Removal

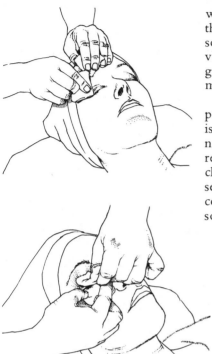

The tissues are held, one in each hand, in such a way that they will not drag the skin or press upon the eye itself and cause discomfort. One pad is held so that it lifts the eyebrow and lifts the eyelashes very slightly, whilst the other pad is used to sweep gently downwards and outwards to remove the eye makeup with small repeating movements.

The tissue is turned at the corner of the eye, to present a clean surface, and the flat area of the tissue is then lightly swept under the lashes towards the nose. Heavy mascara present can be removed by repeating the under eye stroke, and pausing to cleanse the lashes down onto the pad, using the second pad as a wiper. In this way the mascara is contained within the pads and does not spread to soil the skin or irritate the eyes.

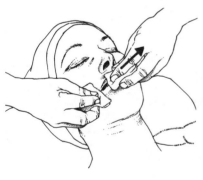

Lipstick Removal

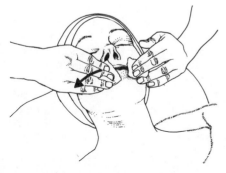

The lipstick is removed by lightly passing across the lips a damp cotton-wool tissue folded into a manageable shape. The pressure must be light and should not cause discomfort or distort the mouth. Care should be taken to avoid touching the nose. The lipstick is removed by first holding one side of the mouth with a cotton-wool tissue, whilst the other hand passes across the mouth, removing the lipstick and cleansing preparation onto another folded shape of cotton-wool. The routine is then reversed, using a fresh surface of the tissues, to complete the entire cleansing sequence for the lips.

Facial Cleansing Removal

The cleansing preparation may be removed either with the hands following each other, or working in unison on both sides of the face at once. The throat is completed before the routine progresses to the face, first on the left cheek, across the chin to the right cheek, then moving up the face to the nose, and on to the forehead, if the hands are following each other. With the hands working in unison, the neck is completed, followed by removal on both cheeks, then the nose and

METHOD A   METHOD B

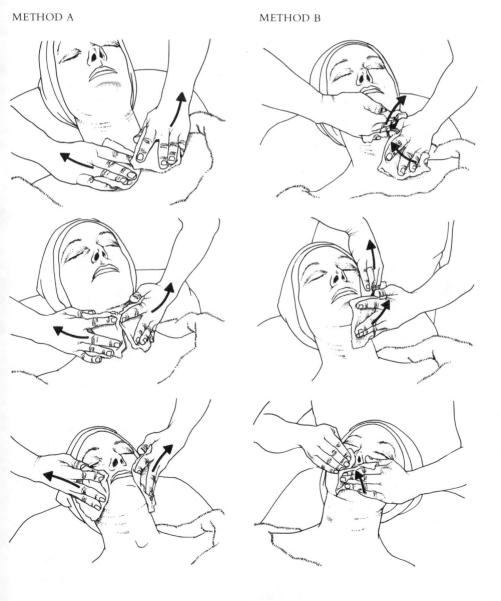

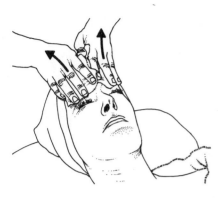

METHOD A (cont.)

forehead. Both methods complete the sequence by circles around the eyes, finishing with gentle pressure on the temples.

Whichever method is chosen, certain points are of importance to achieve an efficient and thorough removal which feels comfortable to the client. The cotton wool used for the pads should be of the very best quality, which should split into layers easily when cut into squares and moistened. It should be free from lumps, scratchy bits, and be evenly split so that it holds together when in use. The pads should be about 4 ins (10 cms) square depending on the size of the therapist's hands, and any oddments can be used to make the eye and lip pads. The pads should be wrung out *firmly* so that they are just *damp* not wet; otherwise they will be incapable of removing the oily makeup and cleansing preparations.

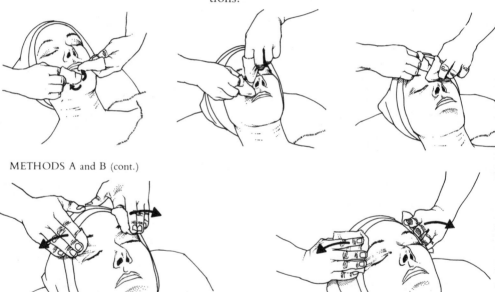

METHODS A and B (cont.)

METHOD A (end)   METHOD B (end)

The pads should be controlled by the therapist during the sequence, and not allowed to flap in the clients face, or tickle, breaking the relaxation. The pads are normally held between the thumb and index fingers, and the fourth finger and the little finger, spread open by the pressure of the hands against the clients skin. Pads may alternatively be wrapped around the fingers. The important thing is that the pads remove the preparations used, without irritating the skin or annoying the client.

Sponge pads can also be used when water-soluble creams are in use, and they are very convenient, but must be sterilized meticulously to avoid the risk of cross-infection. Many pads are necessary to allow for washing and sterilization between clients. Removal on the larger areas of the face and neck is completed, turning the tissues over where necessary, or renewing them, to avoid spreading the tinted makeup preparations around the face. In the case of a heavy makeup application, the removal sequence can be repeated to this stage, to ensure a complete cleansing of the skin.

Either method then proceeds to detailed cleansing of the centre panel. Cleansing pads are firmly tucked around the index finger, and deep rolling movements are applied to the central area of the face where blockage occurs, and makeup becomes trapped, even in the older skin. The strokes move up onto the forehead, become slower, and accomplish the removal gently. Removal should be more thorough in this area in method B as it has not been previously cleansed.

The pads are then opened out under the fingers, and eye arching completes the removal sequence for both methods.

If removal pads are still showing evidence of makeup present at the conclusion of the routine, the entire cleansing sequence and its removal may be repeated. The correct choice of cleansing preparation selected for its ability to remove the makeup present, as well as suit the skin type, should avoid this occurrence.

SKIN INSPECTION

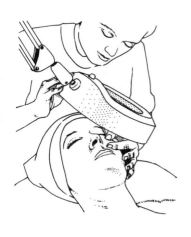

When the skin is sufficiently cleansed, it is then possible to inspect it through an illuminated magnifier to determine as closely as possible the different skin conditions which are present. It may be necessary to wipe the skin gently with a diluted tonic preparation to remove all traces of oiliness left by the cleansing preparation, and to avoid getting a false impression of the skin's balance of natural oil and moisture. Sensitive, easily stimulated skin may present a false picture at this stage of inspection, due to the vascular response created by the activity of the cleansing routine. Certain skins flush extremely easily, and the skin may appear irritated and red at one moment, and completely settled the next. This fast response to stimulation is closely related in action, to the effect of the sensory nerve endings on the blood vessels, as seen in blushing.

After cleansing, the skin can sometimes look mottled, red and irritated, which may be partly at least due to client anxiety as well as to the actual stimulation caused. Mature clients, particularly in the menopause age group are very prone to these red flushes, especially on the neck, which normally fade after a few minutes as the client relaxes. Hormone changes occurring in the body, appear to make the surface capillaries more sensitive to internal and external influences, and dilation (flushing) occurs more readily.

Whether of psychological (emotional) or physiological (physical) origins, evidence of this condition will require that the treatment proceeds with caution till the skins true sensitivity is known.

SKIN DIAGNOSIS

The success of the treatment depends largely on the therapist's ability to recognize facial conditions which are present at the time of treatment and her advice to the client. The number of contributory factors involved in skin diagnosis make it difficult to separate skins into different types, and it is preferable to concentrate on the important factors involved in successful diagnosis, such as age and general health. The reaction of the skin to massage or cosmetic applications can only be learnt by careful observation of differing skin conditions and general experience.

For the purposes of remedial facial therapy it is therefore necessary to have a sound knowledge of general physiology so that the effects of ageing, ill health, and external influences on skin tissue can be understood.

Main Points of Diagnosis

Age
Pigmentation
Skin imperfections
Skin balance (natural oils and moisture)
Skin temperature
Acid/alkaline level

Age   As age is the easiest point to diagnose, it gives the therapist the most immediate guidance as to which treatment will most benefit the client. Skin tissue ages at different rates, according to genetic factors, the care it has received, the external aggravation it has suffered, and the general health of the client. However well the skin has been cared for, nothing can stop the loss of muscle tone in the muscles of facial expression, and it is a softening of both the profile and the skin itself which gives a clear indication of the age of the client.

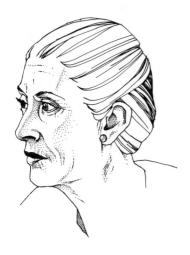

This softening of skin and slight loss of muscle tone combine to cause crêpy loose skin on the sheet-like muscles of the neck and etched lines around the mouth and eyes, where familiar expressions are constantly repeated. It is evident that mature women who retain a fuller face, often due to slight overweight, do not in fact suffer so badly from lines, crêpy skin etc., due to the support that the skin obtains from the adipose (fatty) tissue of the subcutaneous layers. The ageing of the skin can, however, be considerably delayed with correct professional treatment and careful home care routines.

Pigmentation

Easily Stimulated Skin

The increase of colour intensity and reaction brought about by basic skin cleansing is a vital point in diagnosis, as from the reaction observed can be determined the situation of the dermal vascular network and the damage already caused by over-exposure and lack of protection to the surface capillaries. The depth of the epidermal and dermal layers can be judged visually by the skin's colour and by its warmth. Any evident dilated capillaries, either visible through the epidermal layer, or ruptured into it, which assume the appearance of tiny splits or lines of a dark red colour should be noted. The situation and colour of these dilated capillaries will give the therapist valuable information as to the salon treatment possible and the general skin care necessary to prevent the progression into an irreversible skin imperfection.

Balanced Skin

The skin with an even texture, creamy colour, and no visible vascular network, or imperfections, is an excellent skin to treat as its functions are sufficiently balanced to maintain adequate cellular growth. Its biological activity ensures continuous nourishment of the skin's layers. This type of skin is extremely rare, and with working conditions becoming increasingly polluted it requires deep cleansing and a planned home care routine, just as much as any other type of skin.

Discoloured Skin Conditions

If the skin is even-textured but very discoloured, it may be due to a physical condition, and in this case only corrective makeup is advisable. It may, however, be associated with many other causes, one of the most common being ageing, and in this case the condition usually presents itself on several areas of the body, arms, hands, neck etc, and although the process of skin regeneration can be hastened by massage and electrical treatment, it is usually only possible to decrease the intensity of the discolouration.

In younger clients the cause of the problem must be sought in order to eliminate the condition, and here tactful questioning is necessary in order to determine likely reasons for the pigmentation abnormality. It has been seen that some young women taking the female hormone contraception pill do in fact form differing sized patches of pigmented skin on their faces, as in fact do a small number of women in pregnancy, this condition (Chloasma) fortunately disappearing after the birth.

In many cases of over-exposure to ultraviolet, sun-tanned women do also suffer from large patches of pigmentation, and although this condition does respond to treatment it will reappear when the sun-baking is resumed, due to the permanent damage caused.

Sallow Skin   The sallow complexion is often linked with racial tendencies, or general colouring, but it can be improved considerably by stimulatory treatment, both manual and electrical, and corrective facial makeup. The texture of the skin may be even, but rather coarse and heavy in appearance, with no softness apparent. This is due to a slowing down of the replacement rate of the basal layer of the skin, and in consequence a reduced rate of casting off at the skin's surface, causing a compressed, heavy, often oily appearance.

Discoloured, Blemished Skin   If the sallow condition is combined with excessive oil secretion from the sebaceous glands (seborrhoea), usually found in adolescence, it will be easily recognized by the apparent sheen on the skin, and is often associated with a pustular infection of the follicle (acne), where greasy skin, blocked and open pores, pustular infection, and scar tissue are all present at the same time on the face, and, in severe cases, the neck and back. Many treatments are available, some of which require medical approval. If this approval is required your client should be asked to consult her doctor, who can give an accurate diagnosis and advise whether the proposed treatment is suitable.

It is not wise to assume that a sallow skin will be any less sensitive to manual or electrical applications, and care must be taken not to cause an irritant reaction to many of the products used in the treatment of seborrhoea.

Skin Imperfections

When imperfections are evident the therapist must attempt to determine the cause of the condition, and how long it has been present, in order to avoid any repetition of damaging treatment, which could increase the nature of the defect. Many skin conditions become imperfections through neglect or ignoring the problem, until the remedial facial therapy available would no longer be successful.

One of the most common skin imperfections in fine skins is a condition of dilated capillaries, where the blood vessels are bulbous, ruptured into the epidermal layers, assuming a bluish red appearance, with crack-like lines running close to the capillaries themselves. Specialized treatment is available, with varying degrees of success attainable, according to the intensity and site of the condition and how long it has been established.

Pigmentation abnormalities, such as ephelides (freckles), lentigo, vitiligo (partial loss of pigment), should all be noted, as the reaction of the skin in the areas of no pigmentation may be very different from that of the normally coloured parts, and treatment should be given with caution.

Skin tags, fibroma simplex, and other fibrous malformations need attention, and care must be taken when manipulations are being undertaken not to cause discomfort to the client. In cases where several nodules exist in any one area, electrical treatment would not be indicated, and manual skills would be preferable. The facial specialist is often the first person that a client will consult regarding removal of small warts, moles, and other diverse facial imperfections, and here a duty to your client must prevail when your advice is sought, to recommend them to seek medical advice if any condition on the face and body in your limited opinion needs medical scrutiny prior to beauty therapy treatment. It is possible to base your advice to the client on information you gain from her, regarding how long the mole has existed, how rapidly it has grown in recent months, whether it irritates etc., and in this way you can form your opinion of whether or not the client should consult her doctor.

Clients will often seek professional guidance if they desire removal of a prominent mole, particularly if the mole is hairy and darkly coloured, and it is essential that medical permission is given before any treatment is commenced. Many moles can be removed under medical direction at the out-patients department of a hospital, or if they are small in size and medical permission is given, they can be removed by an electrologist, skilled in minor cosmetic surgery.

Skin Texture

The texture of the facial skin depends on several factors, the most important being the rate of secretion from the sebaceous glands found in profusion on the centre part of the face, and in larger quantities on the rest of the face, chest, and shoulders than in any other part of the body. The oily liquid produced contains fatty acids, lipids, and cellular matter, and its rôle of skin protection, both from transient bacteria, and external drying elements, is vital to the well-being of the skin and its appearance.

In a fine textured, older skin, the slower rate of sebaceous secretion is thought to be a contributory factor in the ageing process, and this would seem to be true, as it is observed that older women who have regular facial massage to stimulate the sebaceous secretion level, and who follow a regular routine of daily skin care, do in fact retain a more youthful appearance with firmer contours and soft elastic skin tissue with even texture.

In the middle years of life the sebaceous glands are producing only just sufficient amounts of oily matter to keep the skin in good condition, and so if adequate skin care is given both professionally and at home, the texture of the skin should be even and fine, with the skin in good health with perfect biological activity. However, if the skin is neglected or misused by washing or lack of protective cosmetics, then the natural oil level will be reduced by lack of care, and dry, chapped, flaky skin will result, with fine lines, crêpy skin and loss of firm texture.

In a young skin the normal pattern of sebaceous secretion is over-productive, causing dilated pores, and giving a thickened shiny appearance, due to the build-up of epidermal cells caused by the slowing down of the cellular growth in the basal layer of the skin. This condition of oily and sallow complexion, often leads to an unevenness of texture and over-acidity (a low pH) of the skin.

Skin Moisture

Skin lacking moisture is often referred to as a dry skin, and is easily recognized as a fine skin with no apparent pores and often traced with superficial wrinkles. It is inclined to age prematurely, and its ageing process is hastened by the indiscriminate use of soaps, astringents, and lack of protection. Skin may have the normal sebaceous secretion and still suffer from flaking and tightness over the bony prominences due to loss of surface moisture, a condition of dehydration. Constant hydration of the skin is maintained by a water reserve contained in the lymph circulating between the cells, as well as in the cells themselves. The hydric balance of the skin is maintained by the amount of water in the subcutaneous tissues and the body in general. Dieting is often a prime cause in the diminishing of the hydric element in the subcutaneous tissues. When water is omitted or drastically reduced, dehydration of the skin takes place. As the body needs a certain amount of fluid for efficient blood circulation, it balances the amount from the supply available in the subcutaneous layers of the skin.

The sebaceous secretion level and the moisture balance are very closely allied, and often treatment of one condition will rectify the other as well. However there are individual cases where it can be clearly determined by visual means, or verbal questioning, that the cause of the skin's apparent loss of texture and condition, can be attributed to a loss of moisture through over-stringent dieting, over-exposure to the elements, or neglect. It is important to recognize the difference, as the home care routines and salon treatments would then vary considerably, and the improvement could be accelerated, relieving distress.

Skin Temperature

The most important task of the body and facial skin is control of body temperature through vaso-dilation and constriction of surface capillaries. This is evident by the colour and warmth of the skin's surface, and how efficiently the blood vessels complete this task can be judged by the overall appearance. If the protective epidermal layer overlying the vascular network is fine, then the dilation of surface capillaries can clearly be seen, the face has a pink appearance, and is easily stimulated either by exertion, nervousness, or external aggravation. If the surface capillaries are well covered and protected, then the body temperature would have to be considerably increased before a reaction would become evident, and local stimulation such as manual treatments would have only a moderate effect on the superficial circulation, causing only a slight change in colour and warmth to be evident.

Acid/Alkaline Balance. pH Value of Skin Tissue

The pH value of the horny layer in healthy skin ranges between 5 and 5.6, showing an acid reaction compared to a neutral pH of 7. The secretions resulting from the activities of the sebaceous and sweat glands, and the process known as keratinization of the epidermis, form the so-called acid mantle, covering the entire skin surface. This mantle plays a most important rôle since it acts as a protection against action exerted by bacteria and microorganisms living in the external environment, which is characterized by an alkaline pH. In addition to this, the so-called acid mantle is a determinant factor in the maintenance of the healthy aspect of the skin surface. In fact, a decrease in acidity in the skin tissue results in an unhealthy appearance with uneven texture.

Cutaneous pH varies according to the different layers of the skin; i.e. the pH of the inner layer is similar to that of blood plasma, approximately 7.35, while in the outer epidermal strata it is between 4.8 and 5. Scientific research has revealed that the principal constituents of the acid mantle are represented by acid proteins. The physiological acidity and the pH of the skin tissues (5 to 5.6) may vary greatly, according to external and internal factors such as sunlight, beauty cosmetic applications, skin hygiene, digestion and nutrition, and may change within twenty-four hours. Excessive perspiration can also cause the pH to change. A 6.5 pH favours the development of micro-organisms, causing a number of dermatoses.

CLEANSING PREPARATIONS

In order to accomplish effective cleansing of the skin, without irritation or excessive manipulations, the correct choice of product must be made. Cleansing preparations are made to perform different tasks, and to suit a range of skin conditions and special problems. The products' texture, appearance, and perfume are also important if the client is to enjoy using the items for home care.

Even prior to detailed skin inspection, it is important to have some information about the client, in order to choose the correct preparation to accomplish an effective cleansing sequence, from which the treatment can proceed. Guidance is available from the clients' age, colouring, and the type of makeup that is being worn. Tactful questions to the client help the therapist in her choice, and avoid over stimulation of the skin at this stage.

Cleansing is of more importance to some skin types than others, and this point should reflect in the cleansing preparation choice. Finely pored, easily stimulated skins will need to be cleansed swiftly, gently, and thoroughly all in one application, as they become over stimulated if the process is repeated, which prohibits any further treatment. Blocked or blemished skins need both general and specific cleansing to remove the oily surface build up, so more time can be spent on this aspect of the treatment, to allow following applications to be more effective.

Growing awareness of the importance of deep cleaning the skin has brought about a general increase of products and electrical systems designed specifically for cleansing.

Cleansing Preparations:

can remove the makeup present;

are suitable for the client's skin;

have the correct texture for easy application;

have a pleasant feel on the skin, and a subtle perfume or be unperfumed;

are economic in use.

Cleansing Items

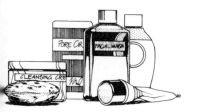

Cleansing Milks
Cleansing Creams
Liquefying Cleansing Creams
Soapless Cleansers and Complexion Soaps
Cleansing Lotions
Pore Grains

Cleansing Milks

Available in many consistencies, most milks are emulsions and are made of differing proportions of water and oil. Cleansing milks may have the appearance of real milk, may have a jelly-like consistency, or be fairly heavy rather like diluted cleansing cream. Essentially, this is the formulation of a cleansing milk, a diluted cleansing cream, made to a formula that is preferred by younger clients, who like a light, and grease-free-feeling product. The advent of polythene flexible bottles greatly increased the popularity of cleansing milks, making them a convenient form of cleansing medium.

The more liquid, thin consistencies normally have a higher proportion of water to oil, and are less effective as cleansers for removing heavy or oily based makeup preparations. In this case repeated use would be necessary, which professionally would not be satisfactory. For light makeup or for the younger client these products would be adequate, as they will remove water-based makeup, and naturally will satisfactorily cleanse a skin that is free from makeup altogether.

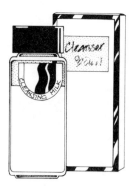

The detergent element in many cleansing milks is effective in removing surface bacteria and oily blockage from the skin, when it is free from makeup. However this detergent element can prove drying to mature or sensitive skins, and they should be advised to use cleansing milks with a high oil content, which will also be more effective removers of makeup.

Cleansing milks with a high fluid content will feel cool on the skin, and feel pleasant in use, particularly to the younger client with oily skins. They also leave the skin free from oil after removal. The fluid proportion may be made up partially by fruit juices, lemon etc., which adds to the fresh feeling, and adds variety.

The middle range of cleansing milks, often sold as 'emulsions', have a wide range of uses, and suit many skin types. They account for a large proportion of total cleansing product sales. These products have a higher percentage of oil to water, have less or no detergent, and are capable of swiftly removing makeup. They are formulated to accomplish deep skin cleansing without stripping the skin of natural oils, or irritating the surface. For the 20-40 years age range they make an alternative to cleansing creams, and may be preferred to creams even in the older age group, because of their pleasant feel and convenience of use. Products for dry, sensitive and allergy prone skins are available within this type of cleansing milk, which may be recognized by its more jelly-like consistency, and slight gloss apparent on application to the skin. Its greater efficiency as a cleanser will also help identification, as will the skins appearance after its removal. The skin will have a slight sheen on it after the removal, and the client will not experience sensations of tautness on the surface. Toning the skin with a mild tonic preparation is necessary in this instance.

Heavy cleansing milks have a high oil-to-water proportion, feel more oily on the skin, and have an evident glossy sheen when on the skin. They are excellent cleansers, able to remove substantial makeup, even theatrical and photographic, and are well suited to the dry and mature skins. They liquefy quickly, so do not drag the skin, and can act as a lubricant where the surface of the skin is dry. The oily film left after their removal requires thorough toning procedures to disperse, a point of importance when advising them for home care use to clients.

Cleansing Creams

Now available in a wide range of textures and consistencies, including whipped-up, mousse-like preparations, creams are increasingly popular for clinic and home use. Always the most efficient of the cleansers, creams were normally confined to clinical treatment as they left a film on the skin, which was hard to remove without completing a mask application. Creams are now available so finely textured that they are similar to milks in application and convenience.

Wherever the skin is dry, stretched, dehydrated, or becoming mature, a cream will prove the best cleanser for removing makeup and suiting the skin as to consistency. The lubricant properties of a cream cleanser dissolve makeup rapidly, making prolonged manipulations unnecessary, and so avoid over stimulating the surface capillaries.

Apart from liquefying cleansing creams, all creams are based on a water in oil, or an oil in water formulation, and contain a percentage of soap. The degree of stiffness in the consistency depends largely on the form of emulsifier used, often beeswax, and the method of manufacture. The more that is understood regarding the ingredients and effects of products the easier will be choice and guidance of these products to clients.

Liquefying Cleansing Creams

Designed for the fast removal of stage or television makeup, the cream appears like petroleum jelly, liquefies rapidly on exposure to the warmth of the skin, and quickly dissolves the makeup present. Liquefying creams contain no water or detergent and may be classed as emollients. As they are made up of oily materials only, they are ideal for dry, loose skins, where skin drag might be a problem. They do require very thorough toning to remove the final traces of the cream. For extremely

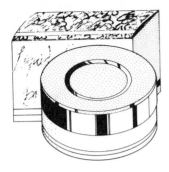

dry and dehydrated skins this feeling of lubrication left after cleansing is desirable, and this type of cleansing agent chosen for daily use and removal of day makeup.

Like all active cleansers, reactions to the product are possible, and skins that are both dry and sensitive should have liquefying creams used on them with caution. They should be tried out extensively in clinic treatment before suggesting them for home use, as they have a strong irritant effect on some skins. Clients who like this type of cleanser will be hard to wean from them, and if they suit the skin type, it should not be attempted.

Soapless Cleansers and Complexion Soaps

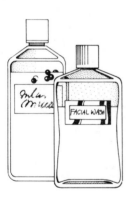

Used on oily skin, or blocked areas, these products are in fact soap, but in a form which does not leave the skin taut or with an extremely altered pH level as normal soap would. The effect is to free the skin from surface oils, reduce the acidity, and leave the skin close to its correct acid/alkaline balance. Ordinary soap can leave the skin over alkaline, tight, and sometimes dehydrated and irritated. In many cases of excessively oily skin this does not matter unduly, as dehydration is not a problem, and ordinary soap plays an important part in the care of the oily skin. For oily or blemished skins that are also sensitive, the soapless cleanser is kinder in action on the skin, and can be used more frequently without irritation resulting. They may also be advised for the very young person for home use, to prevent skin blockage forming. Clients with young children may often seek advice as to the relevant home care for the adolescent skin to avoid blemishes, and soapless products may then be suggested.

Soapless cleansers come in many forms, liquid, semi liquid, in tubes, or as actual soap bars, sometimes incorporating almond meal, or oatmeal chips to increase the skin refining effect. Only by experimenting will the ideal product be discovered and its correct frequency of use be known. If the skin flakes or is irritated, the product needs dilution or less frequent application. Daily use is not always required with specialized cleansers; it is better to let the skin condition guide as to the correct frequency of use. As a skin becomes less oily with age, then use of specialized cleansers can diminish or cease and a new product take over. Clients do not always recognize that their skins have changed, but the therapist must, and advise accordingly.

None of the complexion soaps or soapless cleansers are effective removers of makeup; they are designed to deep cleanse an already clean skin. Professionally they follow traditional methods of skin cleansing, and they should be advised for home use in the same manner. Only young women who do not wear makeup would find them the total cleansing answer for their skin needs. Being unperfumed and rather clinical they may also be used by young men very successfully.

The public love of face-washing, against years of therapists' advice to the contrary, has resulted in manufacturers researching and producing products which keep both sides happy. Now available are soaps that do not dry the skin, deep cleanse the blockage, and please the client. Most cosmetic houses offer a product of this type in their range.

Cleansing Lotions

Useful in the case of oily or blocked skins, or for central areas of the face in the normal skin, these products have a de-greasing action on sebaceous material present on the skins surface, or trapped in the mouth of hair follicles. They may unfortunately also have an effect on stimulating the sebaceous secretion, so increasing the oil flow to the skins surface, worsening matters. Young clients enjoy the stripped feeling the skin suffers after the use of cleansing lotions, but they should be guided to a more rational programme of skin cleansing if possible, to avoid over-stimulation of the skin.

In fact in laboratory tests cleansing lotions have been found to be less effective removers of oily blockage than the traditional creams, but clients' preference of lotions to oily products retains their popularity. As 'fresheners' to remove surface grime and oil, they are useful for daytime use, on young skins free from makeup. The modern trend is for combined cleansing/toning lotions, to use as 'fresheners' or to remove very light makeup. Where normal tinted foundation makeup is worn they can follow the use of basic cleansing milks, creams etc., to leave the skin feeling fresh and pleasant.

Pore Grains

Pore grains still have an important place in the treatment of the extremely oily or blocked skin, although they have been largely superseded by complexion soap bars incorporating almond meal or oatmeal chips. In fact the grains are detergent chips, which are made into a gritty paste in the palm of the hand with a few drops of water, and used like an abrasive rub to free oily blockage. The paste is worked into blocked areas of the skin, on the face and back if needed, kept moist and rinsed off after a few minutes. The paste should be continually worked into the skin, and not allowed to dry as is often recommended, so that it can be deep-acting without being excessively drying. For the detergent grains can easily cause the skin to peel or flake off, as they dehydrate the Stratum Corneum by a de-fatting action. This may not always be a bad thing in moderation, but it can leave the skin sore and irritated, and really offers no permanent solution to the skin blockage. Desquamation is increased, skin debris is removed, scar tissue is gradually removed, but the skin can become sensitized in the process, and lose its natural protection so becoming more liable to infection. There are kinder, more professional and certainly more effective methods of achieving the same results without soreness or skin abrasion.

Used within professional control treatments of the oily and blemished skin, pore grains can be effective to start the removal of the hardened sebum plugs, which can then be freed by following treatment. Galvanic desincrustation produces more effective dissolving of the blockage, and does not involve the general skin so drastically.

Used correctly, pore grains are a useful home back-up to prevent the formation of blocked pores. The client must be advised carefully as to the method of use and the frequency of application, then the pore grains can act as an effective preventative measure. Application may be necessary daily, or weekly, or even monthly, depending on the degree of oiliness, and skin sensitivity. Reaction to the initial application will guide the therapist in her advice to the client.

Product Choice

Clients have very strong personal preferences regarding cleansers, many based entirely on the feel of the preparation on the skin. Young clients with troubled skins cannot bear any oily or greasy feeling items on their skins, fearing it will aggravate matters. They like to feel the skin is stripped clean, free from natural oils. However, if this stripping is stimulating the sebaceous glands to further activity, this point must be explained to the client and a compromise sought.

In the same way clients who feel they must wash their face to feel clean, can be advised to use only gentle acting facial washes, and be advised to compensate the skin for any dehydration caused.

Products can be introduced to clients during treatment, so that they are accustomed to them before purchase. In this way items can be presented to the client so that they sell themselves by feel, smell and action on the skin, rather than by hard sell techniques. The client then feels she has chosen the items, with the therapists guidance.

Any product advised and sold in this way, so that the clients' wishes are accommodated into the cleansing preparations choice is guaranteed a repeat sale.

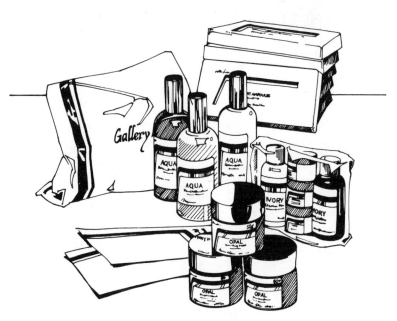

WELL CHOSEN TREATMENT PRODUCTS ENSURE GOOD RESULTS FOR
THE CLIENT AND HIGH PROFITS FOR THE CLINIC

Chapter 3

Facial Anatomy

Before we proceed with further manual or electrical applications, a knowledge of underlying structures, bony supports, and the very nature of the skin itself, is necessary.

FACIAL PROPORTIONS

An ideally proportioned face is thought to be one which has equal measurements, (1) from the tip of the nose to the lowest part of the chin, and (2) from the outer corner of the eye to the tip of the nose.

The facial features and expression are determined by the shape of the bony structures supporting the muscles of facial expression, and the subcutaneous fat overlying the muscles. As an individual ages, or loses weight, the true bone structure emerges and the nose, cheekbones etc. appear more prominent. Differences in the shape and size of the skull, due to national and heredity characteristics, determine the facial features, whilst superficial muscles provide the expression. The position and attachments of facial muscles to fascia and bones of the skull determine the massage technique and sequence of movements required.

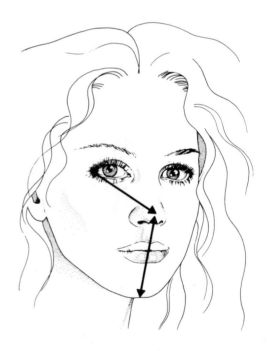

IDEAL FACIAL PROPORTIONS

BONES OF THE SKULL
AND FACE

The bony framework of the head is called the skull. The skull, apart from the lower jaw (the mandible) is usually classed as the cranium. There are 22 bones involved in the formation of the skull, all of which are fixed in position apart from the lower jaw. The skeleton of the face and cavity enclosing the brain are made up of 15 bones, whilst the other 7 are deeply situated and do not affect the contour.

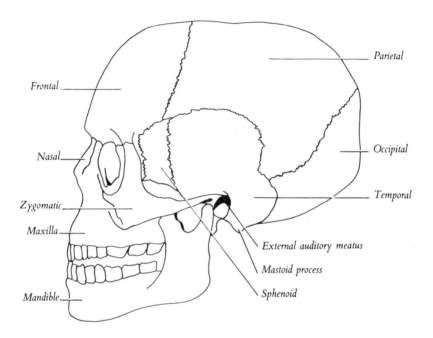

Bones of the Head (Cranium)
1 frontal bone
2 parietal bones (right and left)
2 temporal bones
1 occipital bone
1 sphenoid bone
1 ethmoid bone

Bones of the Face
2 maxillae (single maxilla)
1 mandible (lower jaw)
2 zygomatic (cheek bones)
2 nasal

Internal Facial Bones
2 palatine
1 vomer
2 lacrimal
2 inferior conchae

THE CRANIUM

1 Frontal Bone

The frontal is a large bone which forms the forehead and upper part of the eye socket. It is joined to the 2 parietal bones by a serrated articulation, the coronal suture.

2 Parietal Bones

One on either side of the dome of the skull, these two bones form the largest part of the cranium.

2 Temporal Bones

Situated on the sides and base of the skull. An irregular shaped bone with three main areas; the squamous part, placed vertically at the side of the skull; the petrous part, wedged between the sphenoid and occipital bones, which contains the organs of hearing; and the mastoid part, which contains the projection, the mastoid process.

1 Occipital Bone

At the back and underneath the skull is the occipital bone. It has a large opening called the foramen magnus through which the upper part of the spinal cord passes. At either side of the foramen magnus, the occipital bone articulates with the vertebral column at the condyles of the skull.

1 Sphenoid Bone

Situated at the base of the cranium, with wing-like projections forming the temples. It has a main body from which grow two larger and two smaller wings. The optic nerve and ophthalmic artery pass through a round opening (the optic foramen), situated at the base of the lesser wing.

1 Ethmoid Bone

This lies in front of the sphenoid and below the frontal to form part of the nasal cavities, and parts of the orbits (eye sockets).

BONES OF THE FACE

2 Maxillae (upper jaw bones)

These form a large part of the face, and carry the upper teeth. Each bone forms part of the roof of the mouth, the orbital cavity, and outer wall of the nasal cavity. The maxilla has four processes, zygomatic, frontal, alveolar, and palatine, which arise from the main body. The zygomatic process articulates with the zygomatic bone.

1 Mandible (lower jaw)

The mandible is a large strong bone, forming the chin and sides of the face. It has a main curved body, and two flat broad processes called rami, which project up and back, giving it a horseshoe-shaped appearance. It contains the lower teeth, and is the only bone in the skull that moves. It articulates with the temporal bone, and gives rise to muscles that assist mastication. A perforation (the mental foramen) situated on each side of the main body, provides a passage for the mental nerve and blood vessels.

2 Zygomatic Bones   An irregular-shaped bone, which forms the prominence of the cheek and part of the floor and lateral walls of the orbital cavity. It articulates with the zygomatic process of the temporal bone to form the zygomatic arch. Its other aspects articulate with the maxilla and frontal bones.

2 Nasal Bones   The nasal bones are two small bones which together form the bridge of the nose. They articulate above with the frontal bone.

INTERNAL FACIAL BONES

2 Palatine Bones   These bones aid in the formation of the floor and wall of the nasal cavity, the roof of the mouth, and the floor of the orbital cavity.

1 Vomer   The vomer bone forms the back and lower part of the nasal septum.

2 Lacrimal   Two very small bones within the orbits.

2 Inferior Conchae   These are separate bones forming part of the nose.

The bones of the adult skull, with the exception of the mandible, are joined so tightly to one another that no movement between them is possible. The serrated joints (sutures) become less evident with age, and the bones become fused. The complex nature of the facial bones is seen clearly in the orbital cavity, where 7 bones are involved: the frontal, lacrimal, sphenoid, ethmoid, zygomatic and maxilla.

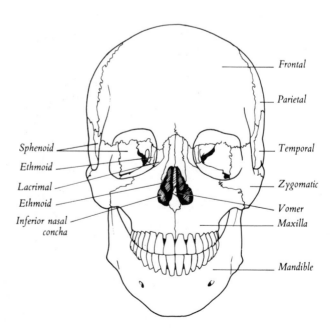

MUSCLES OF FACIAL EXPRESSION AND MASTICATION

Facial Muscles

Occipitofrontalis	Scalp and forehead
Corrugator	
Procerus	Eyelids and forehead
Orbicularis oculi	
Zygomatic minor	
Nasalis	
Orbicularis oris	Nose, mouth and cheek
Risorius	
Zygomatic major	
Buccinator	
Levator labii superioris	
Levator anguli oris	
Depressor labii inferioris	Mouth, chin and
Depressor anguli oris	superficial neck
Mentalis	
Platysma	
Triangularis	

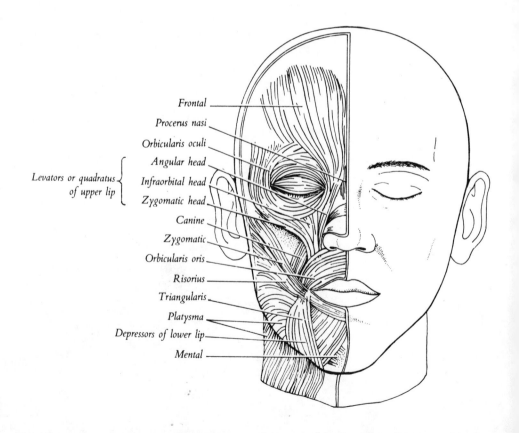

Frontal
Procerus nasi
Orbicularis oculi
Angular head
Levators or quadratus { Infraorbital head
of upper lip   Zygomatic head
Canine
Zygomatic
Orbicularis oris
Risorius
Triangularis
Platysma
Depressors of lower lip
Mental

Muscles of Mastication
Masseter
Temporalis   Mastication
Pterygoideus lateralis

Bone Attachments of Facial Muscles

Many facial muscles originate from and insert into skin and surface fascia, and do not have a bony attachment. Those that do, may both originate and insert into bone, or have one skeleton attachment, with the more flexible portion inserting into other muscles, skin or fascia (see diagram on page 38.)

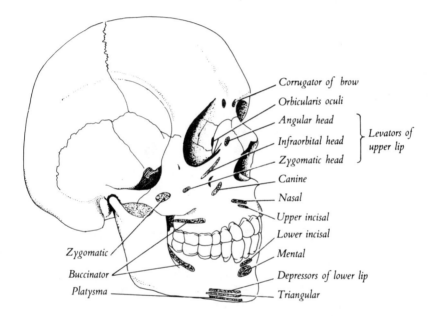

Corrugator of brow
Orbicularis oculi
Angular head   ⎫
Infraorbital head   ⎬ Levators of upper lip
Zygomatic head   ⎭
Canine
Nasal
Upper incisal
Lower incisal
Mental
Depressors of lower lip
Triangular

Zygomatic
Buccinator
Platysma

Muscles of Facial Expression and Mastication

The group of muscles in the head have in common their superficial arrangement and, especially, their attachment to, or their influence upon the skin. Almost all the superficial muscles have an influence upon the facial expression and are, therefore, collectively called the *muscles of facial expression*. Beyond this, however, they perform such major functions as, for instance, closing the eye, and auxiliary functions during the intake of food and its mastication, and in speaking.

The superficial muscles of the head are distinguished by their great variability. The muscles are variable not only in their strength, but also in their shape. In some persons many of these muscles consist only of a few pale muscle bands, whereas they form in others solid though thin muscle plates or bands of a dark red colour. In many cases it is difficult to separate one muscle from the other, either because two neighbouring muscles fuse to one muscular unit, or because they exchange muscle fibres. An added difficulty is that the terminal parts of these muscles are interlaced; e.g. lateral to the corners of the mouth. The difficulties are increased by the peculiar way of insertion of these muscles into the skin. They insert as a rule by isolated, thin, and sometimes elastic tendons which are continuations of the individual muscle bundles. These tendons are frequently separated by lobules

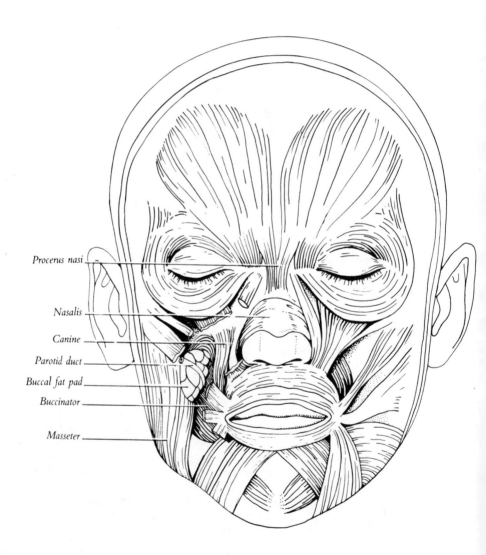

Procerus nasi

Nasalis

Canine

Parotid duct

Buccal fat pad

Buccinator

Masseter

SUPERFICIAL AND DEEPER FACIAL MUSCLES

of fat. Where the tendons are attached to the skin in lines or in small concentrated areas, the skin is either folded or pulled inward to form a small groove which is known as a dimple. The creasing of the skin along certain lines, repeated over and over again, leads finally to the formation of permanent folds. The folds become deeper and sharper with advancing age due to loss of elasticity in the skin. Inconsistent folds are caused by habitual wrinkling of the skin, e.g. on the forehead and between the brows. They too become permanent when, by long repeated action or by advancing age, the elastic fibres of the skin degenerate. The same origin can be established for crow's-feet in elderly persons as well as for those who are used to squinting in bright sunlight.

MUSCLES OF THE SCALP AND FOREHEAD

All the muscles of facial expression are supplied by the facial nerve.

The Occipitofrontalis

Formed from the frontalis and occipital muscles, this is a broad musculo-fibrous sheet that covers the upper part of the cranium from the eyebrows to the back of the head. It has two anterior and two posterior bellies connected by a fibrous sheet. The anterior bellies arise from the frontal bone, and the posterior from the occipital bone and mastoid process of the temporal bones.

These muscles lift the eyebrows, and fold the skin of the forehead into horizontal creases. Fully contracted, an expression of surprise or horror is produced.

MUSCLES OF THE EYELIDS AND FOREHEAD

The Corrugator

The corrugator is a small triangular muscle arising from the frontal bone, lying beneath the inner part of the orbicularis oculi. Its main action is to cause vertical wrinkles between the brows, as in frowning. The corrugator interlaces with the frontal muscle and pulls the eyebrow medially.

Procerus

A slender muscle arising from the nasal bone close to the midline, which runs straight up and is inserted into the skin of the brow and forehead between the eyebrows. Its action is to depress the wider part of the eyebrows.

Orbicularis Oculi (sphincter muscle of the eyelids)

The orbicularis oculi surrounds the opening of the lids in wide sweeping arches. It is located in the upper and lower eyelids, and its fibres extend outwards over the temporal region and downwards over the cheek. Its action is to close the eye, as in sleeping or winking. Firm contraction of the muscle wrinkles the skin around the eye as well as closing the lid.

MUSCLES OF THE NOSE, MOUTH AND CHEEK

Zygomatic Muscles

Some of the most well-developed muscles of the middle face, they arise from the temporal process of the zygomatic bone, and run downwards and forwards to the corner of the mouth. Their action pulls the corner of the mouth upwards and laterally.

Nasalis (nasal muscle)

The dilator naris, which dilates the nostrils, and compressor naris which narrows the nostrils, both arise from the maxilla bone. The dilator naris inserts into the soft tissue of the nostril, and the compressor naris runs upwards and inwards to the bridge of the nose.

Orbicularis Oris (oral sphincter)

The orbicularis oris has no bony attachments, and its fibres occupy the entire width of the lips. Its action is to close or narrow the lips, press them against the teeth, or purse the mouth.

Risorius (grinning muscle)

The risorius arises from the fascia of the masseter muscle, behind its anterior border, and converges towards the corner of the mouth, gaining in thickness. It is a triangular muscle, and is placed horizontally in the cheek. Its action pulls the corner of the mouth laterally, and creates a grinning expression.

Buccinator (cheek muscle)

The buccinator is the principal muscle of the cheek, and forms a mobile, wide rather thin muscle plate, which fills the gap between the upper and lower jaws. It arises from the maxilla and mandible opposite the molar teeth, and is perforated by the parotid duct. Its action pulls the corner of the mouth laterally and posteriorly. Its main function, however, is to keep the cheek stretched during all phases of opening and closing of the mouth. By maintaining tension of the cheek, it prevents injury by the teeth, and by pressing the cheek against the teeth it aids in the mastication process.

MUSCLES OF THE MOUTH, CHIN AND SUPERFICIAL NECK

Levators and depressors

These are: levator labii superioris (elevator of the upper lip); levator anguli oris (elevator of the angle of the mouth); depressor labii inferioris (depressor of the lower lip); depressor anguli oris (depressor of the angle of the mouth).

The actions of these muscles are given by their names. They are also known as the quadratus of the upper lip (quadratus labii superioris) and quadratus of the lower lip (quadratus labii inferioris).

Mentalis (chin muscle)

The mentalis muscle arises in an almost circular area above the mental tuberosity, in a slight depression on the mandible bone. It inserts into the skin and lower borders of the orbicularis oris. Its action is to elevate the skin of the chin, and turn the lower lip outward.

Triangularis (triangular muscle of the lower lip)

The triangularis originates at the lower border of the mandible, at and just above the line of the platysma muscle attachment. It forms a triangular plate, and mingles with the platysma to converge into the corner of the mouth. Its action pulls the corner of the mouth downwards and inwards.

Platysma

(Dealt with in the muscles of the neck.)

MUSCLES OF MASTICATION

Four powerful muscles, the masseter, the temporal, the internal and external pterygoids, are described as muscles of mastication. Three of these, masseter, temporal and internal pterygoid, exert their power in a vertical direction, acting as closing muscles of the jaw. The fourth, the external pterygoid, is situated in a horizontal plane and acts as protracter of the mandible.

Masseter

The most superficial of the masticatory muscles, it stretches as a rectangular plate from the zygomatic arch to the outer surface of the mandibular ramus. It runs downwards and backwards to insert in the angular region of the mandible. Its action is that of a powerful elevator of the lower jaw, closing the jaw and exerting pressure on the teeth, especially in the molar region. The deeper portion of the muscle has a retracting element which is important during the closing movement, a combination of elevation and retrusion.

Temporalis

The temporalis is a strong, fan-shaped muscle which arises from the temporal fossa on the side of the head. Its fibres converge towards the zygomatic arch, and are inserted into the coronoid process and reach down to the ramus of the mandible. Its action is to elevate the mandible and close the mouth, and it aids the mastication process.

The Pterygoideus Lateralis

The internal pterygoid is situated on the medial side of the mandibular ramus, and it is anatomically and functionally a counterpart of the masseter muscle. Its origin is the pterygoid fossa, and its insertion into the medial surface of the mandible. The action is to aid the masseter in elevating and protruding the mandible.

The external pterygoid originates from the greater wing of the sphenoid bone and lateral pterygoid plate, and inserts into the articular disc and mandibular neck. Its action pulls the head of the mandible forward, and both muscles combine to cause a side to side grinding motion, which assists mastication.

All the muscles of mastication are supplied by the branches of the mandibular nerve.

ANATOMY OF THE NECK AND SHOULDER GIRDLE

Muscles of the Neck   Platysma
Trapezius
Sternomastoid

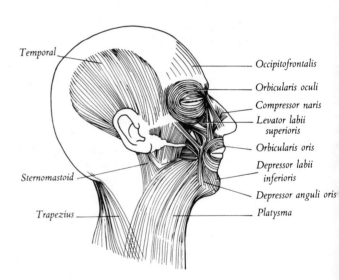

Platysma   The platysma is a weak superficial muscle, which arises from the fascia overlying the upper parts of the pectoralis major and deltoid muscles. It is inserted in the border of the mandible and the subcutaneous tissue and skin. Its action causes wrinkling of the skin of the neck and depression of the lower lip. It is supplied by the facial nerve.

Trapezius   The trapezius is a large, flat, triangular muscle, which covers the back and sides of the neck and the upper part of the back. It arises from the external occipital protuberance, spinous processes of the last cervical and upper six thoracic vertebrae. Its action is to steady the scapula bone during movements of the upper arm, and in combination with other muscles assists in rotating, elevating, or retracting the scapula. The insertion is the lateral third of the clavicle, acromion process, and the spine of the scapula. The nerve supply is the accessory nerve and the third and fourth cervical nerves.

Sternomastoid

The sternocleidomastoideus, usually called sternomastoid, is a powerful muscle of the neck, originating from two heads, one from the sternum and the other from the inner third of the clavicle. It inserts into the mastoid process of the temporal bone. Its action is to flex the neck, aid in rotation and, with both muscles working together, bows the head.

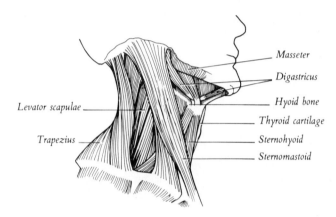

Masseter

Digastricus

Hyoid bone

Thyroid cartilage

Sternohyoid

Sternomastoid

Levator scapulae

Trapezius

SUPERFICIAL AND DEEPER MUSCLES OF THE
NECK (PLATYSMA REMOVED)

THE SHOULDER GIRDLE

Bones of the Upper Limb and Shoulder

The Scapula

The scapula is a large flat triangular bone that occupies the posterior aspect of the shoulder girdle. It has a very prominent ridge across the upper half of the posterior aspect, called the spine of the scapula. The lateral end of the spine is expanded and extends the shoulder joint, forming the acromion process. The head of the humerus positions into a concave area below the acromion process, called the glenoid cavity, and above it a hooked process projects forward to form the coracoid process.

The Clavicle or Collar Bone

The clavicle is a slender elongated bone, lying at the base of the neck. It articulates at its inner end with the manubrium of the sternum.

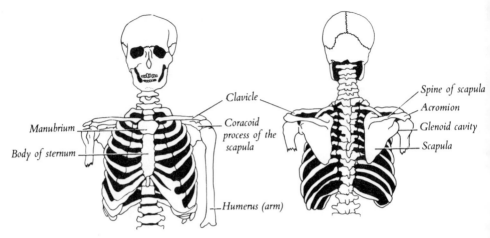

BONES OF THE SHOULDER GIRDLE

Muscles of the Chest and Shoulder Girdle

Pectoralis major
Deltoid
Trapezius

Pectoralis Major

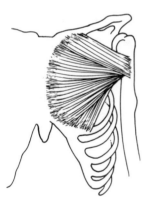

The pectoralis major is a powerful muscle covering the upper half of the chest wall. It originates from the medial half of the clavicle, the anterior surface of the sternum and the cartilages of the first six or seven ribs. The muscle fibres spread out and then converge to end in a tendon inserted into the outer lip of the bicipital groove of the humerus (arm). Its action is to adduct and medially rotate the arm, and draw it forwards and downwards. The muscle is supplied by the fifth to eighth cervical nerves and the first thoracic nerve.

The Deltoid

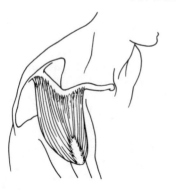

The deltoid muscle covers the shoulder area and gives it shape. It arises from the outer third of the clavicle, the acromion, and spine of the scapula, and converges into a thick tendon inserted into the outer side of the humerus. Its action is abduction, flexion, inward and outward rotation, and extension of the arm. The deltoid is supplied by the circumflex nerve.

The Trapezius

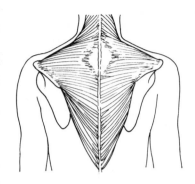

The trapezius is a large, flat, triangular muscle, which covers the back and sides of the neck and the upper part of the back. It arises from the external occipital protuberance, spinous processes of the last cervical and upper six thoracic vertebrae. Its action is to steady the scapula bone during movements of the upper arm, and in combination with other muscles assists in rotating, elevating, or retracting the scapula. The insertion is the lateral third of the clavicle, acromion process, and the spine of the scapula. The nerve supply is the accessory nerve and the third and fourth cervical nerves.

STRUCTURE OF THE SKIN

The skin consists of a superficial layer of stratified epithelium, the epidermis, laid on a foundation of firm connective tissue, the dermis or corium.

A diagrammatic version of the skin anatomy gives a clear indication of important areas for consideration, and shows relative anatomical positioning.

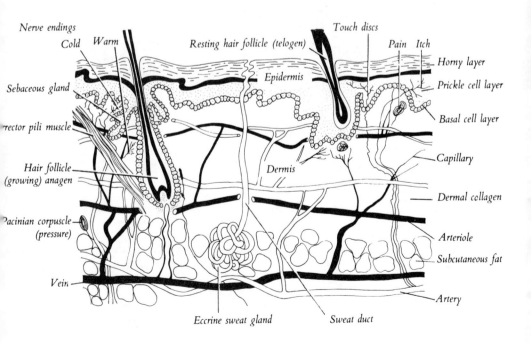

THE EPIDERMIS

The stratified epithelium of the epidermis is superficially converted into cornified material which is continually being worn away by usage, and is continually being replaced by proliferation from the deeper strata. Consequently its layers represent every transition from basal cells with well-defined nuclei, to superficial flaky débris in which the nuclei and all evidence of cell structure have disappeared. The epidermis has five layers, with two main divisions:

Stratum Corneum

Stratum corneum, a dead horny layer
Stratum lucidum, a clear hyaline layer
Stratum granulosum, here cells acquire keratohyaline granules

Living Stratum Malpighii

Stratum spinosum
Stratum germinativum, or basal layer. A living layer, where mitotic activity (cell division) takes place.

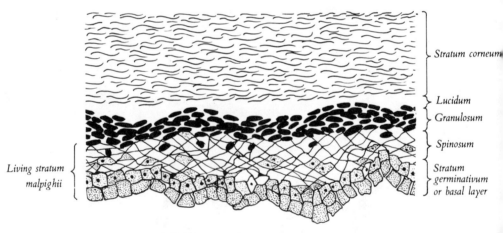

STRATA OF THE EPIDERMIS

The Stratum Germinativum or Basal Layer

This is the deepest section of the epidermis and is in contact with the dermis, from which it derives its nutrient fluid from the capillary blood vessels. In the basal layer the development of new cells leads to a gradual displacement of the older cells towards the surface. In spite of apparent low mitotic activity, the epidermis is a reproductively self-sufficient system that regenerates entirely from cells resident within it.

Melanocytes, melanin-forming cells, are found in abundance in the stratum germinativum, one in every ten cells being a pigment-forming melanocyte. Melanin protects the skin against injury from ultraviolet radiation, and is responsible for differences in skin colouration. Melanin is formed from the amino-acid tyrosine, by a complicated series of chemical reactions. The dendrites of melanocytes are in contact with at least one basal or Malpighian layer cell, and they are the only cells capable of forming and distributing melanin in the epidermis. Melanocytes seem to share the fate of Malpighian cells, being desquamated at the surface of the skin.

Stratum Spinosum

The prickle cell layer is often classed with the stratum germinativum, to form the basal layer. Most mitotic cells which appear to be in the spinous layer are actually found in the basal cells around the dermal papillae of the hair in other layers, and mitotic activity takes place largely if not entirely in the stratum germatinativum. The prickle cells are well-defined polygonal, and the whole layer is in organic connection by means of the prickle-like threads which join up the cells.

Stratum Granulosum or Granular Layer

The thickness of this layer may vary from one to several cells depth and is thickest on the palms of the hands and soles of the feet. The cells are flattened, and evidence of granules of keratohyaline may be seen if the skin is stained. These cells reflect light and give the skin a white appearance.

Keratinization is the change of living cells into dead horny flat cells with no nucleus. Loss of fluids is an essential process in the stages of keratinization, and the stratum granulosum cells are believed to represent the first stage in the transformation of the epidermal cells into horny material, keratin.

Stratum Lucidum

This layer derives its name from its clear translucent almost transparent appearance. It is only a few cells deep and lies between the outer horny layer and inner granular layer. It is thought that the stratum lucidum is the site of the barrier zone controlling the transmission of water through the skin. At this level of their growth towards the surface the cells have lost their clear cut line, and the nuclei are becoming indistinct.

Stratum Corneum

The superficial portion of the horny layer contains mainly layers of dead, flattened cells, which are constantly being shed. The cells contain an epidermal fatty material, which keeps them waterproof and helps prevent the skin cracking and becoming open to bacterial invasion. The surface stratum forms the greater part of the thickness of the epidermis in many parts of the body. Nuclei are no longer evident in these elements, cell structure has become completely obscured, and from below upwards, the flattened remains of cells become gradually converted into cornified flakes. The stratum corneum is transversed by the ducts of sweat glands and by hairs where they are present.

The epidermis rests upon the dermis, a dense fibrous layer beneath it, into which it interlocks by a series of finger like projections called papillae. The irregularity of the basal layer of the epidermis can be clearly seen.

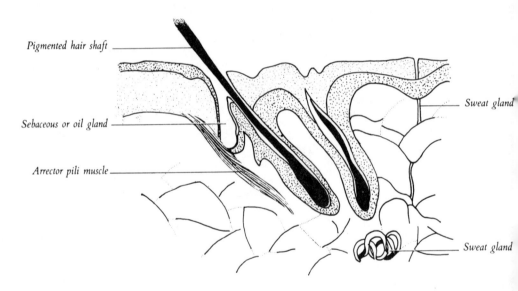

DIAGRAM OF HAIR, SWEAT AND SEBACEOUS GLAND

THE DERMIS

Being a condensed connective tissue, the dermis is unstable and undergoes change, breakdown and renewal. The dermis contains elastic tissue, blood vessels, lymphatics, nerves, tactile corpuscles and hair follicles, and is totally different in structure from the epidermis. The dermis is thicker in men than in women, and thicker on the dorsal and extensory surfaces of the extremities than on the ventral and flexor areas of the same individual. It is thickest on the palms and soles of the feet, but being continuous with the tela subcutanea it lacks exact boundaries, and its thickness cannot be measured accurately. The dermis has a superficial papillary layer and a deep reticular layer.

The Papillary Layer

In the papillary layer, widely separated delicate collagenous, elastic, and reticular fibres, enmeshed with superficial capillaries, are surrounded by abundant, viscous ground substances. The surface of the layer is moulded into intricate valleys, ridges and papillae, whilst the cutaneous appendages that extend into the dermis, piercing the reticular layer, are accompanied by the papillary layer throughout their length. Around hair follicles, the papillary layer forms the connective tissue sheath.

The Reticular Layer

The fibrous reticular layer is composed of dense, coarse, branching collagenous fibre bundles, which form layers mostly directed parallel to the surface. A few fibres can be traced down to the tela subcutanea, where they branch loosely, becoming incorporated into the framework of the fatty layer, and form the retinacula cutis that separate the fat into lobules. Loose networks of elastic fibres between the collagenous fibres are more closely woven around the cutaneous appendages. Around the blood vessels and nerves the connective tissue fibres are always delicate and more widely spaced than they are elsewhere. Connective tissue cells, more of them in the papillary layer than in the reticular layer, are sparsely distributed among the fibres.

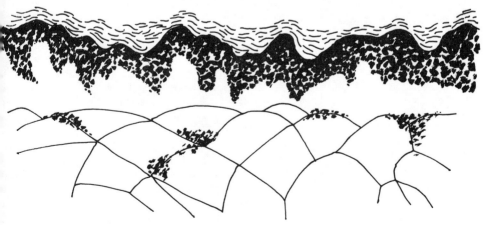

NORMAL SKIN WITH WELL DEVELOPED PAPILLARY PROCESSES

Blood Supply of the Skin

For growth the skin requires amino-acids, vitamins, trace elements, and essential fatty acids. Mitosis in the stratum germinativum gets the necessary energy from the nutrition supplied by the vascular system of the dermis.

Nerves of the Skin

Four primary sensations can be experienced through the skin: touch, cold, warmth and pain. A stimulus applied at any point of the skin evokes not one but a pattern of responses. Our standard concept of the distribution of the cutaneous sensory nerves is that there is a *deep cutaneous plexus* in the panniculus adiposus from which tortuous fibres transverse the dermis to the papillary body, where they form a superficial cutaneous nerve plexus, less complex than the deep one. Many fibres from the deep plexus are also thought to go directly to the papillary ridges of the epidermis. During development the nerve net is the first ordered structure to appear in the dermis, and may influence the development of cutaneous appendages. Smooth muscle, sebaceous glands, sweat glands, and the thickness of the dermis itself, all have a profound influence upon the particular form of the nerve networks.

Temperature, pain, and other sensations are perceived by a variety of different receptors. It would seem that the specialized end organs are modified according to the region in which they grow, and not according to the function which they subserve.

Sweat Glands

Sweat glands are tubular in nature and commence in the deeper layers of the dermis. The coiled body of the gland opens onto the surface of the skin via a long narrow tube passing through the skin's layers. The sweat glands are divided into two types the eccrine, and apocrine or large coil glands. The eccrine or true sweat glands secrete water and water soluble substances, and are found in abundance all over the body, apart from the margin of the lips and certain areas of the sex organs. The main function of the sweat glands is regulation of body temperature by evaporation of their contents from the surface of the skin. The apocrine glands are connected with hair follicles and are found mainly in underarm, breast, and genital areas of the body. Cellular waste, fatty substances, water and salt are secreted and body odour is more connected with these glands, which are thought to play a part in sexual attraction.

Sebaceous Glands

Most sebaceous glands are appendages of hair follicles and open inside the hair follicle cavity via a duct. The size of the gland often varies inversely with the size of the hair follicles with which they are associated. On the face some very large glands, amongst smaller ones, empty into the dilated pilary canals of vellus (downy) hair follicles. Sebaceous glands are most numerous in the scalp, forehead, nose, chin, and cheeks and in decreasing numbers on the back, the rest of the trunk, and the limbs. They are of epidermal origin but lie in the dermis level, forming irregular shaped structures.

These glands secrete a fatty substance, sebum, which helps keep the skin and hair supple, and plays a part in protection against bacteria. Sebum is markedly different from tissue fats, and a number of unusual substances not found elsewhere in the body can be detected in the sebaceous secretion. Cholesterol, free fatty acids, and lipid products of keratinization have been traced in different quantities. The amount of sebaceous lipids on a particular area of skin could be dependent in part upon the number, size, and rate of secretion of the glands, and the thickness and wetness of the skin.

The glands are influenced by the action of the endocrine system, and at puberty become very active, often causing facial blemishes.

FUNCTIONS OF THE SKIN

The skin acts as a covering for the body, and its main function is protection. It does however have other functions:

Heat regulation and elimination
Secretion and absorption
Sensation

Protection

The horny outer layer of the skin, the stratum corneum, is tailored in every detail to protect the body against its environment. The structure, rate of replacement, and physical repair properties of the outer layer protect against bacterial invasion and minor injury. The skin is waterproof and acts to contain body fluid, whilst preventing entry of large quantities of fluid through the epidermis.

Heat Regulation and Elimination

Loss of body heat is mainly controlled by the blood supply and sweat glands of the skin. Evaporation of sweat from the surface is an automatic process, which works efficiently unless the surrounding air is also hot and moist. The complex distribution of blood vessels in the dermis is well adapted to the various changes and stresses to which the skin is exposed. Body temperature regulation is the main function of cutaneous vessels, but blood pressure regulation is also important. Through dilation (expansion) of superficial capillaries, surface heat is lost and body temperature is reduced. The skin changes colour and appearance, becomes pink and warm and, combined with the perspiration loss, reduces discomfort effectively. To retain heat the blood vessels constrict (contract) and become smaller in diameter, and the passage of blood slows, giving a blue or dark red appearance due to loss of oxygen. The skin looks pale, and the arrector pili muscles can cause the hairs to raise to trap air close to the surface.

Secretion and Absorption

Sebaceous secretion, sebum, and perspiration both help to keep the skin supple and intact. Decomposed sebum and perspiration in the presence of bacteria produce 'body odour'. Considerable quantities of water are lost in perspiration as an automatic reflex action in body temperature regulation. As the prime function of the skin is protection its absorption rôle is limited, although there are several routes through which agents may enter. The hair follicle and sebaceous gland opening, and the skin itself, are capable of absorption, as is the sweat duct to a lesser degree. Penetration is affected by the health and condition of the skin, and breaks or irregularities in the surface increase the risk of infection occurring.

Sensation

The skin contains nerve endings which make us aware of our surroundings. They act as a warning system to indicate heat, cold, pain, pressure and other external factors. The nerve receptors are located at different levels in the skin, touch and pain indicators being close to the surface, and closely involved with the reactions received from the hairs. Pacinian corpuscles indicating pressure lie deeper in the skin, so that a certain threshold of pressure would have to be reached before sensation was stimulated. Cold indicators lie at varying depths beneath the surface, and like other organized endings are accompanied by pain receptors.

THE SKIN'S DEFENCE AGAINST BACTERIA

The normal skin is never sterile, its surface being contaminated by a wealth of bacteria. Most of these are non-pathogenic and cause neither harm or inflammatory reaction. Other bacteria, such as staphylococci, and haemolytic streptococci, which in certain circumstances can provoke inflammation, may also be present without exciting any reaction. In its course of evolution the skin has come to accept many such organisms as part of its natural resident bacteria. It has the power of inhibiting or restricting their growth until a state of equilibrium has been reached. When this control fails, or transient bacteria become present, boils, folliculitis or other skin disorders occur. An overwhelming invasion of organisms from some outside source, or a new and virulent strain, may precipitate such attacks. The mechanisms available to the skin to prevent or limit the invasion of these bacilli, are numerous and complex. The most important factors are:

The 'Acid Mantle'

The aqueous fluid bathing the outer surface of the skin is acid in reaction, and acts as a defence mechanism against infection. The pH of the fluid present is part of a total buffer protection of the skin and does not function independently.

Fatty Substances

Sebum secreted from the sebaceous glands contains a complex mixture of lipids and fatty acids, some of which are bacteriostatic and bactericidal. Adult sebum is also fungicidal and can help prevent some types of ringworm. By keeping the surface of the skin smooth and free from cracks, abrasions, etc., the sebum plays an important part in maintaining an intact skin surface.

The Sweat

The sweat exerts a powerful bactericidal effect: by maintaining the surface of the skin at a certain level of acidity it inhibits the growth of organisms. However, excessive perspiration becomes less acid, and encourages their growth, whilst softening the skin's surface, making entry more available.

The Horny Layer

The horny layer itself acts as a protection against invasion. Normally it is impervious to fluids and bacteria, but its protective mechanisms can be damaged by caustic preparations and elements which alter oil, fluid and pH levels of the skin.

Desiccation

There is evidence that simple 'drying out' of bacteria limits their spread. The value of moderate applications of dusting powder can be seen in many skin conditions.

Vascular Reactions

If an organism manages to invade the main body of the epidermis, an inflammatory response is aroused. Histamine is liberated; vascular dilation, oedema and leucocytosis occur. The leucocytes engulf and destroy invading organisms as soon as they pierce the horny layer. The skin may react violently to the external agent in attempt to prevent the spread of infection to surrounding tissues.

It can be seen that many of these mechanisms are mutually antagonistic. The integrity of the normal skin depends upon a balance between them. This protection against infection is remarkably efficient considering the abuses and injuries to which the skin is continually subjected.

ANATOMY OF THE HAIR

Hairs are dead structures, composed of keratinized (horny) cells that are compactly cemented together before they leave the hair follicle cavity. They grow out of tubes of epidermal cells, which are sunken into the dermis, and receive their blood supply from capillary loops situated in the papillae of the dermal layer. Hair is a sensitive tactile organ, and its main rôle now must be to increase awareness of surrounding environment through sensation and touch.

Hair grows at an angle to the surface, so that it follows the natural contours of the body above the surface, soft body hair is termed vellus hair, and coarser more visible hairs, terminal hairs.

The hair consists of a shaft, the part visible above the surface, which is horny in nature, and usually pigmented. The shaft has several sections depending on the hair type, the outer cuticle surrounding the pigmented cells of the cortex, which encloses the central cells of the medulla. The medulla is absent in lanugo or primary hair. The root of the hair, the enclosed area, grows from a papilla area of active cells at its lower end, and forms a column of compressed cells, which gradually harden into the shaft. The concave dermal papilla area derives its blood supply from the capillary loop adjacent to it, and this determines the growth and health of the

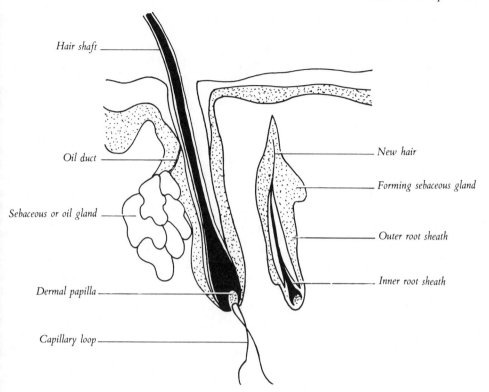

Hair shaft

Oil duct

Sebaceous or oil gland

Dermal papilla

Capillary loop

New hair

Forming sebaceous gland

Outer root sheath

Inner root sheath

THE HAIR STRUCTURE

hair. The hair follicle is a narrow pocket, formed partly by the dermis and partly by the epidermis. The outer sheath is composed of basal layer cells which follow its descent into the dermis, and the inner sheath is formed from the horny epidermal cells. The follicle and the hair are as one, and in removal, i.e. plucking, the inner sheath is visible. Attached to the underside of the sloping hair follicle is a small non-striped muscle, the arrector pili, which under stimulus of fear, cold etc., makes the hair stand on end.

Hair growth is continual in healthy adults, going through a cycle of growth, loss and replacement, which keeps the amount of hair present constant.

THE HAIR GROWTH CYCLE

The Biology of Hair Growth

When follicles cease to produce a hair, they shrivel up and the lower part or bulb, largely degenerates, its rôle fulfilled for the time being. These resting or quiescent follicles are simpler and much shorter structures than active ones. At the base of a resting follicle the hair, if still present, forms a club that is anchored by thin keratinous strands to the epithelial sac around. The club is surrounded by a hyaline capsule, or vestige of the inner root sheath; this continues up to just below the duct of the sebaceous gland, where it becomes wrinkled and fragmented. Around the capsule, the remaining outer root sheath forms a thickened epithelial sac: at the base of which is a peg of cells; at the flattened base of which is the ball of *dermal papilla* cells, no longer incapsulated by a bulb. Close inspection on epilating a hair in the resting stage will show the shallow position results in a hair which sits almost on the skins surface and has a blob like dot or full stop on its root end. This rounded club is the pedicle of cells and the lower part of the epithelial sac called the hair germ, from which the next generation of hairs develops.

Changes in the body can swiftly affect the hair growth pattern, either increasing its renewal rate or decreasing its capacity to regenerate correctly. Endocrine influence on the hair follicles results in unwanted hair in women, and is responsible for male baldness. The hair follicle responds to the messages it receives from the endocrine system and its pattern of growth is altered accordingly. Healthy hair growth in the young person may be found to have few resting follicles, with hairs being replaced before the old club hair is shed naturally. These double-haired follicles are simply skipping the resting stage, and the old club and the new finely pointed hair can be observed emerging from the same follicle. So the new hair is established before the old one is lost.

In a very simplified formula:

Growing hairs are said to be in *Anagen*.

Resting or quiescent follicles are said to be in *Telogen*.

Transitionary follicles in the stage between Anagen and Telogen are said to be in *Catagen*.

So the sequence of events if simplified becomes Anagen, Catagen, Telogen, and repeats constantly until a hair ceases to be formed due to internal influences. It is important to remember that very little that occurs externally has any effect on the hair growth, apart from disease involving the actual follicle structure. The strength, vitality, colour, and texture of the hair is determined from within. Certain treatments are thought to increase the growth of hair follicles, such as plucking or waxing, but this is due to the disruption in the growth cycle rather than any actual increase. If all the hairs present are removed, as with waxing, they will have been at various stages of growth, some resting, some in Catagen and many growing in the Anagen stage. Inspection of a wax strip after removal of hairs is an easy method of determining the different stages of growth, due to obvious differences in length and structure of the hairs present. However, although all the hairs showing were removed at different stages, they have to grow back from a similar stage after the follicle has recovered. It really acts to bring the hair follicles into a regularized pattern of growth which would not be found naturally.

How hairs react to this disruption in their natural cycle gives rise to the widely differing views held about the reaction of waxing etc. on the overall growth. In some cases the hair appears increased, in others slowed down and sparse in character. Insufficient study has been completed to form definite statements regarding alterations in the growth patterns. Experience has shown that the general health, age and hormone influences have the greatest effect on the hair growth overall. Into the same category of undisclosed knowledge come why hairs turn white and why only some men become bald prematurely. If an external application did exist that increased hair growth, bald men would have used it long ago.

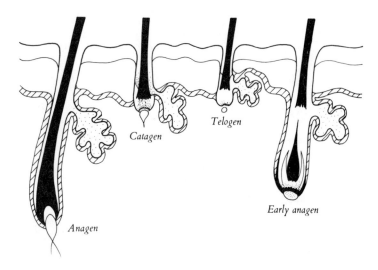

DIFFERENT STAGES OF HAIR GROWTH

GROWTH CYCLE OF THE FOLLICLE

The Resting Hair Follicle. Telogen

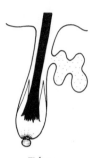

Telogen

Considering the simplest of the stages of the growth cycle first, it is necessary to understand the structure of the follicle, so the following more active stages can be understood. In a resting follicle, two physiological distinct regions are apparent, the one above the level of the duct of the sebaceous gland, and the one below. In the upper region, the cells of which are in direct continuity with the surface epidermis, the mitotic activity of the basal cell layer is similar to that of the basal layer of the epidermis, but in the lower region the cells are mitotically inert. In the upper follicle there is an open space or channel between the follicle wall and the hair shaft. In the lower follicle the walls press closely onto the hair, which at its base has a strong brush-like attachment to the surrounding cell mass. Beneath the follicle base is the small dermal papilla.

The follicle appears collapsed, like an empty stocking, deflated, waiting for further stimulus to be refilled, like filling the stocking with a leg. The follicle may stay in this state for some considerable length of time. Hair does appear to grow less at certain times of the year; whether due to dietary influences or not seems uncertain.

Early Follicle Growth. Anagen Stage I

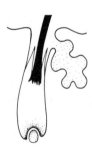

Early anagen stage I

The first sign of that mitotic activity which results in the production of a new hair is seen in the basal cells of the lower follicle, which then grows downwards as a solid column of undifferentiated and dividing cells to surround the dermal papilla. So the lower part of the follicle starts to grow downwards, with the rôle of many of its cells as yet undetermined (undifferentiated cells). There is no mitotic activity in that part of the lower follicle which surrounds the brush or club-like base of the old hair, whilst in the upper follicle normal mitotic activity continues as normal.

Later Follicle Growth. Anagen Stages II and III

As the new follicle elongates rapidly, the inner follicle sheath and the tip of the newly forming hair begins to differentiate, and the cells involved cease to show mitosis. From the base upwards, the sequence is as follows.

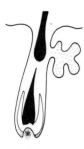

Later follicle growth
Anagen stage II

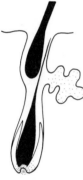

Anagen stage III

1 The basal region of very increased mitotic activity takes the form of a ring which surrounds the dermal papilla.

2 Next a narrow region of differentiation, where no mitosis is seen. The cells are becoming organized but in this section not involved with growing.

3 Then a rapidly elongating region containing centrally the newly differentiating hair, and peripherally (around the outer perimeter) a zone of active mitosis in which are produced many of the new cells involved in the lengthening of the hair follicle. Until the follicle is fully grown, the lengthening of the follicle keeps exact pace with the lengthening of the new hair shaft. Consequently the hair tip remains static beneath the brush-like club attachment of the old hair.

4 The non-mitotic zone surrounding the brush like club attachment of the old hair remains unchanged.

5 The cells of the upper follicle now show an increased rate of mitosis, and a similar increase in the mitotic activity takes place in the overlying surface epidermis.

The Fully Grown Follicle.
Anagen Stages IV and V

When its growth is complete, the follicle is at least six times longer than it was in the resting condition. From the base upwards, the sequence of zones is as follows.

1 The cells of the basal ring-like matrix show violent mitotic activity which, however, ceases abruptly at a point level with the tip of the dermal papilla.

2 Above the dermal papilla is a zone in which the cells arrange themselves into columns, and in which they begin to elongate and differentiate. No mitotic activity is present.

3 Above this is the keratogenous zone in which the cells are keratinized to form a recognizable hair. They lose moisture and harden. No mitotic activity (cellular division) is seen in any of these cells, or in the cells of the surrounding follicle wall.

4 With the point of the new hair now forcing upward, the brush-like attachment of the old

hair and the surrounding cells are pushed to one side, these surrounding cells show no mitotic activity, and are subsequently shed.

5   The cells of the upper follicle show a subnormal mitotic rate, and a similar sub normal mitotic rate is found in the overlying epidermis. The growing process over for the time being the surface skin returns to a near-normal state.

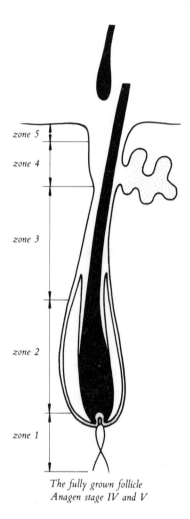

zone 5

zone 4

zone 3

zone 2

zone 1

The fully grown follicle
Anagen stage IV and V

The Final Stage. Catagen

When the new hair is fully grown, mitotic activ ity in the basal ring-like cell matrix suddenly ceases and the new hair develops a brush-like attachmen to the cell mass which surrounds its base. The worl of the follicle now largely completed, that o developing a new hair, its structure again changes

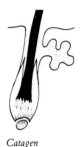

Catagen

its usefulness temporarily over. There follows the rapid degeneration and destruction of a greater part of the lower follicle. The outer root sheath in the upper part of a follicle forms at least part of the 'Hair Germ' and the epidermal sac around the club hair. The inner layers of the vitreous membrane become extremely thick and form a wrinkled sac around the degenerating lower part of the follicle. (In Telogen this becomes fragmented and is re-absorbed.) Resting hair follicles are surrounded by only a thin hyaline membrane which corresponds to the outer layer of the vitreous membrane. The connective tissue sheath becomes wrinkled and thickened. (In quiescent follicles, the connective tissue sheath becomes fragmented and is re-absorbed, leaving only a wispy trail in the area vacated by the follicle.) So the process has come full cycle, and by this complex yet orderly process the follicle returns to its normal resting length, its task of producing a new replacement hair over for the time being.

The fact that hairs have a predetermined cycle is obvious from the length hairs attain in different parts of the body, eyelashes, arm and leg hairs having different length potential to hair on the head. Only individuals with a prolonged growth cycle for example could grow their hair to below the waist, and many people can never achieve more than shoulder-length hair. At an average growth rate of ½ an inch a month, waist-length hair is obviously several years old and must have a very spaced-out replacement growth cycle.

This very simplified description of the growth cycle illustrates the replacement method of hairs in established follicles, and it must not be confused with the initial formation of the follicles in the unborn child.

Chapter 4

Facial Massage: Principles and Techniques

The main purpose of facial massage is to increase the skin's capacity to function more efficiently. The skin's natural protection and regeneration ability has been studied, and it is evident that in good health the skin is well equipped to cope with the effects of bacteria, minor injury, and normal exposure. Stimulating vascular activity with facial massage will increase natural cellular regeneration and maintain the skin's correct oil and fluid balance. The main effects of facial massage are stimulation, relaxation, cleansing, toning and refining.

By planning sequences of varying massage movements, it is possible to devise a routine ideally suited to maintain or correct the existing skin condition, observed during diagnosis. Skilful massage technique, adapted to the minute nature and attachment of the facial muscles, should tone and stimulate the tissues without causing skin distension, irritation or loss of relaxation. Additional benefit is also gained from the relaxing, soothing properties of certain facial routines by clients suffering from nervous tension, fatigue or depression.

MANUAL MASSAGE: CLASSIFICATION OF MOVEMENTS

Facial massage movements can be divided into several different classifications or groups. The purpose and effect of the different movements gives guidance as to suitability of application or contradiction, on any specific skin condition.

Effleurage Movements

Light pressure, flowing movements, including stroking, and rollpatting.

Petrissage Movements

Compression movements, which include kneading, knuckling, lifting, rolling, pinching, frictions and many other techniques involving increased pressure, and vascular stimulation.

Tapotement Movements

Percussion movements, covering all light tapping, whipping movements, performed to increase nervous response to stimulation.

64

These three main classifications cover nearly all the different forms of general facial manipulation, apart from vibrations, which are used for treatment of specific skin conditions, including hypersensitive and delicate skins.

Effleurage Movements

Effleurage or stroking movements are performed with light even pressure, in a rhythmical continuous fashion. The pressure used can vary according to the underlying structures and muscle bulk but should never become unduly heavy. The effleurage strokes prepare the tissues for deeper massage, link up individual manipulations, and complete the facial sequence. The hand contours to the area under treatment, and the maximum palmar surface of the hand maintains contact with the skin, whilst even pressure, rhythm, and rate of movement are established.

The effect of superficial effleurage is a reflex vascular and nervous response from the surface layers of the skin, causing increased skin temperature, warmth, and colour. The client becomes accustomed to the therapist's hands, and relaxation results. Deeper effleurage can be performed when relaxation of muscle tissues has been achieved, after which a more mechanical response is attained, through increased vascular and lymphatic activity, by constriction and dilation of subcutaneous blood and lymphatic vessels.

Effects of Effleurage: Summary

1   Aids venous circulation.

2   Arterial circulation is aided by removal of congestion in the veins.

3   Lymphatic circulation is improved and absorption of waste products hastened.

4   Aids desquamation, so cleansing the skin, freeing surface adhesions.

5   Aids relaxation in preparation for further massage.

6   Relaxes contracted, tense muscle fibres.

Petrissage Movements

Petrissage or compression movements must be performed on relaxed muscle tissue, as the pressure applied is intermittent and deeper than the effleurage movements. The effect of compressing and relaxing the tissues is to bring about surface reaction, increased vascular and lymphatic response, and evident local skin temperature and colour change. The movements may be performed with the palmar surface of the fingers, thumb and fingers, both thumbs working in combination, or the entire palmar surface of the hands. The movements must be performed slowly, rhythmically, and gently, with the part of the hand used conforming to the contour of the area. The increased effect of petrissage movements will contra-indicate (prohibit) them on certain sensitive skin conditions and require adaptation for mature or loose skin conditions. Pressure must be increased or reduced according to muscle bulk and the degree of tension present. Effleurage should be used to link compression movements and maintain or re-establish relaxation. Improved cellular function and surface desquamation of horny cells increases basal layer activity, resulting in a fresher, more refined skin texture. Keratinized, oily surface cells in the younger client are removed, and increased lymphatic and vascular flow improves the skin's nutrition and defence against bacteria.

Effects of Petrissage: Summary

1 Compression and relaxation of muscles cause blood and lymphatic vessels to be filled and emptied, thus increasing circulation and removal of waste products.

2 The skin, superficial and deeper tissues are all stimulated to further activity, improving cellular functions and regeneration.

3 Desquamation removes surface cellular matter and leaves the skin clear, refreshed and refined.

4 Larger contracted muscles are relaxed, and muscle tone is improved through compression and relaxation of muscle fibres.

Tapotement Movements

Tapotement or percussion movements are performed lightly and in a brisk stimulating manner. The rhythm of the strokes is important, as the fingers are continually breaking contact with the skin and the movements could be irritating performed incorrectly. A fast vascular reaction is achieved without compression of the tissues, due to the skin's nervous response to the stimulus. In many instances where petrissage would not be indicated, tapotement may be used to advantage in order to achieve desired results. In any area of the face where skin distension might result from manipulation, i.e. around the eyes, or loose crêpy skin along the mandible (jaw), application of tapotement may be preferable.

Effects of Tapotement: Summary

1 Stimulation of the skin through reflex nervous response.

2 Increased vascular activity. Light tapotement causes blanching of the skin, constriction of vessels, and, if continued, produces erythema, reddening of the skin, due to the interchange of blood.

3 Tightening, toning effect on skin tissue.

Vibrations

Static or running vibrations are performed on delicate skin conditions, or within a general facial sequence, where additional relaxation without over-stimulation of surface tissues is required. Vibrations are applied on a nerve centre, or running along the path of a nerve, and they are produced by a rapid contraction and relaxation of the therapist's arm muscles so that a fine trembling or vibration results. The entire palmar surface of the hand may be used or, for an intensive effect, the tips of the first two fingers, or the thumbs can produce excellent relaxation results.

Facial massage routines for the fine sensitive skin can be based on vibratory movements, which combine gentle stimulation with relaxation, whilst avoiding surface irritation or capillary damage.

Effects of Vibrations: Summary

1 Relaxation, relief of tension.

2 Gentle stimulation of the deeper skin layers.

3 Stimulation of nerves, relieving fatigue and muscular pain.

ROUTINE OF MASSAGE TECHNIQUE

The massage commences with effleurage strokes, and proceeds to petrissage movements when sufficient relaxation has been achieved. All the indicated aspects of compression and tapotement movements follow linked and concluded with effleurage.

REQUIREMENTS FOR CORRECT MASSAGE TECHNIQUE

The most important requirement for massage is thoughtful concentration, based on knowledge of facial anatomy, guiding flexible hands in the facial application. The other requirements are:

1 to maintain an even rhythm;

2 to establish the correct rate of movement;

3   to keep hands flexible, so that they fit the contour of the area;

4   to maintain correct body posture during facial massage;

5   to regulate pressure according to the muscle bulk and specific skin condition observed.

These essential points of correct massage technique have more importance in obtaining satisfactory results, including client relaxation, than the actual movements which make up the different facial routines. Controlled movements of the hands will only be possible if the therapist's body posture is correct, well supported, with a free range of arm movement. Fatigue will be avoided and correct technique maintained if both client and operator are in a comfortable position for the general facial application.

Rhythm and rate of movement can be practised on the cleansing and basic facial routines, and should be established before proceeding to more advanced massage routines.

Flexible hands develop gradually and can be improved by daily hand mobility exercises. Thoughtful awareness of underlying structures, and muscle bulk will develop a sense of touch, important in judging the pressure regulation necessary. Long and careful practice is the only way to develop this sense of touch, so vital to the beauty specialist.

HAND MOBILITY EXERCISES

These exercises must be performed progressively, increasing the range of movement possible gradually over a period of time. General mobility, an increased range of movement, and more flexible, relaxed control of the hands will develop with practice.

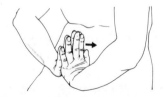

1   Press the fingers back from the palms of the hands to their fullest limits, with the fingers held together.

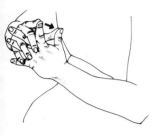

2   Press each finger back separately.

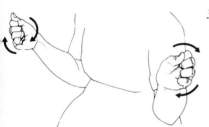

3   Rotate the hands and wrists, with the elbows held close to the sides, and the hands formed into fists. A full rotation should be attempted, with even rhythm, stretching the finger tendons fully.

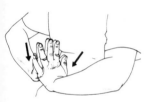

4   Form the hands into a praying position in front of the chest, with palms and fingers in full contact. Press the hands downwards, attempting to keep the palmar surfaces in contact, until the action is felt on the wrists and lower arm muscles.

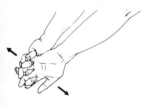

5   With the backs of the hands together, fingers interlocked, press the backs of the wrists together, and pull against the fingers.

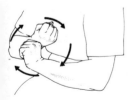

6   With the arms bent at the elbows, wrists held at chest height, revolve the hands around each other, with the hands formed into fists.

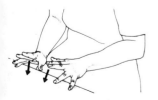

7   Attempt to tap the fingers of both hands, in a co-ordinated rhythm, onto a hard surface. Increase the speed, making both hands keep in rhythm. Increased practice of the slower hand will improve its speed and control. Work first index to little finger, then reverse the sequence.

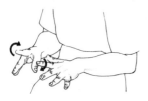

8   Practise making each finger and thumb form rotaries in the air, endeavouring to make each work independently of the others. Attempt full circles, to the left and then to the right.

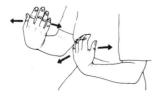

9   Vigorously shake the hands and wrists, to increase general mobility and circulation.

APPLICATION OF MANUAL MASSAGE

For the client to gain the maximum physical and psychological benefit from the facial treatment she must be made to feel at ease in her surroundings by skilful reception and client handling. Correct preparation, positioning and robing will have established a relaxed atmosphere, whilst the cleansing sequence and skin inspection will have indicated the general skin condition and any areas requiring particular attention.

Discussion with the client will indicate which factors cause the most personal worry, and attention should be directed to these problems first, to relieve anxiety and create a feeling of personal interest in the improvement.

Choice of facial massage sequence will be based on skin diagnosis, with age, general health and the emotional state of the client being important considerations.

Applications of Facial Treatment

The classic facial treatment includes cleansing, massage, mask, toning and makeup if desired. There are many additions and variations on this basic pattern, for specific skin conditions, but a one-hour facial treatment will include all or most of these elements within it.

Indications for Treatment

1   Normal skin conditions requiring deep cleansing, skin balancing, and refinement.

2   Dry or dehydrated skin conditions, where stimulation of cellular function is required.

3 Mature, ageing skins, requiring regeneration, deeper stimulation, and surface desquamation.

4 Young, blemished, or greasy skin conditions, which require a cleansing, toning, refining action, to remove surface adhesions and cellular matter.

5 Delicate, sensitive skin conditions, where gentle stimulation, pH stabilizing and oil fluid balancing are required.

6 Conditions of nervous tension, depression, or fatigue, where muscular pain is evident.

Contra-indications to Facial Massage

1 Hyper-sensitive skins prone to allergic reaction.

2 Extremely vascular skin conditions.

3 Any evidence of acute inflammation, bites, stings etc.

4 Skin infection, irritation, or other evidence of sepsis and malfunction requiring medical attention.

5 Diabetics. (Unstable skin condition, and poor healing capacity.)

6 Asthmatic, or sinus disorders.

7 Excessively loose skin.

THE BASIC FACIAL MASSAGE ROUTINE (TRAINING FACIAL)

The basic facial incorporates most simple massage techniques and permits hand flexibility to develop whilst the natural rhythm, rate, and pressure of the movements are established.

The movements are described by (a) their muscle positions, (b) bone proximity, (c) massage classification, and (d) direction and rate of the stroke. In this way the action, and the effect of the movement on the skin and underlying muscle can be easily traced. The purpose of the movements must be understood, so that as experience develops, individual massage routines can be devised to suit individual requirements. All facial routines give a framework, which can be adapted by reducing or increasing repetitions of the movements, or omitting them completely if contra-indicated.

The basic facial routine deep-cleanses the skin, is gently stimulating, and treats all areas of the face and neck equally. It is therefore suitable for younger women who require maintenance of skin texture, muscle tone, and oil, water and pH balance. Being a general routine, it is not designed to deal with specific faults or skin conditions requiring remedial care.

Indications for Treatment

Younger skins, in the twenty to thirty age group, with a tendency to dry, dehydrated skin, sensitivity, or erratic behaviour. Delicate skins in any age range, unable to stand prolonged manipulations, will be able to benefit from the basic facial routine.

Recognition of the Dry, Dehydrated Skin

Seen as a fine-textured skin, which responds easily to stimulation. A tight sometimes flaky skin condition, with evident surface capillaries on the cheeks, and finely etched lines appearing in flexure folds, and areas of repeated expression. The skin may have a dry or rough surface texture if it has been abused, neglected, or wrongly treated, and irritation may be present.

The skin of the neck and face respond quickly to treatment planned to include sensible home care to support the salon programme.

BASIC FACIAL MASSAGE SEQUENCE

Preparation

The client is prepared for general facial treatment. Her skin is cleansed, inspected, and the massage cream applied with superficial effleurage movements, as in cleansing.

Massage Routine

(1) Deep Rollpatting Movement (effleurage)

Rollpatting is applied at the established rate of 7 inches per second. The movement lifts and moulds the platysma muscle from its origin (fascia of the pectoralis major muscle) to its insertion in the mandible bone. The hands follow each other from the left clavicle, across the sternum to the right clavicle, and return, keeping the movement continuous. The hands contour to the mandible, and follow the paths of the left superficial cheek muscles, pass across the chin, cover the right cheek, and, the fingers apply detailed strokes to the nostrils and bridge of the nose. The movement concludes on the forehead with lifting of the occipitofrontalis muscles, performed slowly and lightly, without causing the eyes to open. Both hands return to the sternum via the outer border of the face.

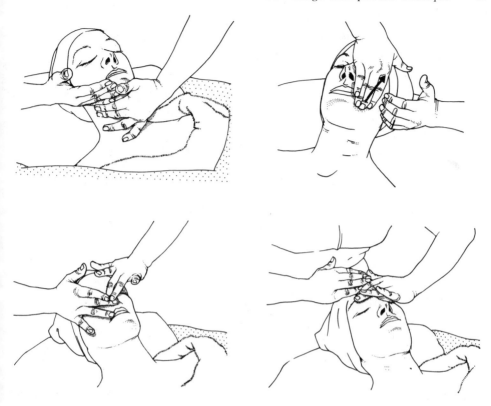

(2) Throat Brace (effleurage and petrissage)

The hands form a relaxed V shape, following the direction of the sternomastoid muscles, over the sternum, with the fingers straight and interlocked at the tips. The movement lifts the platysma and sternomastoid muscles, and forms a brace along the mandible. The pressure is maintained below and onto the lower jaw, back to the mastoid process, in an upward direction, as the hands divide. Link effleurage returns the hands to the sternum and the movement repeats 6 times.

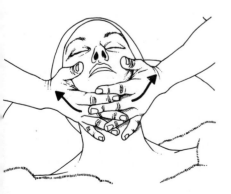

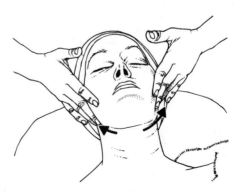

(3) Whipping Movement (tapotement)

This is a continuous, light percussion movement, applied superficially to the platysma and sternomastoid muscle areas of the neck. The hands contour to the throat and follow a rhythm of one longer and two shorter strokes. A flicking, whipping movement develops, as the technique improves and speed is increased. The whipping passes from the left to the right side of the mandible, and back, with the direction of the strokes moving outwards, as they reach the level of the lower jaw. The fingers individually lift, and roll the platysma muscle against the mandible, as they flick off in a fan-like movement. The whipping continues until the required reaction has been achieved.

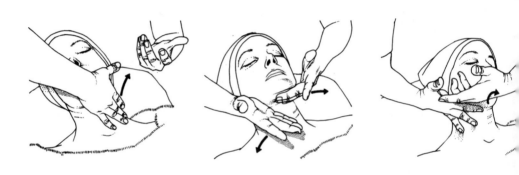

(4) Tapping (tapotement)

A light, fast tapping movement, applied under the mandible, on the subcutaneous tissues and superficial muscles. The strokes pass backwards and forwards across the jaw, with the direction of the taps being upwards, lifting the muscles against the bone. The duration and intensity of this percussion movement will depend on the degree of muscle tone and adipose (fatty) tissue present along the contour. The hands divide at the point of the mandible and return to the mastoid process.

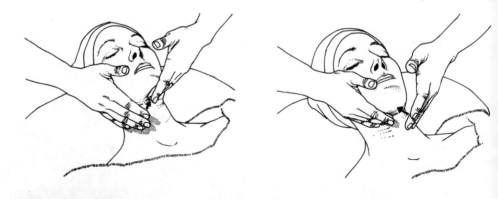

(5) Broad Sweeping (effleurage linking movement)

A deeper effleurage link movement, to re-establish relaxation and break the activity of the sequence. The movement sweeps down the sternomastoid muscles, over the upper fibres of the pectoralis major, contours around the deltoid, and lifts the upper fibres of the trapezius forward to return to the starting position. The hands contour to the area, and the maximum palmar surface is kept in contact with the client. The established rate and an even rhythm will increase relaxation. Pressure must be regulated according to muscle bulk and tension. Repeat 6 times.

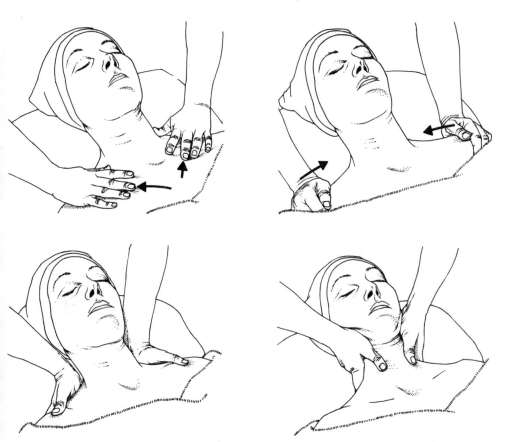

(6) Knuckling (petrissage)

The knuckling strokes are performed on areas of adequate muscle bulk by hands formed into loose fists, with the fingers working independently to give a circular compression movement. The wrists complete a half rotation, and the fingers form circular compression and relaxation actions applied slowly and deeply on the larger muscles and superficially on surface tissues. The movement commences at the mastoid process, the hands form into fists as they move down the sternomastoid muscles, and knuckling commences on the bulk of these muscles. The strokes move to the trapezius muscle, with deeper pressure, and reverse rotations, returning via the sternomastoid to the start position. Repeat 3 times.

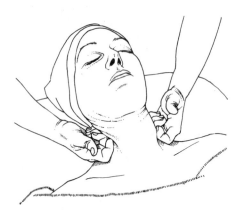
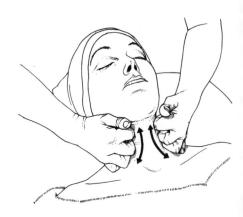

(7) Facial Lift (effleurage and petrissage)

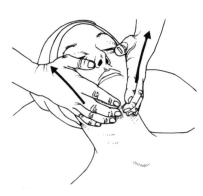

This movement links the neck and facial sections of the routine, and commences as an effleurage stroke, changing to a compression movement as it reaches the face. The facial lift begins as in the throat brace, with the hands moulding the mandible. It changes into the facial lift at the triangularis muscle position, by losing palmar contact, and lifts the superfical cheek muscles with the heel of the hand. Upward pressure is applied at the mandible, and immediately decreased as the hands pass upwards, losing contact with the face. The heels of the hands pick up the occipitofrontalis, whilst retaining contact with the levators of the lips, and the hands move into an effleurage movement of the forehead, decreasing the pressure and speed of the strokes. The hands return to the start position via the outer borders of the face, and the movement repeats 3 to 6 times.

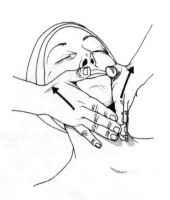
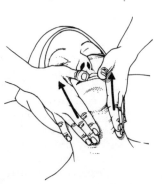
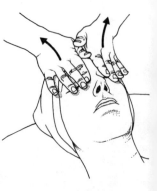

(8) Cheek Lifting, Zygomatic Movement (petrissage)

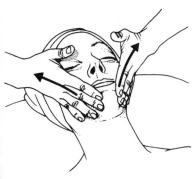

The hands lift from the point of the mandible, drop down and pick up the zygomatic muscles from the corner of the mouth attachments, and lift upward and outward to the zygomatic arch. The face is supported by the hands, and care must be taken to avoid distortion of the eyes or any general discomfort. Repeat 6 times linking the strokes with effleurage.

(9) Cheek Rollpatting (deep effleurage)

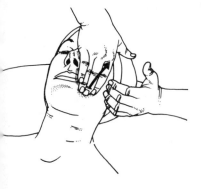

The hands follow each other, with the index and second fingers in contact with the superficial cheek muscles. The position of the zygomatic, risorius, and levators are picked out, with specific rollpatting strokes in a fan-shaped pattern, from the mouth to the outer borders of the left cheek. The movement crosses the chin rolling deeply into the cleft, and repeats on the right side. The hands divide and complete on the mastoid process. One continuous movement.

(10) Frictions on the Centre Panel (petrissage)

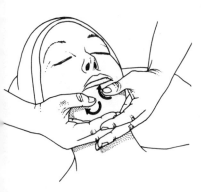

Thumbs are used to move the surface tissues over the underlying bony structures, in a circular and brisk manner, to remove surface adhesions and aid desquamation (skin shedding). Thumbs work in opposing rotaries on the chin area, with firm pressure forming between them to create a stimulating effect. The movement is applied around the orbicularis oris to the nostrils and bridge of the nose, and completes with effleurage to the temples area. Link effleurage returns the hands to the start position, and the movement repeats 3 to 6 times, depending on skin blockage in the central area and the reaction produced. The last repeat ends on the temples.

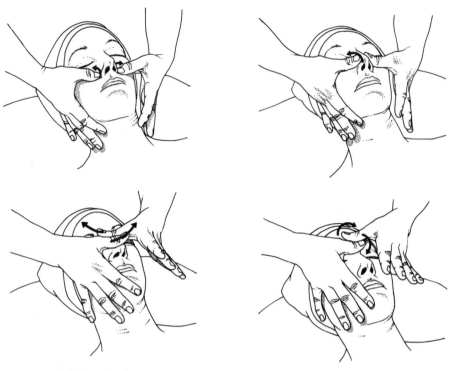

(11) Forehead Frictions
(petrissage)   Light but brisk friction movements cover the occipitofrontalis area, using the finger tips in semicircular movements against each other. The stimulating action of the movement helps prevent the formation of permanent expression lines horizontally across the forehead. The duration of the application will depend on the vascular response of the skin and the amount of subcutaneous adipose (fatty) tissue present. Downward pressure must be avoided to prevent client discomfort. The movement concludes at the temples, the hands dividing at the centre brow.

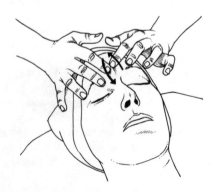
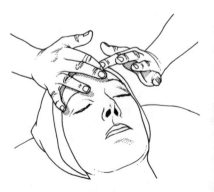

(12) Forehead Rollpatting
(effleurage)

A slow gentle rollpatting rhythm is established, with the hands moving continuously, from the left to the right temple and back, lifting the frontalis and upper fibres of the orbicularis oculi muscles. The strokes are applied at half the established rate, and the movement finishes with upward strokes over the corrugator muscle. The hands divide and finish at the temples. One continuous flowing movement.

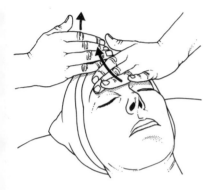
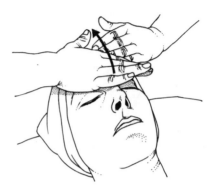

(13) Circles around the Eyes
(effleurage)

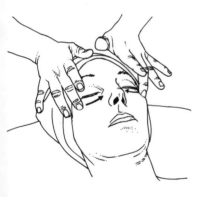

With the longest or index fingers bent, the movement sweeps under the eye, then inwards towards the nose, following the orbicularis oculi (eye sphincter) muscles. The movement is light on the under-eye tissues, but changes at the nose to lift firmly with the palmar surface of the index finger, to raise the inner eye corner, and changing direction again, lifts the upper fibres of the eye muscle and the frontalis. The lift is maintained as the movement passes along the eyebrows to the temples. The wrists and forearms control the movement, with the lifting and holding elements being applied from the arm positions of the therapist. The movement repeats 6 times.

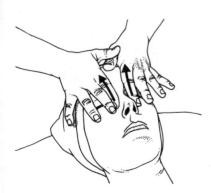
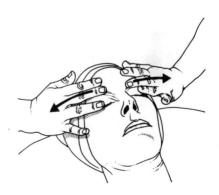

(14) Reinforced Eye Circling
(effleurage)

The movement commences as previously, but the movement is reinforced at the forehead by all the fingers lifting the orbicularis oculi and occipitofrontalis muscles. The movement is stronger and the eye sphincter more involved.

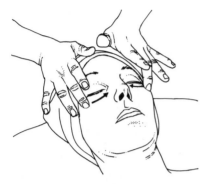

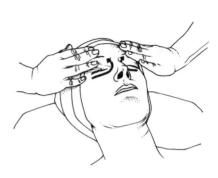

(15) Tapping on the Cheeks
(tapotement)

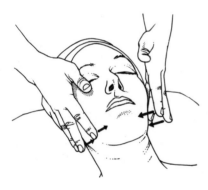

The hands commence light sharp tapping above the mandible, with the fingers working in unison. The movement covers the entire cheek area, up to the eyes, and changes into effleurage to link back to the temples. The taps must be rhythmical, and fast, with pressure adapted to the skin's sensitivity, and reaction to the application. This tapotement movement may be repeated 3 to 6 times.

(16) Facial Lift

As in movement (7). Repeat 6 times, with even pressure and rate of movement.

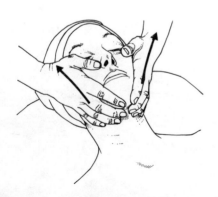

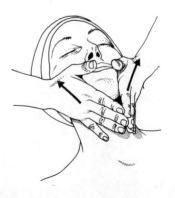

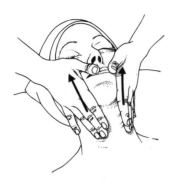
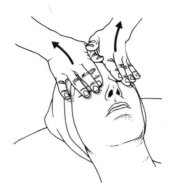

(17) General Rollpatting   As in movement (1), but performed more deeply on the resulting relaxed muscle fibres, caused by the massage routine. The massage concludes with gentle upward pressure on the temples.

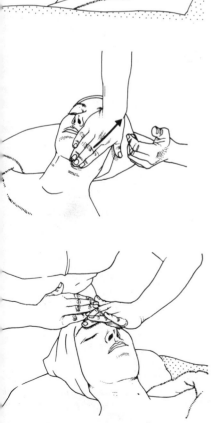

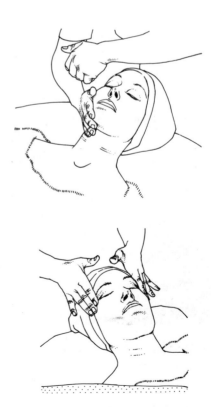

Completion

The massage cream is then removed in the same manner as for the cleansing sequence, and the skin inspected to determine the mask choice. Application of the mask follows, over the face area, and the neck if indicated.

The skin may be wiped over with mild tonic solution, or refreshed with a vaporizer spray between the massage and mask stages, if the skin appears excessively oily. This is not really necessary as the mask removes all surface oil from the skin, but it is pleasant and cooling after the massage. If a mask was not following the massage, then toning would have to be really thorough and performed with the correct toning lotion, to settle the skin and free it from massage cream.

THE PORE TREATMENT MASSAGE ROUTINE

The pore treatment routine is a facial sequence designed to stimulate the skin, increase desquamation, and refine the surface texture. The movements remove surface cellular matter and permit the skin to function more efficiently. Removal of scar tissue and control of oily secretions can be accomplished with regular treatment.

The pore treatment is not a relaxing facial routine, as its main function is to remove overabundant sebaceous secretions, and to deep cleanse and stimulate the skin. Its effect is mainly superficial and it is not designed to affect or tone the muscles of facial expression.

Indications for Treatment

1   Adolescent skin conditions, where overactivity of the sebaceous glands causes blocked pores and a coarse skin texture.

2   Blemished skin may be treated, once medical permission has been granted, by combining the massage in a treatment routine of manual and electrical applications.

3   The pore treatment has several applications for removal of pigmentation (skin discoloration) scar tissue, or for general refining effects, or many varied age groups.

Recognition of Skin Conditions

Hard compacted surface skin layers, with a glassy, oily appearance, coarse texture and uneven colour, are usually apparent. The hair follicles may be blocked, or have formed into comedones (blackheads). Evidence of skin infection, pustules, irritation etc., require medical permission prior to treatment, as manual massage may spread, not restrict, the nature of the condition. A general overactivity of the sebaceous glands may persist into the 20 to 30 age range, gradually becoming more restricted into the centre of the face where the oil glands are most abundant. The slightly older skins may require more refining due to scar tissue, uneven texture and colour, left as an aftermath of acne vulgaris or over-exposure.

Heavily pigmented skins, found in all age groups and nationalities, respond well to this form of stimulating massage, and the compacted, hyperkeratinization of the skin benefits both from the desquamation and cellular regeneration aspects of the pore treatment massage.

Preparation

The client is prepared for general facial therapy, with hair and clothing well protected against the medicated creams and solutions to be employed.

General cleansing may be followed by specialized cleansing in the case of adolescent skin (see Chapter 7, Control Treatments) to remove all oily matter.

Suitable creams are applied to the face: medicated, sulphur or zinc oxide based cream for the oily or blocked areas, and bland cream for the neck and other unaffected parts of the face.

(1) Pinchment Movement (light petrissage)

The thumb and index fingers of both hands pick up a small amount of subcutaneous tissue, and release it sharply. The movement covers the entire neck and face areas, wherever sufficient tissue bulk permits the pinchment to be applied. A rhythmical and planned pattern of strokes increases vascular and lymphatic flow and prepares the face for further massage. The movement ends at the temples, and the hands return to the angle of the mandible.

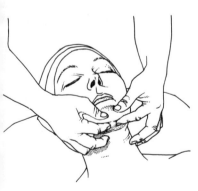

(2) General Rotaries on the Lower Face (petrissage)

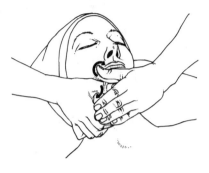

The subcutaneous tissues and superficial muscles are involved in this compression and relaxation movement. The thumbs of both hands compress and release the tissues of the neck and lower face, causing mechanical constriction and dilation of surface vessels. The effect is immediate, and care must be taken to avoid sensitive skin areas, split capillaries, etc. Pressure is applied and released smoothly, and the tissue bulk and skin area under treatment will determine the pressure and rate of the application. This circular movement is repeated over suitable areas, until the desired result (erythema, skin reddening) has been achieved. The hands conclude at the mandible, and change to chin frictions.

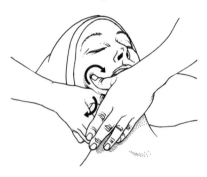

(3) Chin Frictions (petrissage)

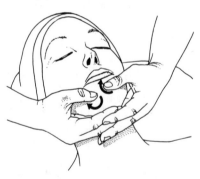

With the fingers loosely placed under the mandible, the thumbs complete small, brisk rotaries on the chin, moving the surface skin layers over the underlying bony structures with the pads of the thumbs. The skin is compressed and released between the thumbs, and desquamation and stimulation should result. The whole chin area is covered with continuous moving rotaries so that the skin does not become irritated, and the movement completes with a flick up of the thumbs over the oral sphincter. The movement may be repeated according to skin blockage and general sensitivity and scar tissue present.

(4) Rotaries on the Nose (petrissage)

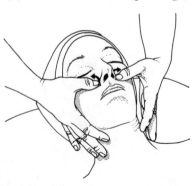

The movement commences on the chin, moves over the orbicularis oris muscle, and works deeply in the nostril area, each thumb working independently with firm rotaries over the surface of the skin. This superficial movement concludes with a sweeping stroke, under the eyes, returning to the chin, via the sides of the face.

(5) Frictions on the Nose and Centre Forehead (petrissage)

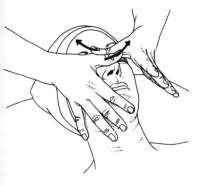

With the fingers loosely held under the mandible, the movement commences on the nose tip, with firm rotaries, moving up and over the tip, to the bridge of the nose. The hands change direction and the thumbs exert pressure towards each other, in a criss-crossing motion up to the corrugator muscle between the brows. Firm rotaries recommence on this area, and the movement concludes with effleurage back to the start position.

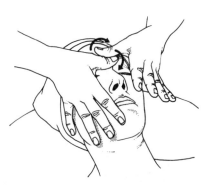

(6) Rollpatting and Whipping (effleurage and tapotement)

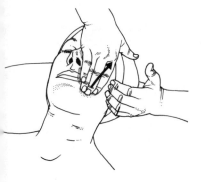

The movement commences at the mandible, with deep rollpatting cheek strokes, then changes to a one-finger whipping movement on the risorius muscle, with increased pressure and rate of movement. The fingers roll deeply into the chin fold, passing backwards and forwards several times, and the pattern is repeated on the right cheek. From the risorius position, the fingers move to the nose, and light whipping movements are applied over the nostrils, bridge of the nose, and the levators of the upper lip. The hands work together, first covering one side, then the other of the nose, concluding with gentle forehead rollpatting, finishing on the temples.

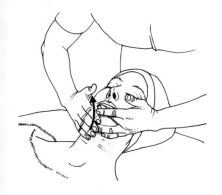

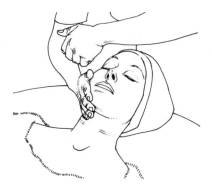

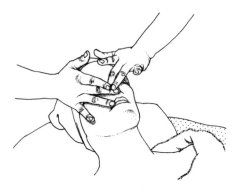
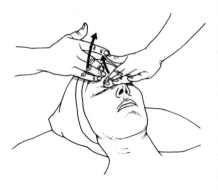

(7) Forehead Frictions (petrissage)

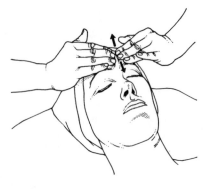

The hands face each other, and friction movements are applied to the entire forehead area. Compression is maintained between the fingers, and care must be taken to avoid downward pressure onto the frontal bone. The left hand moves backwards and forwards, forming a ridge of subcutaneous tissue, which the right hand presses against. When the left hand moves backwards, it has to release and contact the skin, with smooth and controlled movements, to avoid moving the head and causing discomfort. The right hand moves up and down against the compressed ridge, and creates a very stimulating movement with immediate effect. The hands divide at the centre of the forehead, and repeat the friction, 3 times.

(8) Forehead Frictions (petrissage)

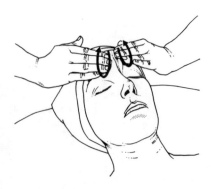

The movement commences as in (7), but the hands both move in opposition to each other, working in close connection to create the friction effect on the occipitofrontalis muscle area.

(9) Forehead Frictions, Circular
(petrissage)

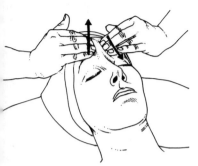

The movement commences as in (7), but the fingers form opposing circular strokes, to create the stimulating effect.

(10) Tapping (tapotement)

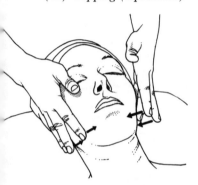

A tapotement movement covering the entire facial area, commencing at the mandible, progressing up the face, to the forehead, concluding at the temples.

(11) Soothing Static Movement
(effleurage)

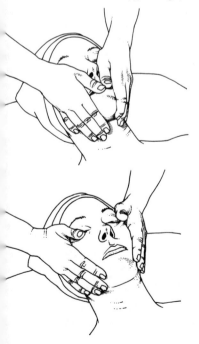

A soothing contact movement of the cheeks and forehead, used to calm sensory nerve endings after the vigorous pore treatment sequence. The hands contour to the mandible, remain static, then progress to the cheeks, and hold the superficial cheek muscles in a relaxed position for a few seconds. The movement is repeated on the forehead area, and the routine concludes with gentle upward pressure on the temples.

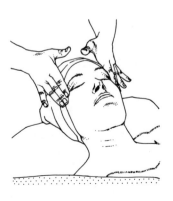

Conclusion

The pore treatment massage movements are extremely stimulating and skin inspection is essential after cream removal to ascertain the degree of sensitivity present, prior to mask choice, and application.

THE CONTINENTAL FACIAL MASSAGE ROUTINE (Face, Neck, and Shoulder Girdle)

The continental facial sequence is more extensive in its application than the basic facial, covering the face, neck and shoulder girdle areas. Its action on the muscles of facial expression, and the larger muscles of the shoulder girdle, makes it more suitable for the mature client in the 40 years upwards age range. Massage technique is more advanced and increased strength, hand control, and flexibility is necessary before the continental massage routine should be attempted by the therapist.

The relaxing elements of the routine bring increased psychological benefit to tense, fatigued, depressed, or highly strung clients of all age groups, and this should be a major consideration in the choice of application. Physical effects of the massage include relaxation of tense muscle fibres, improved vascular and lymphatic circulation, and increased cellular activity of the skin's basal layers. This regeneration process produces a finer, softer skin texture, avoids the formation of dry or crêpy skin conditions, and delays the effects of ageing considerably. The surface tissues are maintained in good health, delaying or preventing the formation of pigmentation, skin thickening, or fibrous malformations frequently associated with the menopausal age group.

Indications for Treatment

1   Mature skin conditions, with dry, crêpy or loose texture, and evident expression lines around the mouth and eyes, and between the nose and mouth.

2   Neglected or abused younger skin conditions where lack of care or exposure to the elements has caused dehydration of surface tissues and premature ageing.

3   Physical conditions of depression, worry or fatigue, or following a period of ill health.

4   As a preventative measure on younger clients to delay the ageing process.

Recognition of Skin Conditions

A combination of facial conditions may be present, which will indicate application of the continental facial routine. Loss of skin tone and elasticity due to the ageing process create a looser skin texture and soften the facial profile. Flexure lines of muscles are firmly etched, and expression lines become a permanent feature, particularly between the brows, from the nose to the mouth and around the eyes. The skin's natural secretions, desquamation, and biological activity decrease, and surface cells build up to give a thickened appearance in the mouth and chin areas. Continual exposure on a fine skin many have caused surface capillaries to dilate and rupture into the surface skin layers, presenting a general vascular appearance on the upper cheeks and nose. Dehydration of the skin, due to incorrect care, exposure, or an incorrect dietary balance, is evident by dry flakey patches, a crêpy skin texture, and fine lining of poorly supported muscles, i.e. platysma.

Preparation

The client is prepared for the more extensive massage sequence by robing being placed across the breasts, under the arms, leaving the upper arms, shoulders, and upper back available for massage. Adequate protection of blankets around the chest, arms, and back must be observed, as these areas would not normally be involved in the massage sequence and can easily be soiled.

The entire face, neck, shoulder, upper arm and back areas must be cleansed throroughly with an extended form of cleansing and removal sequence. Client relaxation should be established during the cleansing section in preparation for the deeper movements which follow in the massage routine.

Application of suitable nourishing, hormone, hydrating, or toning creams should be accomplished with rollpatting strokes applied with varying pressure according to muscle bulk.

CONTINENTAL FACIAL MASSAGE ROUTINE

(1) Broad Sweeping Effleurage

Superficial followed by deep effleurage over the sterno-mastoid, pectoralis, deltoid and trapezius muscles, up to the occipital cavity, at the base of the skull, returning to the angle of the mandible. Repeat 6 times.

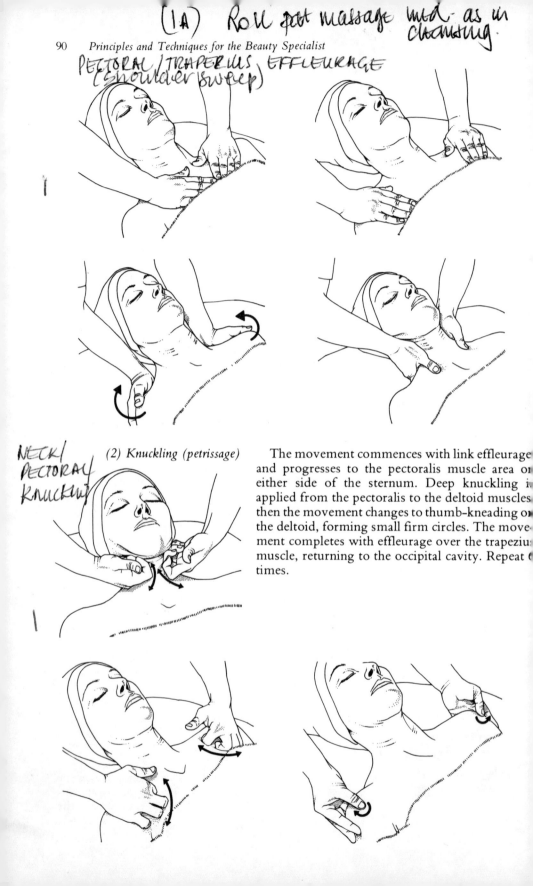

(1A) Roll get massage med· as in cleansing.

PECTORAL (TRAPEZIUS) EFFLEURAGE (shoulder sweep)

NECK/ PECTORAL Knuckling

(2) Knuckling (petrissage)

The movement commences with link effleurage and progresses to the pectoralis muscle area on either side of the sternum. Deep knuckling is applied from the pectoralis to the deltoid muscles then the movement changes to thumb-kneading on the deltoid, forming small firm circles. The movement completes with effleurage over the trapezius muscle, returning to the occipital cavity. Repeat 6 times.

(3) Throat Brace   As in the Basic Facial.

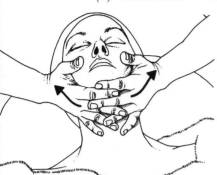 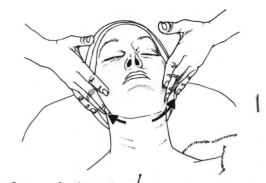

(4) Trapezius Rolling (petrissage, kneading)

TRAPEZIUS KNEAD/EFFLEURAGE

The head is placed slightly to the right, and both hands alternately lift and knead the trapezius muscle, from the shoulder to the occipital cavity on the left side. The right hand commences, completes 4 to 6 repetitions and links across to the right side, whilst the left hand follows. The sequence is repeated on the right side, with the head turned to the left, and the left hand commencing. On completion both hands return to the mastoid process area, and the head is placed centrally.

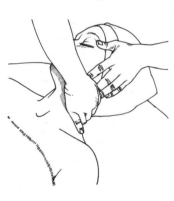

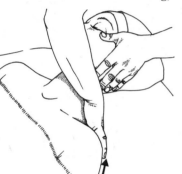 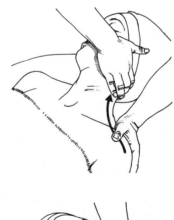

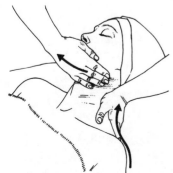 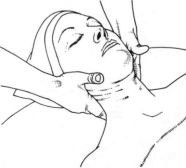

(5) Broad Sweeping Effleurage

(6) Kneading on the Trapezius
                    (petrissage)

As in movement (1), repeated 6 times.

The movement begins as in (1), and changes into firm kneading of the trapezius, with a forward lifting movement, using the palmar surface of the hand, with the thumbs abducted. The entire muscle bulk is covered with varying pressure, right up to its insertion in the occipital cavity. Repeat 3 times.

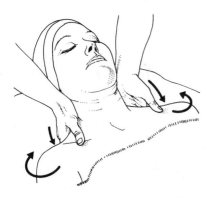

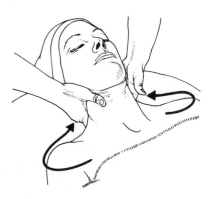

(7) Triangular Movement
(effleurage lifting movement)

Each hand works separately, forming a triangular-shaped movement over the chest and neck. Superficial effleurage moves down the sterno-mastoid muscle, changing into broad sweeping over the pectoralis, and sternum areas, and contoured lifting effleurage from the origin to the insertion of the platysma, finishing each stroke in a firm upward direction on the point of the mandible. The superficial neck muscle is held against the lower jaw, and then the movement relaxes, the hand returns to the angle of the mandible, the alternate hand repeats the movement. Four slow repeats on each side.

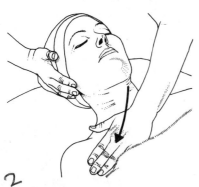

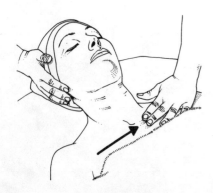

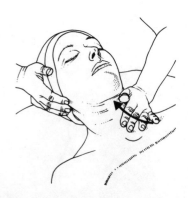

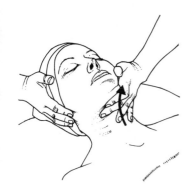 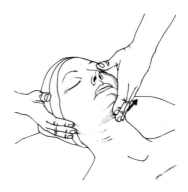

(8) *Deep Kneading on the Shoulder Girdle Muscles (petrissage)*

Deep Knuckle – Shoulder Girdle

The movement commences with sweeping effleurage, and progresses to deep kneading on the biceps, triceps, deltoid and trapezius muscles. The maximum area of the hand should be in contact, with pressure maintained between the fingers and thumbs wherever possible. The arms must be free to accomplish the movements deeply, and the hand control and sustained strength necessary will develop gradually. The sequence may be applied in three stages with linking effleurage, or as one long active movement, as experience of the routine grows. The therapist should have a relaxed posture and a steady breathing rhythm to avoid fatigue and maintain satisfactory technique.

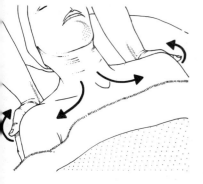

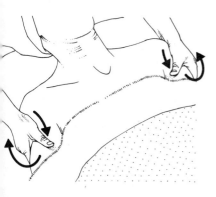 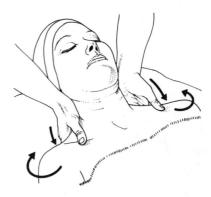

(9) *Sweeping Effleurage and Vibration*

As in movement (1) with the addition of vibrations in the occipital cavity. The forearm muscles contract and relax, to produce a fine trembling

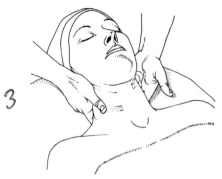

3

vibration at the finger tips placed at the base of the skull. The vibration is held for a few seconds, and the movement repeats 6 times.

(10) Kneading along the Mandible (petrissage)

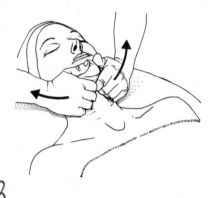

3

The movement commences with link effleurage, with the mandible passing between the thumb and bent index finger to the point of the chin. The kneading movement progresses back towards the ears, compressing and relaxing along the jaw, with smooth rhythmical strokes, to the angle of the mandible. Repeat 6 times.

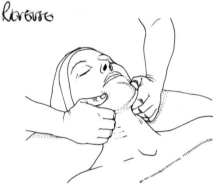

(11) Lifting Movement under the Mandible (petrissage, for lymphatic drainage)

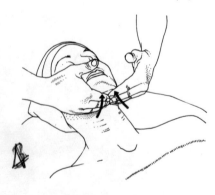

A lifting compression movement along the mandible; linked with effleurage, using the palmar surface of the fingers, with the thumbs abducted. The movement progresses from the point to the angle of the jaw, with four compression strokes in the direction of the lymphatic nodes.

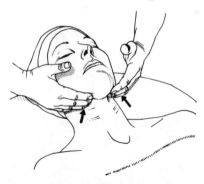

(12) Chin Crossing Movement
      (effleurage and petrissage)

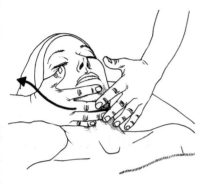

Both hands commence at the angle of the mandible: the right hand crosses the chin and lifts the left superficial cheek muscles, and returns to the right cheek to lift the massater muscle from the mandible to the zygomatic arch. The left hand replaces the right, continuing and then releasing the compression, to link with effleurage across the chin, and repeat the movement on the left side. The hands alternate, making and breaking contact smoothly, with the main emphasis being placed at the mandible level, whilst compressing and lifting the massater muscle with the heel of the hand, moving backwards. To finish the continuous movement, the hands divide at the point of the chin, and return to the angle of the jaw. Repeat the movement until the desired result is achieved.

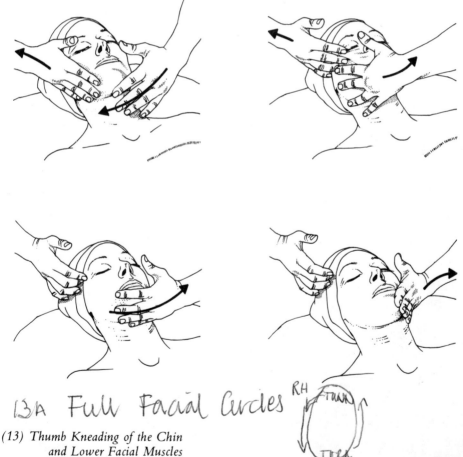

13A Full Facial Circles RH

(13) Thumb Kneading of the Chin
      and Lower Facial Muscles
                  (petrissage)

Compression and relaxation of the lower facial muscles, the triangularis, depressor of the lower lip, and platysma, using both thumbs working in

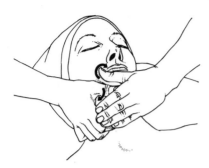

opposition in order to form kneading movements
along the mandible. The pressure and rate of application are dictated by the tissue bulk and sensitivity
present. A continuous movement.

(14) Lip Bracing Movements
(effleurage)

old - Centre mandible, Rock, split, R
out to

The hands form a cradle over the orbicularis
oris muscle, and lightly follow the shape of the oral
sphincter to the corners of the mouth. The index
and second fingers of both hands smooth out superficial lines gently and the movement repeats 6
times.

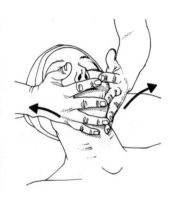
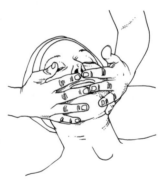
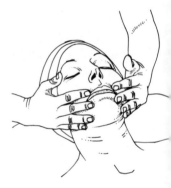

(15) Facial Lift (effleurage and
petrissage)

As in the basic training facial. The facial lift links
the lower and upper facial movements, and is
repeated 6 times.

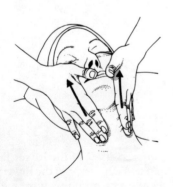

*(16) Forehead Rollpatting
(effleurage)*

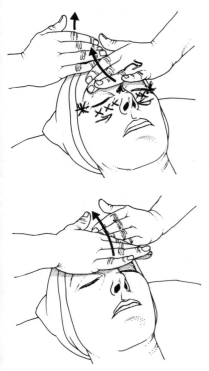

Slow deep rollpatting, lifting the orbicularis oculi muscles, from the left to the right temples and back, completing 16 rollpatting strokes across the forehead. At the left temple, the movement changes to superficial effleurage on first the crows feet area, then under the eye, and back to the outer eye area, using the index or second finger for 4 strokes on each section. The movement links across the forehead and with slow rollpatting, repeats on the right eye, and returns to the central brow, and divides to return to the temples.

This movement is performed slowly, carefully, and increases the relaxation aspects of the massage sequence. The bony nature of the underlying structures dictates the pressure and rate of movement necessary.

*(17) Eye Circling, and Lifting
(effleurage)*

From the temples the second fingers perform superficial circles under the eyes, towards the nose, following the orbicularis oculi muscle fibres. The index fingers join the movement at the nose to form a lifting stroke at the corrugator muscle. The direction of the hands changes to lift the upper fibres of the orbicularis oculi and frontalis muscles, along the length of the eyebrow back to the temples. The upward lifting movement is maintained along the upper fibres of the eye muscle, raising the upper lids, but not opening the eyes. The movement is repeated 6 times.

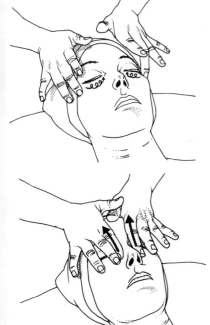

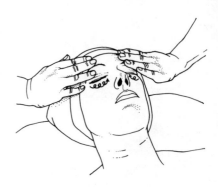

(18) Forehead Frictions (petrissage)   As in the basic facial No 11 movement.

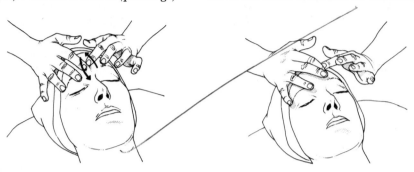

(19) Eye Lifting Movement
(effleurage)

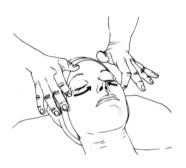

Effleurage under the eye progresses to lifting of the corrugator muscle, with the index finger. The lifting pressure is maintained by the index finger, and then transferred first to the fourth, third, second and index fingers, moving outwards to the temples, keeping the upper lids and eyebrows lifted. The movement repeats 6 times.

Finger control and evenness of rhythm are important points of technique in this movement if relaxation is to be maintained.

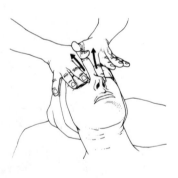

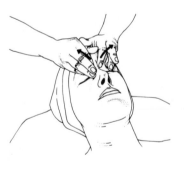

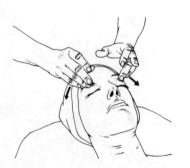

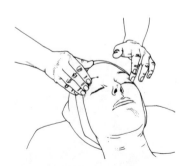

(20) Praying Movement (effleurage and petrissage)

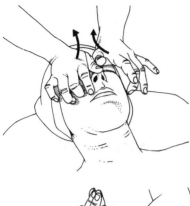

Effleurage under the eyes progresses to a lifting movement of the frontalis muscle, where the hands pivot on the central brow. The hands form a praying position, which stretches and lifts the occipito-frontalis muscles towards the temporal areas of the skull. Repeat 6 times.

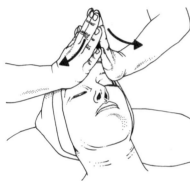
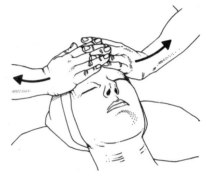

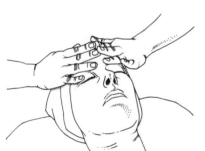
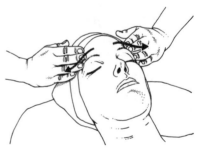

(21) Tapotement along the Mandible

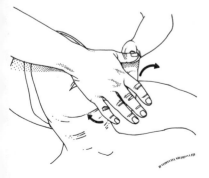

Effleurage from the temples to the mandible brings the hands into a tapotement position under the mandible. The fingers work in a tapping sequence, backwards and forwards along the jaw. The intensity of the taps increases, and the fingers form outward fan-like strokes, concentrating on the central area under the point of the mandible, where adipose tissue accumulates. The lower area of the massater muscle may be included in the movement, if the muscle tone of the lower facial muscles indicates its inclusion. A continual tapotement movement, which is applied until the necessary reaction is achieved.

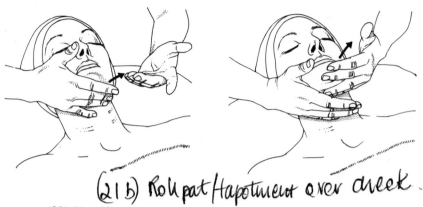

(21 b) Roll pat Hapotinent over cheek.

(22) Knuckling on the Sternomastoid (petrissage)

The movement commences on the clavicle area, with knuckling of the sternomastoid muscle up to the mastoid process. It progresses along the mandible and is linked by effleurage back to the clavicle. Repeat 6 times.

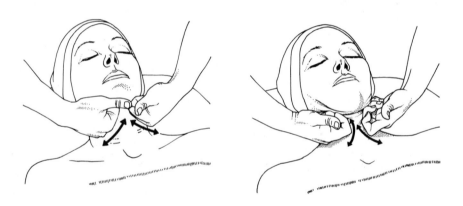

(23) Facial Lift   As in the basic facial.

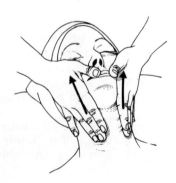

(24) Rollpatting (effleurage)

Deep slow rollpatting over the entire shoulder, neck, and face areas, concludes the massage sequence, finishing with gentle upward pressure on the temples.

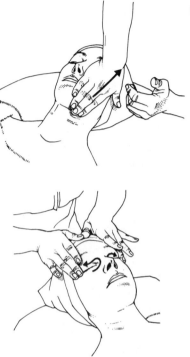

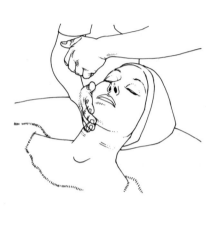

Conclusion

After removal of the massage cream and skin inspection, the appropriate mask and a throat pad may be applied.

These three facial massage routines cover all general facial conditions and age groups. Specialized skin treatments combining massage and electrical applications for specific conditions will be dealt with in later chapters.

Chapter 5

Skin Disorders and Minor Imperfections

Very few skins on magnified inspection are found to be perfect in texture and general appearance. Recognition of skin disorders and blemishes is important as they may contra-indicate (prohibit) or limit the treatment planned. Medical agreement is necessary in the treatment of certain stages of adolescent skin disturbance and other conditions where sepsis is present. Knowledge of the skin's physiology gives guidance as to the reasons for malfunction and possible causes of imperfections. However, recognition is the most important aspect for the therapist, preventing her from treating, cosmetically, conditions which require medical attention. Whilst it is within a beauty specialist's competence to treat minor skin complaints, she must, as a professional person, refer acute and chronic skin disorders to the client's personal physician.

Many minor skin imperfections can be cured or controlled by salon treatment and cosmetic home care sequences, and success in these applications will increase client confidence and the operator's professional status. Acceptance of the limitations in cases which are outside the field of reference will prevent client disappointment. Suspected infectious conditions on the face, hands and feet should be referred for medical attention, and must be noticed prior to treatment. Primary inspection is vital if cross-infection is to be avoided, and due to the exposed position of the therapist, regarding the client's personal circumstances, and the open method of appointment booking, she should take additional care to safeguard herself, her clinic, and her other clients from the risk of infection.

Common sense and a sound knowledge of skin diseases, minor blemishes, and pigmentation abnormalities will guide the therapist in her decision regarding the application of salon treatment. Any condition which appears irritated, inflamed, or where secondary infection is present should be referred for medical attention. As the client may consult her beauty specialist first, it is a duty to her to see not only that she receives the most suitable attention but also that the treatments should not increase or prolong her skin complaint.

DERMATOLOGICAL TERMS IN USE

Erythema, redness of the skin.

Macule, a mark or discoloration of the skin, which can be seen but not felt.

Wheal, the fully developed wheal is red, raised above the surface, has a whitish centre, and a superficial lumpy feel. It may vary in size from a centimetre in diameter to a plaque many centimetres in surface area.

Papule, a firm lump, which does not contain fluid. It may be vascular in appearance and varies in size from a pin-head to half a centimetre.

Vesicle, a small elevation in the skin, containing fluid.

Bulla, a larger blister.

Pustule, a pustule is a lesion which commences as a papule, and becomes purulent in the centre (containing pus). Pustules develop at the mouths of hair follicles, appearing as an inflamed, red area, with a central core of pus, from which a hair may project.

SKIN DISORDERS REQUIRING MEDICAL ATTENTION OR LIMITED THERAPY

The Facial Area

Eczema (dermatitis)
Inflammation of the Skin

A skin condition which commences as an itching red area, with pin-head sized vesicles, and progresses to a scaly, dry patchiness, or continued vesicle formation and weeping. Eczema is a tissue reaction involving the epidermis and upper layers of the dermis, caused by

1 External contact with a substance to which the skin is allergic (exogenous).

2 Internal stimulus via the blood stream (endogenous).

Herpes Simplex (cold sore)

Vesicles grouped in a cluster around the mouth and nostril areas are apparent. The eruption commences as an itchy patch of erythema, which develops into weeping vesicles if scratched. Herpes simplex is a recurring disease, which lasts for a few days, usually leaving no trace. The area should be left alone, and salon facial treatment postponed until the condition has cleared.

Urticaria (hives)   An elevation of the skin into red wheals, from the size of a dot to a few centimetres, forming itchy patches. The distribution of the eruption may be local or widespread, and individual lesions subside in a few hours. Urticaria may be caused by an allergic reaction from internal or external sources. The most common cause is the introduction of a foreign protein, which causes the tissue cells to release histamine, brings out the dilatation of surface blood vessels, and creates the itchy swollen patches. The condition usually corrects itself, but in some extreme cases medical opinion is needed to determine the cause of the attack and eliminate it.

Rosacea   Rosacea, like acne, is an eruption which affects the face, and is associated with seborrhoea (excessive oiliness). The cutaneous vessels of the nose and cheeks are the most affected, giving a red flushed appearance, particularly after the intake of food, or due to a change in temperature. The disease may be of long standing, and is disfiguring as the skin surface becomes lumpy and thickened with papules and pustules. Rosacea is sometimes confused with acne, due to its location, but rosacea seldom appears before the age of 30, whilst acne has usually regressed by that age.

Seborrhoea   Seborrhoea is caused by over-activity of the sebaceous glands, secretion, an excess of sebum, and abnormal oiliness of the skin's surface. The situation and density of the sebaceous glands in the scalp, face, centre of the chest and back cause the seborrhoea to be most evident in these areas. During puberty the activity of the glands is increased due to hormonal changes, and the sebaceous gland ducts and hair follicles become enlarged, the skin becomes coarser, and open pores are evident. The excessive oily secretion blocks the outward flow of sebum to the surface, and it becomes lodged in the follicle and sebaceous duct. The retained sebum increases in amount, and the external area hardens and becomes overlaid with epidermal cells to form a comedone (blackhead). Seborrhoea is the basis of several skin diseases, particularly acne vulgaris.

Acne Vulgaris   In acne vulgaris the skin appears greasy, has a dull sallow colour, and blackheads, papules, pustules, and scars are often present at the same time. Acne vulgaris is most commonly found in adolescents, and it may involve the entire face, chest, and shoulder girdle, or be confined in any one of these areas. Seborrhoea is present and forms comedones in varying intensities depending on the influence of the endocrine glands on the sebaceous secretion. The dark colour of the blackhead is due to the development of sulphides in the keratinized cells of the surface blockage. Not all follicles become blocked, but removal of surface oiliness and skin blockage reduces the possibility of the acne condition increasing in area. Secondary infection is sometimes present due to staphylococcal infection, with inflammation and pustules forming around the horny blackhead. The infection may spread to involve the sebaceous gland, and a deep seated pustular condition becomes established. Many acne eruptions leave disfiguring scars, and so must be dealt with medically if secondary infection is present. Therapy treatment can be applied to good effect if medical agreement is given to control the condition and improve its management. See Chapter 9, Control Treatments.

MINOR SKIN BLEMISHES

PIGMENTATION ABNORMALITIES

Naevi (Vascular and Pigmented Birthmarks)

Spider Naevus (telangiectatic angioma)

The spider naevus consists of a central dilated vessel, with smaller capillaries radiating from it like the legs of a spider. It is often called a broken vein, and may be isolated or in an area of vascular skin such as the cheeks. The spider naevus usually develops in adult life, and is commonly found on the face, particularly on the upper cheek and eye areas. They respond well to diathermy coagulation treatment, performed by a skilled electrologist.

Port Wine Stain (capillary angioma)

The port wine stain consists of a large area of dilated capillaries, causing a pink to dark red skin colour, which makes it contrast vividly with the surrounding skin. The stain is commonly found on the face and, as the skin texture is usually normal, application of cosmetic masking camouflage is very successful in alleviating embarrassment and distress. (See Chapter 7, Makeup Techniques). The port wine stain does not usually regress, and its treatment is limited.

Strawberry Mark (superficial cavernous angioma)

A brightly pigmented skin area, seen at birth or developing soon afterwards, which usually disappears before adult life.

Pigmented Naevi   Pigmented naevi may occur on any part of the body and are often found on the neck and face being sometimes associated with strong hair growth (pigmented hairy naevi). They vary in size from a pin-head to several centimetres normally, but in rare cases may be extremely large. The pigmentation present may be light brown to very dark or black. Pigmented naevi, with the exception of the coal black variety, are classed as benign tumours, and their removal is usually for cosmetic reasons. Small pigmented naevi can be removed by an electrologist using diathermy (heat) coagulation, if medical agreement is given, or they can be surgically excised, with very successful results.

Freckles (ephelides)   Ephelides are small pigmented areas of skin, which become more evident on exposure to sunlight and are found in greatest abundance on the face, arms and legs. Fair-skinned individuals suffer most from the condition, which can be cosmetically disfiguring, especially on red-haired women, where the freckles join up to form large patches. The intensity of the colour can be reduced by bleaching creams, and peeling pastes, but will re-appear on exposure to sunlight.

Lentigo   Darker areas of pigmentation, which appear more distinct than freckles, and have a slightly raised appearance, and more scattered distribution. They do not increase in colour density or number on exposure to sunlight.

Chloasma   A condition of pigmentation most freqently associated with pregnancy, involving the upper cheeks, nose, and occasionally the forehead areas of the face. The discoloration usually disappears spontaneously with the termination of the pregnancy, but if it persists the usual desquamation therapy methods will affect a cure.

Vitiligo   A complete loss of colour in the skin and hairs in well-defined areas of the body, face and limbs. Commencing as small patches, which may converge to form fairly large areas. The skin around the patches sometimes appear hyper-pigmented, and the condition is most obvious on darker-skinned individuals. The basal cells are no longer able to manufacture melanin, and so the areas must be protected from ultraviolet exposure, or irritation will result. Cosmetic camouflage can be used to disguise prominent areas on the face, neck or hands, which cause anxiety or embarrassment to the client.

SKIN IMPERFECTIONS

Papilloma (moles)   Moles are a common occurrence on the face and body, and present several different forms, varying in size, colour, and vascular appearance. Flat colourless moles are termed as 'sessile', whilst those which are raised above the surface, attached by a stalk, are said to be 'pedunculated'. All raised and pigmented moles require medical agreement prior to electrology treatment, or they can be removed surgically if they cause distress.

Skin Tags   A common fibrous skin condition, associated with ageing and most frequently found on the neck and major flexures of the middle-aged and elderly. The tags form a single or multiple distribution, and they are of a soft pedunculated form, being made up of loose fibrous tissue. The colour may be unchanged, but is often hyper-pigmented, making them more obvious. The most common situation is the sides of the neck, where they form a tear drop arrangement. The stalks of the tags can be treated successfully with diathermy coagulation by a skilled electrologist, trained in minor cosmetic surgery, once medical approval has been granted. Therapy treatment will be limited by the presence of skin tags, to avoid catching them and causing discomfort.

Split Capillaries   Dilated capillaries on a fine skin texture assume a general vascular appearance, often affecting large areas of the face. The skin responds fiercely to stimulation and permanent dilated vessels are apparent, particularly on the upper cheeks and nose. The fineness of the skin and its general sensitivity, give guidance as to the probability of split capillary formation, and limit the range of possible treatments. Ruptured blood vessels assume a line-like appearance in surface tissues, and can become bulbous and blue in colour due to the congestion of vascular circulation in the area.

Treatment varies in success, depending on the location, intensity, and establishment of the condition, but can be very satisfactory in certain cases. Early stages of capillary damage can be arrested by cosmetic means, and additional protective measures, including avoidance of exposure to ultravoilet rays. Ruptured or dilated vessels can only be reduced by diathermy or chemical coagulation methods, applied with caution, and attention to the general skin condition present. Removal of minor skin blemishes by diathermy is a specialized field of epilation, which requires additional training and experience in order to ensure success.

The presence of split capillaries limits and alters treatment routines, and generalized conditions require specialized applications to prevent causing further damage. See Chapter 6, Specialized Skin Treatments.

Whiteheads (milia)   A whitehead is formed when sebum becomes trapped in a blind duct, with no surface opening. The condition is most common on dry skin, and the milia appear frequently on the orbicularis oculi muscle area, and between the brows. Milia can form after injury, i.e. sunburn, on the face or shoulders, and are sometimes widespread in their location. Recently formed whiteheads can disappear spontaneously after a period of regular massage treatment, appearing to be reabsorbed by the body. Well established milia have to be pierced, with a sterile probe or by diathermy, to create an opening to the surface, and release the contents. The whiteheads appear as pearly, rounded lumps under the skin, or raised above it, depending on their size. When the skin is stretched, the milia becomes more obvious and white in colour. The delicate nature of their location and the risk of infection require an experienced approach to the removal to prevent discomfort. Strict attention must be given to personal and salon hygiene, and to the aftercare advice to the client.

Crow's-feet   Fine lining around the eyes is caused by habitual expressions and normal flexure folds associated with ageing of muscle tissue. Premature formation may be due to eye strain, and is often associated with oedema (swelling) around and under the eyes. Dislike of spectacles in the mature client may be a contributory factor in crow's-feet lining, and should be considered as a prime cause for the condition in this age group. Skin which has been continually exposed to excessive amounts of sunlight is most susceptible to fine wrinkling, as are dry, fine skins lacking in natural oils and moisture. By early recognition of the fine eye skin, and its predisposition to crow's-feet, formation of the condition can be delayed by reduction of eye strain and application of herbal eye treatments and a revised skin care sequence.

Crêpy Skin   Crêpy skin can be due to several causes, and is most evident on dry skins, which have been neglected or abused by over exposure or insufficient cosmetic care. Ill-health or an extreme weight loss, causing a reduction in the subcutaneous adipose tissue, can cause crêpy skin to be very marked and unpleasant in appearance. Prevention of the condition is more successful than treatment after its formation, but results can be achieved with specialized forms of therapy, which stimulate the skin and hydrate the surface layers.

The condition presents a loose, soft lined appearance in which fine lines criss-cross to form a network of superficial wrinkles. The elastic fibres of the skin are altered in their action, and loss of adipose tissue gives the skin the appearance of being too large for the underlying muscles. Poorly supported muscles are the first to be affected, i.e. the platysma, and orbicularis oculi, but the condition can affect the whole facial and body skin.

Superfluous Hair (hypertrichosis)

The growth of strong hairs in an abnormal situation is termed hypertrichosis. The condition is extremely distressing and causes embarrassment, particularly when a heavy facial growth is formed. The upper lip hairs are the most commonly involved, changing from a vellus to a superfluous or terminal form, and becoming coarse and apparent. Hypertrichosis may develop at any age, and is seen with increasing frequency after the menopause. A disturbance in hormonal balance often appears to be associated with superfluous hair formation, and a degree of endocrine disorder would appear to be responsible. Diathermy (heat) coagulation is the most successful method for permanent removal of the hair, whilst temporary measures involving waxing the area offer a short-term solution if the growth is not extensive.

The common occurrence of this condition will bring it frequently to the notice of the beauty specialist, who, if she is also trained as an electrologist, should undertake treatment on the understanding that, although the treatment may be long term, the final result will be very satisfactory to the client.

The study of epilation (permanent removal of hair by diathermy coagulation) is a specialized field of remedial work, requiring additional training and knowledge, and extensive practical tuition before proficiency is reached. The risks of scarring are high, and repeated regrowth and permanent damage can easily result from inexperienced technique.

The work of the facial specialist and electrologist are closely allied, and qualification in both fields extends the range of treatments that may be offered.

ALLERGIC SKIN
CONDITIONS

An allergic reaction is seen as an abnormal response to a specific substance, brought about by antibodies in the blood, formed after a previous exposure to the substance concerned. There are many forms of allergy, which appear as an urticaria or eczematous dermatitis reaction, though these conditions may be due to other causes. The allergic reaction may be due to ingestion of a foreign protein, inhalation as in hay fever, or due to contact with a sensitizing agent. Detecting the underlying cause of an allergic reaction is a medical responsibility, and should not be attempted by the therapist. However, due to the complex nature of allergic reactions in clients, it is necessary for the therapist to be cautious in her cosmetic applications, particularly on any individual who has a history of previous allergy.

On many occasions what appears to be a mild allergic reaction, may in fact be a primary irritation caused by application of an unsuitable item. Primary irritants, such as caustic preparations, highly perfumed creams, and alcohol-based lotions should be avoided, and hypo-allergenic or neutral products used.

The true allergy is a specific type of reaction, and is said to be a specific, acquired, altered capacity to react. It usually follows the same pattern of exposure to the substance or item, a period of time elapsing in which the blood forms antibodies, and lastly, a re-application or re-exposure to the sensitizer causing an allergic reaction.

Use of hypo-allergenic products on difficult skin conditions will relieve some of the problems of allergy or irritation, as all known sensitizing elements have been screened out, leaving a bland preparation. In all salon treatments involving skin care preparations and cosmetic applications special attention during skin inspection and discussion with the client will help to avoid the risk of both primary and allergic reactions being formed. Greater responsibility has been placed on the therapist regarding skin care and cosmetic advice to her clients, due to the increasing complexity of cosmetic formulations, causing an additional risk of allergic reaction.

SKIN DISEASES AND DISORDERS OF THE LIMBS, FEET AND HANDS

Psoriasis

Psoriasis can affect the entire body and facial areas, but is often seen on the limbs, situated on the knees and elbow areas. The lesions of psoriasis commence as dull red papules, the size of pinheads, and they develop into plaques which are bright red in colour, with sharply defined margins. The patches of psoriasis may have flaky silvery-white scales, overlying the surface, which give the condition a distinct appearance. The cause of the condition is not known, but it does appear to be a recurring complaint, and in some cases may be present in small areas most of an individual's life.

Psoriasis may attack the nail fold, or the nail bed, and causes pitting of the nail plate, and a build up of cells under the free edge.

All psoriasis conditions of the skin and nails require medical attention, although a small proportion of salon clients may have small areas which appear at times of stress and which may not prohibit treatment as long as the area involved is completely avoided, and the client's doctor is in agreement with the treatment being undertaken. Soothing salon applications and a feeling of well being achieved through relaxation may be useful in preventing a recurrence of the condition, as it is thought to be connected with the nervous state of the individual.

Eczema

Eczema can develop on the lower part of the legs when varicose veins are present. The skin has a shiny, glazed appearance, with a congestion of the blood supply, giving a bluish red colour, and evident split capillaries. The condition could develop into a varicose ulcer, and as the skin cracks easily, due to its impaired blood supply, no treatment must be attempted.

Ringworm

Ringworm infections account for a large part of all skin infections likely to need medical help for their cure. There are three main genera of Ringworm—Microsporum
—Trichophyton (endothrix and ectothrix)
—Epidermophyton,
but there are many species, some of which will be considered.

Ringworm is a fungus infection and comes within the Dermatophytes group of fungi, which produce superficial infection (termed Dermatomycoses) of the skin, hair and nails. The well known names Ringworm and Tinea do not unfortunately cover all varieties of fungus infection, as there are many other types of fungus involvement apart from these.

Within the Ringworm group the Microsporon fungus affects the surface of the skin and grows within the hair shaft bringing about the condition known as *Tinea Capitis* (Ringworm of the scalp). The vast majority of cases are due to the Microsporon Audouini (a variety peculiar to the human species) or Microsporon Canis, (animal origin). Tinea Capitis is seen as round scaly patches, with the hairs broken off, giving a bald appearance. The condition is most common in children, but does affect adults.

Bald patches on the scalp where the hairs assume a dot-like appearance may be due to the Trichophton fungus, though this is much less common. The 'black dot' ringworm is in fact a condition where the hairs only are attacked, and break off at the surface showing a pigmented stump. The species involved is the Trichophyton endothrix, mostly of human origin.

Where the condition is more inflammatory, the patches more scaly and clearly defined, the fungus may be the Trichophyton Ectothrix, of animal origin, horses, cattle, cats and dogs. This uncommon condition often leaves the patches without hairs after treatment is completed (Alopecia), so is extremely disfiguring.

Ringworm of the beard, Tinea Barbae, is also due to the endothrix and ectothrix Trichophytons, taking superficial and deep forms, depending on severity. The superficial type shows scaly patches, with partial hair loss in the affected patches. The hairs are brittle, and show enlarged white bulbous roots on removal. Alopecia can result in the affected areas, making this an extremely disfiguring but uncommon problem. The deep form of the condition produces deep pustules, nodules, in addition to the hair loss, and is mainly found affecting the lower cheeks and neck. The condition may be localized along the jawline, and is complicated by the process of shaving, which normally has to cease in the affected areas.

Ringworm of the skin is caused by various forms of Trichophyton and Microsporon and is described as *Tinea Circinata*. The lesions are ringed, single or multiple, and vary in severity, from mild scaling to inflamed itching areas. The primary lesion is a small red macule which spreads outwards as it heals in the centre. The ringed appearance is often distinctive. Most common in children, the patches affect the face, shoulders and neck areas most frequently.

The Epidermophyton genera of ringworm is a fungus closely related to the Trichophyton variety, but it does not affect the hair, only the skin, hence the name Epidermophyton, an epidermal fungus. The conditions Tinea Cruris, Tinea Pedis and Tinea Unguium may all be traced to this genera through different species.

Tinea Cruris is an acute eruption involving the groin, and inside thigh area, and is more common in males. The Epidermophyton Inguinale (floccosum) form is the most common cause, but occasionally it can be traced to forms of Trichophyton. The scaly lesions often have the appearance of eczema, and are extremely irritating.

Tinea Pedis is mainly caused by the Epidermophyton Inguinale (floccosum) and involves the toes and the sole of the foot. The lesion on the foot may be the primary one, and elsewhere on the body may be seen other eruptions of a fungus type. Tinea Pedis is extremely common, and infectious, but is fairly easy to control. The skin between the toes assumes a sodden appearance, and when rubbed off shows deep splits in the skin, and a raw reddened area.

Tinea Unguium, ringworm of the nails, can be caused by the Trichophyton or Epidermophyton types, but it may have other causes. The nails are attacked from either the free edge, or from the nail fold, and assume a distorted horny appearance. The nail plate is discoloured, rough, opaque and very disfigured. In most cases the nails of the feet will have been affected prior to the hands becoming involved.

Athlete's Foot (tinea pedis)

Athlete's Foot is a fungus infection which affects the spaces between the toes, assuming a sodden white appearance, with deep splits at the base of the macerated tissue. It is an extremely infectious condition, which can also affect the hands, and it is difficult to eliminate completely due to continual re-exposure to contact. Athlete's Foot can be acquired by contact with objects which have previously been in contact themselves with the disease. Communal living, swimming baths, residential schools, and family contact are all sources of the infection. No salon treatment must be given to an individual suffering from Athlete's Foot, and the risks of cross-infection if the condition is undetected, are extremely high. Sterilization of tools and bowls etc. in foot treatments, is essential, to maintain salon hygiene.

Onychia (hands) Inflammation of the Nail Fold and Nail Bed

The nail fold becomes swollen, tender and inflamed, and pus is discharged between the fold and the nail plate. The cuticle disappears, and one or more nails may be affected over a period of time. The structure of the nail becomes altered around the base and sides, the cells become yellowish in colour, and transverse and longitudinal ridges appear. The entire nail plate may be shed, causing great discomfort and personal nuisance.

Onychia mainly affects women, and is usually due to prolonged wet work involving contact with detergent or alkaline solutions, which affect the cuticle. The condition may, however, have originated in rough manicuring procedures, or use of dirty implements, and so attention must be paid to scrupulous salon hygiene, and application of correct practical techniques.

Warts

Common Warts (verruca vulgaris)

Common warts are firm papules with a rough horny surface, which range in size from less than a millimetre to over a centimetre in diameter. Warts are due to a virus infection and can be acquired by contact with another person suffering from the condition, as they are highly contagious. Common warts occur most frequently on the hands, but can be found in all areas of the face and body. The warts are often dark in colour, and form groups on the backs of the hands, around the nail fold and sometimes under the nail. They often have a multiple formation, and after varying periods of time tend to disappear spontaneously.

Flat Warts (verruca plana)

Flat warts appear as smooth, pearly epidermal elevations, about the size of pin-heads, usually found in groups, and most frequently situated on the face and hands.

All kinds of warts can be removed surgically, or with diathermy, and often plantar warts respond to treatment which excludes the air, e.g. Elastoplast. Many warts have been seen to disappear with simple psycho-therapy techniques.

Verruca Plantaris (affecting the soles of the feet)

Warts on the soles of the feet become flattened by pressure so that they do not project beyond the surface. They may be single or multiple, and usually occur on the ball or heel of the foot. Plantar warts usually become painful at some stage of their development, and they should be attended to as early as possible in order to avoid spreading the condition, or causing unnecessary discomfort for the individual.

Corns   The corn is a thickened dense area of skin, forming a raised appearance, situated on pressure areas, such as the toes. Treatment of corns is outside the work of the beauty specialist, who must refer her clients either to a chiropodist or, if the corn is painful and inflamed, to her own doctor.

Chapter 6

Basic and Specialized Mask Therapy, Toning and Minor Skin Treatments

MASK APPLICATIONS

The beneficial effects of the manual sections of the facial routine can be reinforced by a specific mask application chosen to increase the cleansing and toning aspects of the treatment. Masks can have different actions depending on their formulation, and the choice relies mainly on skilful skin diagnosis observation and knowledge of the effects of the basic mask ingredients.

The most important actions of a mask are general refining and stimulation, but they can be used in many other applications to good effect. A mask is a preparation that contains various ingredients, to which active substances are added to form a paste or emulsion. The product is smoothed over the face (and neck if required), avoiding the eyes, lips and nostrils, and is left to act for 5–15 minutes, according to type.

Actions of Masks

Stimulation. Refining. Cleansing (desquamation). Peeling. Soothing. Nourishing (specialized forms of masks).

Types of Masks

Setting Masks, including clay, sulphur, peeling and astringent masks.

Non-setting Masks, including biological masks (fruit, plant, herbal and vegetable based), natural product masks (eggs, fruits, honey etc.), and oatmeal packs.

Specialized Masks, including plastic type masks, thermal masks, paraffin wax, and hot oil masks (involving electrical and cosmetic applications).

SETTING MASKS

Effects of Basic Mask Ingredients

Knowledge of basic ingredients will enable mask formulations to be individually prepared, specifically for the client. The choice will depend on the skin condition observed after completion of the massage section of the facial treatment prior to the mask application. The complexity of diagnosis prevents the use of standard formulations in most cases, and the intensity of action required and duration of the application must be decided by the therapist in consultation with the client.

Clay Masks

Clay masks, which offer excellent cleansing, toning, and stimulation effects, require skill in ingredient choice, blending, and application, but the range of possible actions and low cost make them a popular salon choice.

Basic Clay Mask Ingredients

Calamine which produces a soothing action on surface capillaries, reducing the skin's vascular appearance. A very mild, gentle effect is achieved.

Magnesium Carbonate creates an astringent action for stimulation and toning effects.

Kaolin brings about a stronger response, which cleanses the skin and removes impurities. An improved vascular and lymphatic flow increases nutrition to the skin's surface and hastens the removal of waste products.

Fuller's Earth creates a fast vascular response, and interchange of tissue fluids, a very stimulating effect. The desquamation and cleansing actions make this an ideal mask ingredient for seborrhoea conditions, but its use should be restricted for general skin textures.

Active Ingredients

(Solutions, Oils etc.) **Rose Water** gives a mild toning effect, which increases the action of the basic mask items.

Orange Flower Water gives a stimulating and tonic effect, used in combination with the refining mask formulations

Witch Hazel a drying and extremely stimulating, refining effect is achieved. Witch hazel is contra-indicated on fine, sensitive skin conditions, but successful for its desquamation action on seborrhoea or acne vulgaris.

Almond Oil used in combination with basic mask ingredients, when a stimulating but not very drying effect is desired, i.e. dehydrated or neglected younger skin conditions and mature skins.

Sulphur, Peeling and Astringent Masks

These more active forms of setting masks have one common purpose: refining, through increased desquamation. As the mask sets and tightens, the dead horny surface layers (stratum corneum), and oily secretions (sebum), combine with the mask ingredients, and are removed together. Blocked pores and blackhead formation is controlled, and the drying effect reduces the action of seborrhoea on the skin. Many of these masks can be obtained pre-prepared from treatment and cosmetic firms, or the basic dry ingredients purchased, requiring the addition of the active solutions to create a progressive effect. Use of proprietary masks requires additional caution, as the exact formulations are unknown, and the effect on the client can only be determined by verbal and visual contact during the application.

Indications for Setting Masks

Recognition of the existing skin condition and any minor imperfections will be the decisive factor in the mask choice, applied within a treatment sequence. The cleansing, toning, and stimulation effects of setting masks give them a wide range of applications, particularly among the younger age groups. The tightening, drying actions will contra-indicate them on mature and hyper-sensitive skins, where more specialized forms of mask therapy are preferable.

Applications for Treatment

1 Cleansing, desquamation action on younger, pigmented skin conditions.

2 General stimulation, for maintenance of oil, moisture and pH balance, in the 20–30 age group.

3 Refining, toning, stimulating effects on a sluggish circulation.

4 Dehydrated, neglected skin conditions, requiring stimulation, and an improvement in cellular function.

5 Soothing, stabilizing effect on delicate or unstable skin conditions.

6 Cleansing, drying, stimulating effect on the acne skin.

Basic Mask Formulations

As every facial diagnosis differs slightly, no exact formulations can be assumed to be suitable for all skin conditions that fall within a certain grouping or type. As it has been seen, skins cannot be classified in this way, apart from the most superficial of applications, i.e. makeup, and so only guide lines can be given for mask ingredients for any specific condition.

Normal Skin Mask   1 part kaolin, 1 part Fuller's earth, mixed with water and a few drops of witch hazel, to form a smooth paste. Application time 8-12 minutes, according to effect.

Dry Skin Mask   1 part kaolin, 1 part magnesium, mixed with rose water or orange flower water, to form a smooth, thin paste. Application time 10-15 minutes, according to effect.

Oily Skin Mask   Fuller's earth and witch hazel, mixed to a smooth paste, and spread thinly over the face. Application time 5-15 minutes according to vascular reaction.

Sensitive Skin Mask   1 part calamine, and 1 part magnesium, mixed with rose water and spread thinly over the face. Application 5-10 minutes according to reaction.

Sulphur Mask (drying and desquamation action)   Flowers of sulphur, mixed into a smooth paste with the addition of water and active ingredients if indicated. Application time 10-15 minutes, according to skin reaction and the client's tolerance.

Stimulating Mask   Magnesium 6 parts, combined with Fuller's earth 2 parts, mixed to a fine paste with rose water, or almond oil according to the moisture content of the epidermal layers. Application time 5-15 minutes, according to reaction and the client's tolerance.

It can be clearly seen that no rules can apply in mask therapy, due to the variety of mask products and the different actions they are capable of producing. A flexible approach to the blending and duration of the mask application is necessary. Observation and client discussion regarding tolerance to the mask will increase knowledge of the skin's reaction to the basic ingredients, and avoid unsuitable or harmful applications.

Method of Use: Setting Masks

Preparation and Application

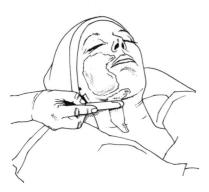

BASIC MASK APPLICATION

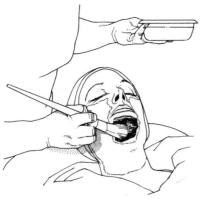

COMBINED FORMULA MASK

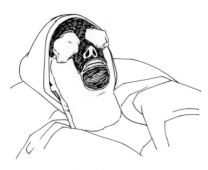

THE COMPLETED MASK SETTING

The mask must be applied on a clean skin, free from oil, cream, etc., to gain maximum benefit. Its action of closing the pores, places the application most effectively at the end of the treatment sequence, prior to the toning and makeup aspects. The protective facial preparation should be checked, particularly around the hair line, to prevent soiling, and the mask applied in a thin even film all over the face, and throat if required with a spatula or brush. The eyes, nostrils and mouth areas must be avoided, and eye pads applied to refresh the eyes and aid relaxation. A combination of skin conditions may require use of two or three different masks on the varying skin areas. Applications must be accomplished neatly and quickly, with the areas requiring the maximum duration covered first, so that the complete mask is ready for removal simultaneously.

Spatulas (tongue depressors) or brushes may be used to apply the mask. The advantage of spatulas is that they are disposable, so reducing maintenance between treatments. If brushes are used they must be carefully cleaned before sterilization, as the mask ingredients make an ideal breeding ground for bacteria. Any mask powder trapped down between the bristles will decompose and stain the brush.

Natural mask ingredients cannot be made up and stored for use for the same reason, as being from natural origins they go off and smell unpleasant. In a busy clinic some of the basic masks can be made up for the day to save time, but 24 hours is the limit of their freshness and effectiveness. As most masks have to be made specifically for the clients individual skin condition they are usually mixed just prior to use, which also adds a very personal touch to the treatment.

Setting masks do not have to become concrete hard to be effective, but they have their greatest effect on cleansing the skin's surface if allowed to dry rather than being removed whilst still moist. It is preferable to apply a mask in a very thin layer and let it set, rather than thickly applied and removed before it can be effective. It should be remembered that it is only the surface of the mask that touches the skin that has any effect on it. Applying thick masks is time-wasting, both for the client and the therapist, and ineffective, quite apart from making the removal laborious and irritating.

Masks can be useful for improving the colour of the skin on the neck, but should not be used on every occasion if the treatment is weekly, especially on the older client. It is more beneficial to alternate masks with oil or neck packs designed to nourish the skin rather than tone it. If a throat pad is to be used, the cream is left on the neck, and more applied as necessary. A fairly warm pad is applied, and it is tucked round firmly to keep it snug and stop the heat escaping. The protective towels are used, moved up into position to keep the throat pad in place, and then moved back after the pad is removed, and the mask rinsed off. The actual pad is made from a large wad of cotton wool, protected both sides by a thin split tissue to allow the heat to penetrate, and make the pad re-useable. Any warm surface can be used to heat the pad, radiator, bulb heat lamp, etc. that is close to the working position.

The relaxation that the throat pack gives to the resting period of the mask, makes it a very popular treatment with clients.

Removal   After the necessary period has elapsed, the eye pads (and throat pads if used) are removed. This awakens the client, and prepares her for the removal of the face mask. The mask substance is removed with damp cotton-wool tissues or sponges, using tepid water, and fast flowing strokes in order to clean the skin. Care and forethought in the removal will avoid mask fragments or water reaching the facial apertures, and should prevent unnecessary soiling of robes, towels etc. Use of disposable tissues is particularly important in the case of highly coloured mask ingredients, but can be used to advantage in all setting mask applications to avoid client discomfort and soiling of chair coverings.

NON-SETTING MASKS

All natural ingredient masks can be classified as non-setting, as although they form a film over the skin, which becomes firm and dry, they do not have a tightening effect on skin tissue, and so do not affect the surface moisture content. The substance of the mask remains flexible, and the client's features are not immobilized. All fruit, plant, herbal, and natural products masks can be termed non-setting, although they have very different action and methods of application.

Biological Mask Treatment

Recent development of specialized biological mask therapy has added a new dimension to beauty treatments increasing the effectiveness of this aspect of the routine for many facial conditions. Certain unstable facial conditions benefit particularly from this form of therapy, as the effectiveness of the action can be achieved without alteration of the skin's moisture level, a side effect of most setting masks. Products based on natural rather than chemical sources are classed as biological, and within this group of treatment items come flower plant, and vegetable extract masks. For ease of application the ingredients are combined into a jelly, cream or emulsion medium, which is applied in a thin film over the face and throat, and left to dry and tighten slightly to form a second skin.

Response to the action of the biological elements is through the vascular network of the dermal layers of the skin, where the trace elements of the ingredients create increased cellular activity in the basal layer of the skin. Refinement of skin texture is the result of improvement in respiration, and elimination, rather than from the tightening, toning action experienced with clay or setting masks.

Fruit Extract Masks

Fruit extracts are available from widely differing sources, and the action obtained from the base varies according to the nature of the natural fruit Many soft fruits have an acid reaction on the skin used in their natural state, but when used as an active mask concentrate, mixed into a jelly base medium, the results are very satisfactory, particularly for dry and normal skin conditions. The fruit mask has a stabilizing action on the skin's pH, and water level, and may be used within a weekly facial treatment, with excellent results.

Plants and Fruits

A combination of plant and fruit extract increases the effect, and is desirable when a dual action is required, such as stimulation and deep cleansing, on a sluggish complexion. A stronger circulation stimulation effect is possible with plant-based masks, and increased cellular regeneration and skin respiration creates a rapid movement in seborrhoea and neglected or dehydrated skin conditions. Because of its effect of encouraging the skin to function more efficiently, it is possible to choose the ingredients to accomplish many different results.

Herbal and Vegetable Masks

For more specialized effects the vegetable and herbal extracts offer the greatest choice of action ranging from cucumber for sensitive, delicate skin to rosemary for a tonic reaction on a dry dehydrated complexion. Regenerating products are often based on mixtures of vegetable extracts, and improvement in a blotchy complexion can be achieved by stimulation of the small capillaries under the surface, using a circulation stimulant such as horse chestnut. Herbal and seaweed products offer a more gentle method of treating the blemished or unbalanced complexion, and create a satisfactory skin texture, without flaking or irritation, whilst permitting the infection of the follicle or seborrhoea present to disperse naturally. This avoids introducing additional products to alter the skin's respiration or decrease its defence against bacteria. The action on the vascular network of the skin is stronger in these masks than in any other variety, with a response occurring in the deeper subcutaneous layers of the skin. This is a counter-irritation response to the surface stimulation of the sensory nerve endings.

Indications for Biological Mask Treatment

1 Hyper-sensitive skin conditions.
2 Dehydrated and dry skin conditions.
3 Mature skin, requiring a regeneration action.
4 Oily or blemished skin conditions, particularly where the skin is also sensitive.
5 Dry, flaky, unstable skin conditions, especially where the pH requires stabilizing.
6 Skin congestion, due to incorrect cosmetic care, over-exposure, or ill-health.

Recognition of Facial Conditions

Recognition of skin conditions that will benefit from this specialized form of cosmetic treatment is vitally important, and for the application to be truly effective the therapist must make an accurate analysis of the client's skin and be able to recognize signs of irregularity. General background information can be gained from the client on past skin behaviour, cosmetic routines, and general health, which help the therapist to form an opinion on the most beneficial routine of treatment. There are many specific skin conditions which benefit particularly from biological therapy, although it is becoming an increasingly popular method of alternative mask treatment, which creates no harmful side effects as it adjusts to the client's skin temperature, water and oil level, forming an individual reaction.

Hyper-sensitive Skins

Hyper-sensitive skins previously contra-indicated to most forms of mask application can now have specially formulated mask concentrates to gently freshen and refine the skin, whilst keeping the acid/alkaline balance constant and improving skin function. Several treatment ranges offer biological masks to stabilize the sensitive, fine, often dry skins. For a soothing action or for a dehydrated complexion, orange blossom in a base medium allows natural regeneration to improve without over-stimulation or irritation of the epidermis.

Inspection of this type of skin under the magnifier will show a fine textured skin, with tiny blood vessels close to the surface, giving a pink appearance. The skin may be tight over the bony areas of the face, and in a mature client the softening of skin tissue will result in a crêpy skin texture and fine lines in areas poorly supported by adipose tissue, such as around the eyes and on the throat. Increased cellular function to improve skin tone and elasticity is an important task in treatment, but due to the danger of over-stimulation through facial applications and massage observed in normal treatment a satisfactory result has previously been hard to achieve.

Dry Skin

Dry skins lacking natural oils, and dehydrated conditions where surface moisture has diminished, both respond to biological mask therapy as stimulation is possible without any further loss of moisture yet leaving the skin fresh and soft, free from surface adhesions and fine textured. Recognition of the dry skin is more possible by conversation with the client as to the reaction of various external and internal factors on the skin. Dieting or poor health, over-exposure to sun and wind, or abuse and neglect of the complexion can all result in a dry, dehydrated or combined skin reaction. The skin will appear uneven in epidermal depth, the colour will vary, and fine lines and general loss of texture will be apparent, particularly in the finest textured skin around the eyes and in the platysma muscle area of the neck. A dehydrated skin may be a temporary condition, and careful choice of biological mask therapy and a revised home care sequence should facilitate a swift response and alleviate the condition.

Mature Skins

Mature skins benefit most of all from biological treatment as they gain from the regenerating effects of the active ingredients, whilst avoiding all the drying, irritating effects of classic mask treatment. Tissue extract masks for cellular stimulation and flower extracts for general refining and toning purposes combine to keep the mature skin in an ideal condition, well nourished, and with sufficient biological cellular function. Skin thickening and discoloration around the mouth and chin area can be successfully treated, without the usual drying or irritant reaction resulting from harsh chemical preparations. Witch hazel or thyme based masks refine the skin, deep cleanse and free any blocked cellular matter, and hasten desquamation in the chin area, resulting in a refined texture and improved skin colour.

Oily and Blemished Skins

This cleansing and desquamation effect can be used to advantage in treating the young, oily or blemished skin by freeing it from adhesions and removing the acid, oily film from the surface. This leaves the skin more able to protect itself from bacteria, which thrive on the acid build-up on the surface. Dry acne conditions can be treated and controlled biologically, and they can be distinguished from acne vulgaris by the extreme flaking irritation and broken surface peculiar to this form of acne. Both forms of acne affect the follicle and, although removing surface oils does not present a cure, it controls the condition, whilst the client's physical and mental health improves. Different treatment is advisable for the varying types and stages of the blemished or oily skin. Yeast packs for cleansing and herbal action masks to refine and balance the pH both give excellent results and avoid over-stimulation on the oily but delicate skin conditions so often found in combination.

Method of Application

Preparation of the skin prior to the mask application is important, and neutral cleansing preparations should be used to avoid changing the moisture balance of the skin or causing over-stimulation of the surface capillaries. Mature or delicate skins should be cleansed with light textured creams or oil-based cleansing milks, so that makeup is removed satisfactorily and the skin left free and able to benefit from biological mask therapy. Younger skins may be further prepared with biological 'soap', which helps to remove cellular adhesions and leaves the skin free from its oily deposit and receptive to the therapeutic action of the sea weed or herbal mask treatment. If the mask is to be used within the normal facial treatment for the dry, normal, or mature skins, it concludes the therapy after the massage routine, and should remain on the skin for 10-20 minutes, according to skin reaction.

The jelly or cream-based masks can be mixed at the time of application, combining the active ingredient with the base medium to form an emulsion, or masks can be obtained ready prepared in a range of substances for salon use. The masks should be spread finely over the face, and throat if necessary, and allowed to dry until sufficient activity can be felt by the client. The removal of the mask should be thorough and gentle, using warm water, taking care to remove every particle because it is transparent and difficult to see.

The skill of biological mask therapy is in accurate skin diagnosis and recognition of abnormal skin conditions. The ease of the mask application makes them an ideal choice for busy salon practice, allowing the maximum application period in which the skin can gain full effect from the active ingredients present in the mask.

NATURAL PRODUCT MASKS

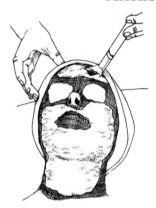

FRUIT MASK ON GAUZE

Masks comprised of basic raw materials, fruits, eggs, honey, cucumber, etc., are termed natural product treatments. The items utilized are left as close to their natural state as possible, and their basic actions used to advantage to correct or maintain differing skin conditions. Gauze may be used to enclose the soft crushed fruits for ease of application and removal, and to avoid client discomfort.

The action of certain natural products can be very effective, but in the normal salon situation their use is restricted due to the additional preparation time required and the availability of the ingredients. Natural product masks are a specialized form of mask therapy, and should be promoted as such if offered in the clinic's range of available treatments.

Dry Skin Egg Mask

Add a small amount of clear warm honey or almond oil to an egg yolk, and mix thoroughly. Apply thinly all over the face and leave for 15-20 minutes. Its action softens and refines the skin texture. Remove with tepid water, rinsing thoroughly, using cotton-wool tissues.

Oily Skin Egg Mask

Add a few drops of fresh lemon juice to a beaten egg white, and mix thoroughly to make a frothy consistency. Apply all over the face, apart from the under eye skin, on oily and coarse-textured complexions. Its action is to tighten the skin and have a stimulating effect, so it is ideal as a pre-makeup mask.

Honey Mask (for mature or dehydrated skin)

Add a few drops of orange or lemon juice to a spoonful of honey, and warm until it is fluid in consistency. Apply all over the face, and include the under-eye skin in the treatment. Leave for 15-20 minutes, and then remove thoroughly with tepid water and cotton-wool pads. Its action is to soften and refresh the skin, whilst delaying the formation of fine lines.

Cucumber Pack

Finely sliced and crushed cucumber pieces are combined with a teaspoonful of thick cream and a few drops of tincture of benzoin and rose water to form a soft mixture. The pack is applied between two layers of gauze, and left for 20-25 minutes depending on skin reaction. The rejuvenating and toning effects of the mask can be increased by the addition of whisked egg white to the mixture, or reduced by increasing the cream content. The action of the cucumber pack is to stimulate the skin, increase cellular function, and refine skin texture. It may be applied on different skin conditions by varying the proportions of the ingredients until the desired effect is achieved.

Fruit Based Natural Masks

Many soft fruits may be used, applied in the same manner as the cucumber pack, to create a variety of actions. Strawberry and raspberry fruits are acid in reaction, and can cause a strong effect unless combined with a neutralizing agent such as cream. The basic actions of fruits can be increased or reduced according to the additional ingredients combined in the mixture. The natural sugar content of fruit, and the acid or alkaline reaction created, mean that many fruits are useful in mask therapy, as long as their action is known. Tropical fruits such as pawpaw, avocado, etc. are well known for their excellent skin effects, and in countries where these items are readily available they may be included in mask therapy treatments to achieve good effects.

Oatmeal Packs

The refining, calming and cleansing effects of oatmeal masks are well known, and they can be used in the treatment of normal and oily skin conditions to maintain or improve skin texture. Fine oatmeal can be mixed to a paste with water, rose water, or lemon juice, depending on the intensity of action required. The paste may be applied directly onto the skin, or between gauze for convenience, and left for 10-15 minutes, to achieve maximum effect. Removal should be thorough, as the oatmeal adheres to the skin and forms a film which is difficult to remove completely.

ESSENTIAL OILS AROMATHERAPY

The choice and application of essential oils to the face and body is an advanced area of work closely allied to the natural and biological forms of skin treatment. The essential oils are chosen for their specific effect, i.e. calming, antiseptic, regenerating actions, and they are applied via an oil medium to the pressure points of the body. The supporting massage routine speeds the absorption of the essential oils, and creates a relaxed atmosphere, increasing the subsequent effectiveness of the treatment on the body system. The use of essential oils is known as Aromatherapy due to the powerful aromas emitted by the concentrated flower and plant essences on contact with the warmth of the client's body. A large variety of oils are available, and skill is required in choosing the correct product and judging its effect on the individual. Many plants, herbs, and flowers are employed, including lemon grass, rose, thyme, bergamot, and camomile.

The essential oils or essences are obtained from a wide variety of sources, as with the active ingredients of biological masks. Their concentrated nature make application and use in therapy a subject requiring further advanced training and experience.

SPECIALIZED MASKS

Hot Oil and Paraffin Wax Masks

Although termed masks, both oil and paraffin masks are a specialized form of therapy, involving the use of electrical apparatus within the application. When their use is indicated they form the basis of the facial routine, and not just a section of the sequence. The principles and techniques of these treatments will be covered in later chapters, when the facts relating to electrical treatments and equipment have been studied.

Warm Masks

Warm masks are a form of mask therapy that has been available for several years, but is enjoying popularity due to improved textures and ease of application. The effects of the masks were always immediately evident, but application was difficult. Now product improvement has made it possible to apply warm masks without any special heating equipment, and they are becoming increasingly important to the beauty industry.

Warm masks are designed to regenerate the skin, create a tightening effect on skin tissues, and delay the formation of surface lines. They are available in a form that hardens into a firm crust which may be removed like a plaster cast in one piece (normally termed 'thermal' masks), or as a thin rubbery film which tightens as it sets, and can be peeled off, also in one piece ('warm' or 'peel-off' masks).

Warm or Peel-off Masks

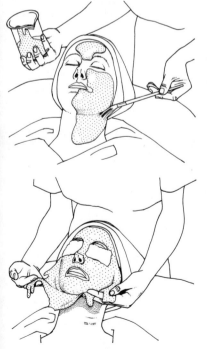

The peel-off or waxy type of cosmetic mask requires warming to facilitate its application. The cream or pellet form of the product permits economy and ease of preparation, in a double saucepan, waxing unit, or simply a container placed to warm in a basin of hot water. A cream or oil may be applied to the skin prior to the masks application to increase the total effect of the routine.

The product is smoothed quickly over the face as for basic masks, and allowed to form a solid mask, which immobilizes the features and softens harsh lines. Removal after 10 minutes is accomplished by peeling away the borders and apertures, and lifting off in a complete film. The cleansing, stimulating and refining effects of the masks make them an ideal choice for the dry, dehydrated and mature skin conditions.

Thermal Masks

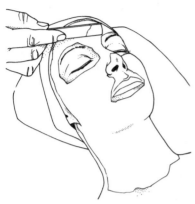

UNDERLYING CREAM APPLICATION

There are several different types of thermal masks, so manufacturers' instructions should be followed as to individual application. However, most are designed on the principle of producing heat within the surface tissues by a chemical reaction caused by the ingredients themselves, rather than by electrical means. The heat produced stimulates the skin and improves its function, whilst aiding the absorption of the associated cream preparation.

So the treatment has the advantage of being complete, requiring no source of external heating, which makes it a useful and novel extension to cosmetic and manual applications.

Application

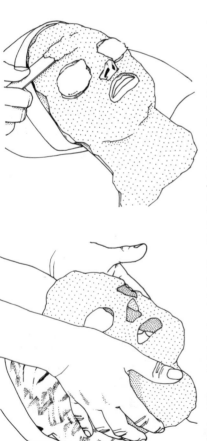

The skin is cleansed thoroughly, and massage applied if desired; then the skin is covered with an even layer of the special cream designed to work in conjunction with the mask paste. The eyes, nostrils and mouth should be left free. The thermal mask paste is then applied, in a fairly thick layer, with the nostrils left free so that the client can breathe. The eyes and lips can be covered, but if the client feels at all claustrophobic it is wiser to leave these free of paste as well. The eyes should be covered with pads, and the client allowed to rest. The heat effect starts to develop as the paste hardens, which takes just a few minutes, and the pulsing warmth then suffuses the facial and neck areas. The heat gradually disperses and after 20 minutes the treatment is complete. At no time does the heat reach an uncomfortable level which would worry the client.

After removal of the eye pads, the rigid mask can be lifted off in one piece, and the skin cleared of any remaining cream. The heat produced stimulates the circulation and the local blood supply is increased, bringing fresh nutrients to the area. The underlying cream is absorbed into the surface of the skin, and the tissues seem refreshed and taut. Small surface lines appear relaxed, and the skin has a smooth, fresh appearance.

Apart from clients with highly vascular complexions, and those of a nervous disposition who would not be happy being immobilized by a rigid mask, thermal masks present few contra-indications for general stimulatory and toning purposes.

SKIN TONING

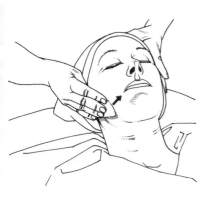

MANUAL SKIN TONING

Skin toning concludes the treatment sequence and prepares the skin for the makeup application. It is completed as a final step to ensure thorough mask removal and maintain a fine skin texture. The skin is refreshed and prepared for the protective aspect of the makeup section by a stimulating, toning sequence, using suitable lotions. A dampened cotton-wool pad, folded into a spatula shape, accomplishes the toning procedure, using light, fast, tapping movements to create the effect.

The entire neck and facial areas are toned in this way, and any surplus solution is smoothed into the skin, by a rolling movement of the hand, with the opened toning pad.

The skin may also be toned electrically using a vaporizer, (see Chapter 8, Specialized Electrical Treatments) or by use of an aerosol spray, normally containing a natural mineral water such as Evian water. Both methods provide a finely distributed mist of fluid, produced under pressure, which is easily absorbed into the skin. The vaporizer apparatus can be used with a range of different lotions for varying skin conditions. Presentation to the client with both methods is very professional, and pressure toning is growing in popularity as treatments become more electrically biased.

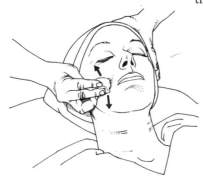

ROLLING IN TONING
LOTION

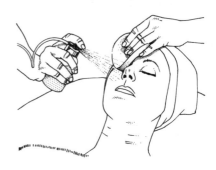

ELECTRICAL SPRAY
TONING

Effects of Skin Toning Lotions

Skin Tonic   A tonic has a mild effect and removes all traces of oil, cream, mask, etc. whilst gently toning the skin. The refining but mild action of the lotion makes it suitable for delicate, dry, dehydrated or mature skin conditions. Different varieties are available, based on natural items, or chemical formulations. A dilution of rose water makes a general purpose skin tonic.

Astringent   The drying and stimulating action of an astringent limits its use to oily and coarse skin conditions with no evidence of sensitivity. The astringent removes surface oil and can disturb the pH balance, so its application is contra-indicated on delicate or blemished skins, due to the risk of skin irritation. Witch hazel is classed as an astringent lotion of strong effect.

Corrective or Acne Lotion   Seborrhoea or blemished skin conditions require a corrective or acne lotion application, either prior to or replacing a medicated makeup sequence. The action of the lotion is to dry and heal pustules, remove oily matter from the skin's surface, and prevent the formation of blackheads. The strong action of the lotion can be reduced for different areas of the face by using a moist toning pad to dilute the effect of the preparation. Acne or corrective lotions are usually chemical formulations of a spirit base, with the addition of germicidal elements to counteract infection.

The skin should feel slightly tacky to the touch after toning, and be calm and stable in appearance. When the lotion has completely settled into the skin, the makeup may be applied.

MINOR FACIAL TREATMENTS

General Preparation Points

Many minor facial treatments are combined in the facial routine for convenience and to save time for the client. All slightly irritating or uncomfortable small treatments, i.e. waxing, tinting, and plucking, are completed after cleansing prior to the relaxing manual aspects of the routine. In the combined application very little additional preparation is required, specifically for the minor treatment.

Independently applied small facial treatments may be undertaken in a semi-upright chair position, with the client remaining fully clothed and prepared just for the specific application. The minimum of necessary preparation, and use of disposable tissues etc., will increase efficiency and permit the treatment to be completed in the allocated time.

EYEBROW SHAPING

Well-shaped eyebrows give definition to the face and form a frame for the eyes, which accentuates them. Plucking the eyebrow hairs is a minor treatment which ideally should be applied within a facial routine, after cleansing, or combined with another grooming aspect such as eyelash and brow tinting, or waxing of the lip or chin.

Any changes to the shape of the brows must be discussed with the client, and suggestions made on the basis of their natural shape and the client's facial proportions: see Chapter 7.

Equipment Required   The equipment required should become part of the normal trolley preparations, i.e. ordinary or automatic tweezers, antiseptic solution, soothing lotion, cotton-wool, small bowls, and a hand mirror. Natural daylight or illuminated magnification is essential to produce a neat fast shaping, with the minimum of client discomfort and operator strain.

Method   With all eyebrow makeup removed, the plucking commences between the brows, removing stray hairs and spacing the inner corners. A routine of wiping over the brows with a cooling, antiseptic pad between the pluckings should be established. This will remove the loose hairs, cool the skin, and give protection against infection. The shape of the brows is formed by removing hairs below the brow, plucking in the direction of the growth, and supporting and stretching the skin with the other hand.

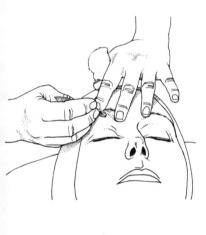

Stray hairs above the brow and at the temple area should be removed, as long as they do not form part of the main eyebrow growth. Strong individual coarse hairs within the eyebrow itself may be removed if they detract from the finished line and do not leave uncovered skin areas. The finished shape of the eyebrows should not be determined if major reshaping is undertaken until the client has agreed to both brows in their approximate form. Final shaping can then be concluded, with client satisfaction assured. Extremely heavy brows can be gradually reduced over two or three shapings, in this way reducing client discomfort and allowing her to get accustomed to her new image slowly.

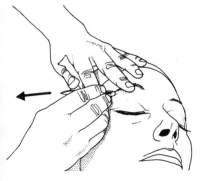

Over-plucked brows must be allowed to grow, and be kept tidy until sufficient hair is available to form a new line. Eyebrow tinting can be used to advantage to increase the apparent bulk of insignificant brows.

Although classed as a minor treatment, eyebrow shaping can be an extremely important part of the client's overall grooming routine. So care should be taken to develop the best shape possible initially, which can then be followed in subsequent shapings. It is worth the time and effort to create a shape that flatters the face, and looks correct to the client.

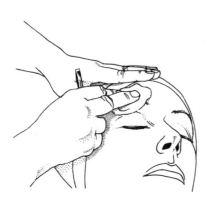

So it is important to stand away from the client periodically whilst shaping the brows, to assess the overall effect, and to judge whether the brows are even, at the same level, and not becoming too thin. Brows that are not matched naturally, for curve or position on the face, can be made to appear similar by skilful shaping and removal of unwanted hairs. Linked with tinting, brows can be formed out of almost nothing, to the great joy of the client. White hairs and tough spiky hairs can be removed if they are spoiling the overall shape, and their removal does not make the brows uneven. Constant checking, and an overall idea of the finished shape to be created, should guard against disasters. Once plucked, the hair cannot be replaced, although of course it will grow back in time. Whilst gaining experience in shaping brows, one is wise to consult frequently with the client, so that she is happy with the finished effect. Taking the trouble to consult with the client, apart from being a fundamental courtesy, is good business sense. On such small treatments as eyebrow shaping, a client will try out the therapist's ability to perform the task quickly and efficiently, and also their willingness to work in accord with the client's wishes. Satisfaction on such a relatively minor treatment, could result in further clinic treatment of a much more profitable type.

Conclusion of the Treatment   The finished brow should be smoothed into shape and soothing lotion applied to prevent infection resulting from treatment and reduce the increased colour.

EYEBROW AND LASH TINTING

The cosmetic effect of brow or lash tinting is to enhance the general appearance, define or correct brow shapes, and emphasize the lashes with intensified colour. The convenience of permanent colour makes tinting a very popular salon treatment for all age groups, and a profitable area of business if applied correctly. If tinting is combined with a facial treatment, it is applied after cleansing, prior to massage.

Equipment Required

Different forms of permanent eye lash and brow tint include cream, jelly and liquid formulas, all of which require combination with 10 vol. peroxide to activate them prior to application. The colour choice of blue, grey, brown, and black, permits many shades and colour tones to be produced,

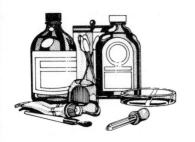

individually suited to the client. The base colour of the hairs affects the density of the finished result, and care must be taken not to over-tint or a strong harsh effect will be created.

The items required for tinting are the chosen type of tint, 10 vol. peroxide, water, a small brush, and mixing palette. Soothing eye solution should also be available in case of irritation resulting from the tint.

Contra-indications to Brow and Lash Tinting

Although modern tint products are mainly of vegetable origin, they are still activated by a peroxide solution, and for that reason will occasionally cause skin irritation. Even patch testing does not rule out completely the possibility of eye irritation, if the tint substance comes into contact with the delicate skin of the eye itself. Certain points can be followed to minimize the risk of this popular treatment. These include checking contra-indications with the client, patch testing, and performing the tint application meticulously, with attention to protection of the skin and scrupulous removal of the tint on conclusion.

Any history of sensitivity or allergy to eye makeup contra-indicates tinting, as does conjunctivitis, eczema in the brow or lash hairs, or psoriasis in the eye area. Skin irritation from any source which affects the area is classed as a contra-indication to tinting at that time. The increased skin proliferation (shedding), seen in eczema and dermatitis conditions, leaves the skin exposed and open to bacterial invasion, and a reaction and swelling or irritation could result.

The therapist must use her own judgement as to who is suitable for tinting, the risks to the clinic's reputation being considerable if a client suffers pain or distress from an eye infection. Any excessively dry flaky skin should be treated with caution, whether from neglect or through systematic causes such as thyroid abnormality. Clients with normally difficult skin, prone to cosmetic reactions, and a tendency to an unstable skin texture, should be patch tested before each application, to check changes occurring in the client's system. Some clients are very highly strung and of a nervous disposition, and will have periods of high and low sensitivity, which must be checked.

Clients who normally wear glasses, and so have hyper-sensitive skin around the eyes, should be treated gently and cream tints used for greater control. Clients totally unable to keep their eyes still, either from some nervous problem, old age, or from a dislike of having their eyes touched could prove difficult in treatment. Success with these clients would depend largely on the therapist's client-handling abilities, and steadiness of hand.

Not a great many clients are contra-indicated to tinting, but the therapist must have the confidence to say when tinting is not suitable. One treatment lost is a small price to pay to safeguard a professional reputation. The legal position regarding tinting and the clinic's liability would be that every reasonable care had been seen to have been taken, to safeguard the client's well being. Keeping clients' records, checking contra-indications, patch testing, and performing the treatment only if suitable would appear to meet these criteria.

Patch Testing

Patch testing is performed on a previous occasion to the tinting, ideally a day or two, and not longer than a week before. The patch can be completed when the initial inquiry is made, or within an eyebrow shaping, where it has been suggested by the therapist, or during a normal regular facial treatment as an extension into related treatments. If the therapist suggests and completes the preparation for the tint, a subsequent booking for the treatment is assured.

A small quantity of tint is mixed, and painted or rubbed onto the skin with a brush or cotton wool bud, in an area immediately behind the ear, so that it is unobtrusive. After 24 hours, if no irritation results, it may be washed off and the client considered suitable for tinting. Only an area the size of a five pence piece need be covered. If irritation does result, the tint should be washed off, and soothing antiseptic cream used to calm the skin. Once the offending tint is removed the irritation normally disappears.

The importance of patch testing reasonably close to the actual time of tinting, is due to changes occurring in the body, particularly if medication is taken or the client is on hormone therapy. For the same reason patch testing should be undertaken if the lashes and brows have not been tinted for a long period. Pregnant clients often produce strange reactions to tinting procedures, even if they normally have regular tinting with no problems. A client's lack of sensitivity a year before is no guide to her immediate reaction, nor is regular hair tinting, as the tints employed in hairdressing are differently formulated from the lash tints. Also the skin around the eyes is considerably more sensitive than the scalp.

Reaction to tinting, if it occurs even after careful checking, can include swelling of the eye skin, irritation and inflammation of the eyeball itself, causing weeping and conjunctivitis if severe. Although tinting is freely available in salons and stores, sometimes with scant regard to safety or procedure, therapists have a professional duty to safeguard their clients, and must follow sensible guide lines to ensure a satisfactory level of proficiency.

Method of Application: Cream Tint

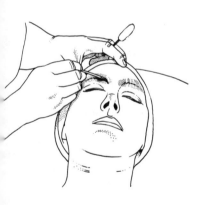

Brows. The cream tints are the most manageable, and so are ideal for delicate or mature skins, where the risks of skin irritation or staining are highest. The softer colour combinations possible, suit the mature or fair-skinned individual, and avoid an artificial appearance being produced.

If brows and lashes are to be tinted, the whole area is cleansed, thoroughly, to remove any oil etc., and the brows are shaped if necessary.

Although ideally the brows should be shaped on a previous occasion, in commercial practice this is seldom the case, and they are plucked just prior to tinting. As long as the skin is completely covered with protective cream in the areas not to be tinted, no tint will be able to penetrate the open hair follicles, and cause skin irritation. Major re-shaping, likely to cause skin irritation, should naturally not be combined with the tinting sequence.

PREPARATION AND
APPLICATION OF TINT

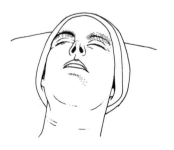

The brows and lashes are surrounded by a light film of cream or oil, applied on a cotton-wool tipped orange stick, to prevent skin staining. A small amount of tint is mixed with two drops of 10 volume peroxide to form an even-coloured emulsion of smooth texture. This is applied first to the underneath brow hairs to ensure complete coverage, working towards the centre brow, and then to the surface eyebrow, smoothing and shaping the finished line. The second brow is completed, and a visual and time check kept on the first to determine colour formation. Removal after 3-5 minutes is accomplished by firm wiping strokes with a damp pad to ensure no tint remains on the brows or skin.

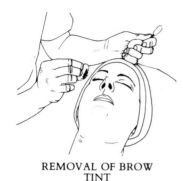

REMOVAL OF BROW
TINT

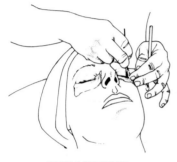

EYELASH TINT
APPLICATION

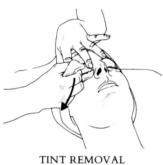

TINT REMOVAL

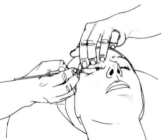

Fine blonde hair colours easily, and should be checked at regular intervals to prevent over colouration. The inner corner tint can be removed for checking purposes, and reapplied if necessary if insufficient colour is present.

Red hair is very resistant to tinting, and may require double the exposure time to achieve a satisfactory result.

Darker brows may only require definition at the outer areas, or to blend in white hairs, and so a natural shade can be used to give a uniform tone to the whole brow, and produce a more distinct profile aspect to the brow.

Lashes. The lashes should be tinted after the brows in a combined sequence, as the timing is not so critical due to the deeper tones preferred. Any tint remaining from the brows may be used for the lashes, with the addition if necessary of a small quantity of a darker tone.

The under-eye skin should be protected with fine damp cotton-wool pieces, shaped to fit snugly under the lower lashes. Once the upper and lower lashes are in place, the client must be advised not to open her eyes to reduce the risks of irritation resulting from tint entering the eye. The tint mixture is applied carefully, and coats and encloses the lashes right down to the skin of the lids. Any tint, however, touching the skin must be removed promptly to avoid skin staining (which can occur even through the film of cream or petroleum jelly which has been applied as a protective measure). The second eye is completed, and 5-8 minutes development time is allowed, depending on natural colouring and the finished tone required. The tint is removed with downward strokes on to the protective pad, and care must be taken not to open the eyes until all the tint substance has been removed. The procedure is repeated gently till the lashes are clean and no tint remains to be a source of irritation. A final check with the eyes open will reveal any tint present in the roots of the lashes, and this must be removed gently with a cotton-wool tip, with the eye skin supported with the other hand. The eyes may be bathed with a soothing Optrex solution if any irritation is present, or to relieve discomfort caused by the extra contact to which the eyes have been subjected.

Jelly Tints

The method of use for jelly tints is identical to cream tints, but greater care is necessary to avoid skin staining as the more fluid consistency is liable to seep onto the skin and cause irritation. The jelly tints are ideal for younger clients with firm unwrinkled skins who require a fashion effect, and do not need the subtle colour blending possible with cream tints. Jelly tints are increasing in popularity due to their economy of use and speed of application. Both creams and jellies have fairly long lasting colour effects, and normally require repeating every 6–8 weeks as the natural growth cycle of the hairs and general sunlight exposure reduces the colour intensity gradually.

Liquid Tints

Liquid tints are composed of two solutions which are applied, one after the other, to produce a colour change. The limited range of colour and the dangers of seepage restricts their professional use, and places them on the retail market for home use. The results achieved with liquid tints are not sufficiently reliable for them to be offered as a salon treatment but, as many customers may have used them at some time, it is necessary for the therapist to have a knowledge of their action.

General Points on Tinting

Neat, fast, and careful application is necessary in tinting to achieve complete coverage, without causing client discomfort or skin staining. A half-hour period should be sufficient for shaping the brows and tinting both the brows and lashes. Lashes tinted separately should not exceed 15 minutes, once proficiency has been reached. Client guidance regarding a reduction in the amount of eye makeup worn when coming for a tinting treatment should be stressed at the time of booking the tint. This can save unnecessary time wastage, caused by the need to remove heavy mascara applications, before the tinting can commence.

It also avoids causing aggravation to the area, skin reddening or irritation from the actual mascara removal itself, which could increase the risk of subsequent skin irritation within the tinting sequence.

APPLICATIONS OF SEMI-PERMANENT INDIVIDUAL LASHES

The individual lash application is classed as a treatment, due to the time involved and the semi-permanent nature of the lashes. The more recent natural makeup fashions have increased the demand for a more personal, less obvious form of lash emphasis. Personally tailored top and bottom lashes are attached individually, and have to be replaced regularly to maintain the full effect. It is a successful salon treatment, with its need for regular attention and secondary sales element.

Equipment   The lash kit comprises the different sized lashes, and adhesive specifically formulated to maintain attachment without causing irritation. Tweezers and scissors are also needed to fix and shape the lashes. All other items should be present as part of the normal trolley preparation.

Contra-indications   Sensitive and delicate skin texture around the eye will be found to be irritated by any artifical form of lash, especially semi-permanent forms. However some clients can tolerate individual lashes, whilst normal false lashes on a backing strip, prove irritating due to the weight involved.

Method of Application   With the client in a relaxed semi-reclining position, the eyes are cleansed, and all traces of oil etc., removed. The individual lashes are shaped and attached with special adhesive to the roots of the natural lashes. A natural sweep, filling out and lengthening of the lash line is achieved by constant checking with the eyes open and then closed, until first the top, then the bottom, set of lashes is finished. The individual lashes must follow the curve of the natural lashes, and if these are very straight they should be curled slightly with eyelash curling tools, before attachment commences. The lashes may be cut if necessary to give a personalized finish, but careful choice of the correct sized lash from the kit should prevent a lot of unnecessary shaping.

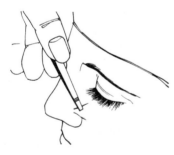

APPLICATION OF
SEMI-PERMANENT LASHES

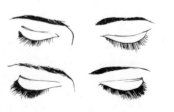

TREATED AND UNTREATED EYES

The use of mascara should not be necessary after the lash applications, as the client must be advised to handle the lashes as little as possible to minimize natural displacement. Even without mascara application and removal, the normal wear and tear on the lashes will demand that they receive attention every two to three weeks, depending on the effect desired.

LIP AND CHIN WAXING
(Warm Wax Method)

Evident vellus hair on the face can be removed with depilatory wax treatment, which, as a form of mass plucking, removes the hair shaft and root areas, leaving the active matrix area of the follicle behind to produce another hair. As a temporary solution to superfluous hair growth, it is popular as it gives instant results, and produces fine, tapered regrowth hairs after a time gap of 3-6 weeks, depending on the rate of growth. A strong hair growth of coarse texture is not suitable for waxing therapy, and a permanent form of removal is indicated (epilation). Fine hairs which regrow extremely quickly, and may at some stage require permanent removal, are also not suitable for waxing, as it does not give sufficiently good results, and epilation is the only answer. However, many fine facial growths, particularly on dark-haired women, respond well and are controlled by regular applications of depilatory waxing treatment. Facial waxing is completed after cleansing in the full facial treatment routine.

Equipment Required

A waxing unit, containing a small quantity of facial depilatory wax, soothing lotion, talc, tweezers, and a spatula or brush for the application.

Contra-indications to Waxing

Hyper-sensitive skins, herpes (cold sores), and any cuts, pustules or irritation of the surface are classed as contra-indications to waxing.

Method: Lip Waxing

The waxing unit is switched on, and the wax allowed to attain a liquid working consistency, which is then maintained by a thermostatically controlled regulator whilst the skin is being prepared. The skin area is cleansed and inspected for contra-indications, and then removal is completed and talc applied lightly against the growth. This lifts the hairs and eases the removal of the wax. Only the facial areas involved must be waxed, as otherwise bald extended sections of the face give a strange appearance.

The wax temperature should be comfortable to the client, and liquid enough to sink around the hairs and affect their removal. Small manageable quantities of wax are applied against the growth from the outer corner of the mouth, over the lip, to the central area under the nose. The second side is covered so that the central portion overlaps to form a solid moustache-shaped piece of wax, extending from the lip line, over the superfluous hair area. Care must be taken to avoid getting wax in the nostrils and mouth area. The wax is pressed firmly but gently onto the skin, and allowed to set, until touching one corner moves the entire piece. Removal is accomplished by first flicking up the outer corners with one firm stroke, whilst supporting the face with the other hand, and then removing the wax in one piece with a firm swift movement, contoured to the shape of the face. The second hand gives immediate relief to the area by firmly placing the index finger on the waxed section, until the smarting passes. Skill in removal depends on being decisive in the actions used, and having the wax the correct consistency, not too soft or over set and brittle. Any loose hairs will be removed with the soothing lotion, and if the borders of the wax piece have been neat, and not fragmented, there should be the minimum of tidying to do. Stray hairs may be removed with tweezers, but any patches of hair missed by the wax or left due to incorrect technique must be rewaxed, either after a short rest or, if the skin is irritated, on another occasion. A successful waxing procedure should remove all the hairs with roots intact, and not cause breakage resulting in hairs being evident soon after the treatment.

Chin Waxing

The preparation and contra-indications to chin waxing are identical to lip waxing. The method of application depends on the strength and situation of the hairs. Vellus hair growth along the jaw can be treated as for lip wax, from side to side, with larger sized pieces being applied. Application and removal are the same, but care must be taken not to break the wax due to the contoured area under treatment. Patches of hair should be dealt with individually, with the wax applied against the growth, normally upwards towards the lip. The same removal methods and after care procedures are used.

The complete treatment may be accomplished swiftly and with minimum client discomfort if attention is given to preparation of the equipment and wax, and the application is neatly performed. After-care of the area should be to apply soothing antiseptic products, and if makeup is to be reapplied over the area it must be of a medicated type. A flesh coloured antiseptic dusting powder is preferable to avoid the risk of infection resulting from the waxing treatment.

Wax Maintenance

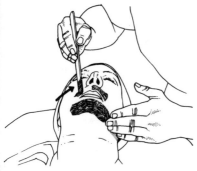

COMBINED LIP AND CHIN WAX

The depilatory wax must be cleansed by filtering to remove the hairs whilst the consistency is fluid. Constant addition or replacement of the facial wax will maintain its adhering properties, and produce constant results without causing skin irritation or infection. The wax is a mixture of beeswax and resins, and so it must not be overheated, otherwise its removal properties diminish and the colour darkens.

The risks of cross infection from lip and chin waxing are high, and so wax maintenance and general salon hygiene are important considerations on the successful applications of this popular service.

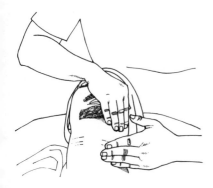

FLICKING UP CHIN WAX

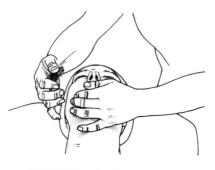

CHIN WAX REMOVAL

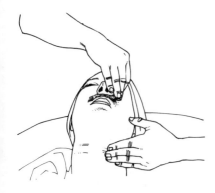

FLICKING UP LIP WAX

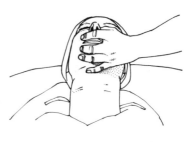

LIP WAX REMOVAL

Chapter 7

Makeup Techniques and Cosmetic Sales Psychology

BASIC MAKEUP TECHNIQUES

Modern makeup is definitely an art form, capable of creating on any woman many different faces, to reflect her mood or personality. A client can have a number of natural or high fashion makeup looks, which a skilful therapist can develop to suit the time of year, fashion trends, or specific occasions.

Basic techniques of colour blending, application, and client suitability remain constant, regardless of the continual introduction of new cosmetic preparations to maintain client interest. The simplification of application methods in products designed for the retail market has increased the client's skill in personal makeup, and requires that the professional service given should be supreme in developing attractive features and minimizing faults.

Day makeup is the most difficult type to apply, as it must stand inspection in natural or artificial light and is subject to close scrutiny. Points on technique mastered in basic day makeup permit maximum concentration on artistic development, to be achieved in evening and photographic aspects of the skill.

Makeup based on correction of facial shapes is outdated for the modern makeup artist, who thinks more in terms of colour, and natural and reflective contouring, to achieve full personality development through the makeup application for her clients.

MAKEUP PRODUCTS

Pre-makeup Base (moisturizers)

The outer layers of skin need to maintain adequate moisture levels if they are to remain smooth and supple, and application of suitable moisture retaining products, prior to makeup, will help to accomplish this task. The skin loses a lot of its natural moisture through evaporation, and is particularly affected by extremes of temperature, sun exposure, and low humidity conditions found in centrally heated surroundings. A condition of dehydration soon becomes evident if a suitable barrier product is not used regularly as a protective safeguard against the effects of the elements on the skin.

Moisture preparations come in many forms, creams, emulsions, and liquids, which have different proportions of water to oil in their formulation, in this way providing suitable products for all skin conditions. Cream moisturizers give the greatest protection and provide a daily treatment product for the dry, mature skins, which supports the nightly skin care sequence. Emulsions and liquids offer a wide range of applications, from the non-greasy protective film for the oily skin, to the hydro-emulsion form, containing active ingredients, which may be applied on many different skin conditions to good effect.

Colourless and tinted pre-makeup bases are available to protect the skin, retain natural moisture, and correct skin tone irregularities. Highly coloured or sallow complexions can be improved, or a glow given to the face by the blush effect of the naturally toned tinted bases. Sun-tanned or even coloured skin can be protected and enhanced simply by a base tint, precluding the need for further tinted foundation items.

Application   The moisturizer should be applied thinly all over the face and throat, with smooth flowing movements, and allowed to settle into a slightly tacky film before the foundation is applied. A well-chosen and applied moisture base prolongs the lasting properties of a basic makeup, and helps to prevent colour change occurring.

Tinted Foundation

Obtaining the correct texture of foundation product is as important as choosing the most flattering colour tone. Unsuitable textures will result in irregularities of appearance ranging from shiny emphasis of faults, to a dry parched complexion, with areas of colour change. For a tinted foundation to be long-lasting, without colour or texture changes occurring, it must be chosen to suit the skin condition as well as enhancing the complexion.

Foundations which improve the appearance and maintain skin texture can be grouped by their consistency as a rough guide to their best application.

Skin 'Type'	Choice of Foundation
Dry and mature	Cream or moisturized emulsion
Dry and sensitive	Cream or oil-based

(cont.)

Skin 'Type'	Choice of Foundation
Combination skin (oily centre panel area)	Liquid, semi-liquid, all-in-one foundation (fluid and powder combined
Oily	Non-oily, astringent or water-based (combined) Cake or block type, suspended liquid (combined)
Blemished, acne	Medicated liquid or block (drying and germicidal)
Allergic/ hypersensitive	Hypo-allergenic (with all known irritants screened out)

Foundations for Special Purposes

1 Tinted foundations for improving facial colouring, i.e. green, mauve, apricot, which have a limited use in professional makeup applications.
2 Treatment foundations, combining tinted preparations and additional nutrient elements, for the mature, crêpy or lined skin.
3 Concealing foundations, to disguise and heal facial blemishes, scars, acne etc., which are applied directly over the blemish, prior to the medicated foundation application, or replacing it. The products are opaque, firm in texture, and have excellent covering properties.
4 Sun-screening foundations, available as tinted jellies, which act as an ultraviolet screen, protecting the skin, whilst adding colour.
5 Cosmetic camouflage products, which disguise disfigurements, birth marks etc., and include covering creams and a variety of foundation items.
6 Theatrical foundations, which are forms of exaggerated colour, for use with the lighting and distance involved in stage productions.

Colour Choice, Uses and Application

The foundation base in day makeup is the most important aspect of general improvement, providing a means of regulating colour tone, concealing minor imperfections, and accentuating attractive facial features. The principles of colour-blending to achieve individual effects have to be practised until a good eye for colour is developed. The foundation application should be viewed as a basic canvas on which the makeup artist will build to create the total illusion. The light reflective properties of many foundations increase the luminous appearance of lighter foundations, and help to bring areas of the face into prominence, whilst darker tones can be used to recess and diminish unattractive features present.

Tones of foundation can be used to accentuate the angular planes of the face, correct facial proportions, and disguise discoloured skin areas. Extensive facial contouring with light and dark shaders should be restricted in day makeup, due to the time involved and obvious nature of the finished result.

The client should be placed in a semi-upright position, and the foundation chosen to suit the age, skin texture, and purpose of the application. The general colouring and personality of the client will determine the range of possible colour tones. A successful approach to makeup will give attention to the animated nature of the client's features, and should reflect her life style and personal makeup tastes. The rôle of the makeup should be determined, whether it is to promote a new image, maintain an established look, or be experimental in its approach. If the client seeks makeup advice for her daily use, over-artistic interpretation by the therapist of her foundation and general colour needs will be confusing and discouraging to the client, and simple techniques are preferable. If however the client appears in need of morale-boosting, for a special occasion, full expression can be given to artistic makeup abilities, to create a flattering and exquisite effect, tailored to the client's desires.

Foundation Colours and Uses

Colour-blending to achieve individual effects is possible with all textures of facial foundations. If a wide range of tones is available it will normally be found that one or two colours give useful medium-toning effects, which alter slightly depending on the base skin tone, and these colours will be used more frequently than the others in the range. Mid-beige and medium tawny peach are two popular colours, found in most ranges under different names, which offer this ability to adapt to many different skin colours.

Client conversation will determine the individual effect desired, and it is extremely important that this preference should be listened to, in order to devise a look which incorporates or interprets some of her wishes. A beautifully applied makeup which does not satisfy the client's demands is unsuccessful, and can spoil the enjoyment of the whole facial treatment.

Colour Suggestions

Skin Tones	Foundation Tones
Light and pale translucent skins	Light warm beige. Soft peach. Creamy, pinky/beige.
Medium skin tones	Cool beige. Rose beige. Warm peach. Soft beige(tan). Pink/tan. Sun bronze.
Dark skin tones	Dark beige. Deep peach (corrective). Sun bronze (to accentuate a tan). Luminous light olive (also suitable for coloured skins).

Corrective Foundation Colours

Complexion	Colour Tone
Highly coloured, vascular complexion	Flat beige or olive, to tone down the colour, may be used as a correction prior to the general foundation application, on affected areas only.
Uneven, blotchy, or veined complexions	Medium beige and tawny tones may be used to regulate the basic colour, and minimize irregularities. Covering cream in medium beige may be applied over particularly prominent veins or areas of discoloration.
Sallow, discoloured or pigmented complexions	Medium pink/beige or pink tawny tones may be used depending on general colouring. The darker the base skin tone the more colour lifting effect is required. Vivid areas of pigmentation may be covered with masking creams prior to the general foundation application.

Foundation Application

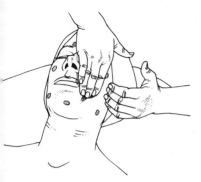

FOUNDATION DOTTING
AND BLENDING

The tinted foundation may be applied in many ways according to consistency, and a flexible approach to blending will achieve satisfactory results with the minimum of fuss or waste. Cream products may be applied with light effleurage movements, keeping the finger tips in contact, and the residue of foundation in the palm of the hand. The application should commence at the throat, and work swiftly over the face and eye areas, to form an even film. Semi-liquid and all-in-one combined foundations are more difficult to apply, and can tend to drag the skin so small deposits on the chin, cheeks, and forehead areas before general blending will facilitate a neater and swifter application.

As these foundations do not require fixing with powder, their finish is drier, and careful checking is necessary to avoid harsh lines around the jaw and a tinted build-up on vellus facial hair, on the cheeks and hairlines.

Liquid foundations are more difficult to control, and a cosmetic sponge may be used to achieve good coverage and prevent accidental soiling. The liquid sets to a matt film, which can give an unnatural appearance unless the skin texture is re-established by hand contact with the face to bring out its natural gloss and life. The staying properties of liquid foundations provide the ideal coverage for oily and blemished complexions, camouflaging and protecting them without aggravating the existing conditions. Excessive oil secretion can cause a colour change in tinted foundations, so oil-free preparations are preferable to avoid this occurrence.

Cake or block foundations should be applied with a clean cosmetic sponge and water to achieve good coverage and a matt texture. The principles of block foundations are similar to liquids, but they have a greater variety of colour tones and applications, due to the increased coverage possible by altering the thickness of the application. The convenience of a compact block has made them a more popular choice for younger clients, combining economy of time and cost.

Medicated foundations may be obtained in liquid, semi-liquid, all-in-one, and block forms, and should be chosen to suit individual needs and life style. Clients with blemished skin should be encouraged to leave their skin free from makeup whenever possible, but the demoralizing effect of an acne skin on the client should be weighed against this advice and a compromise sought. If a foundation is to be worn, it must help to dry and heal the

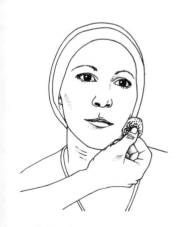

SPONGE METHOD
FOUNDATION APPLICATION

skin, camouflage effectively, and so be light textured, to give excellent coverage, and be anti-
bacterial in action.

Cheek Colour

Rouge, Blushers, Shaders   Cheek shapers, shaders, and highlighters may be
be applied at this stage of the routine, prior to the
loose powder, or they may be the most
superficial of the cosmetic items, concluding the
sequence, depending on the effect required. All
cream-textured products required to have long-
lasting properties, i.e. cheek colour, eye shadows,
highlighters, need to be set with loose powder to
avoid colour loss and evident creasing into facial
lines. The powder application also softens the
appearance if applied correctly, and makes the substance of the preparations less obvious under close
scrutiny.

Types of Rouges, Shaders,
and Blushers   Liquids, emulsions, creams and powders are
available to suit all skin types and occasions. Compact stick and powder blushers in transparent and
frosted versions have re-established the popularity
of additional cheek colour, due to their ease of
application and high fashion effect. Both the solid
stick and powder versions may be applied after
loose powder if used, but as they are normally the
choice of the younger client they will tend to be
used to accentuate the features on top of an all-in-
one foundation base as a final touch. Cream products are softer in effect for the dry and mature skins,
and give lasting colour and convenience of application, avoiding skin distension.

Colour Choice   All colours from pink, tawny rose, bright red,
through to russet brown and yellow are available in
rouges and blushers. Shaders and highlighters used
to accentuate and develop the principle of
illuminating and diminishing the facial features are
available in colour tones ranging from blank or
pearlized white, cream, beige, through to darkest
brown.

Application   The method of use depends on the type of
product, and the effect to be created. In day wear,
accentuation of facial contours and the addition of
flattering colour are all that are required for all but
the youngest clients. The colour should be applied
sparingly to prevent colour build up and an
unnatural appearance resulting. On the younger
client facial contouring to develop the angular
nature of the cheek may be undertaken, whilst on
the slightly older person accentuation on the upper

cheek and zygomatic arch area will be more flattering and will bring the eyes into prominence.

Most skin tones, apart from florid complexions, gain some improvement from the controlled warmth and facial lift of additional colour. Over-emphasis in the older client, however, should be restrained to prevent an artificially young appearance being created, which is extremely unattractive and obvious.

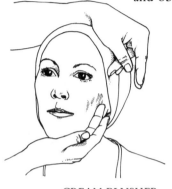

CREAM BLUSHER

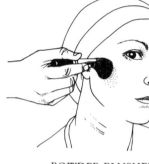

POWDER BLUSHER

EYE MAKEUP

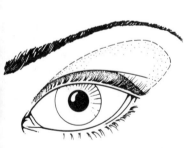

BASIC EYE MAKEUP

Eye makeup may be used to correct faults, accentuate the eyes, and by bringing colour to the face can detract from other poor features. The texture of the products used must be flattering to the eye and suitable for the client's age and skin condition.

The classic eye makeup sequence is to first shape and colour the brows, providing a frame for the eye, then to apply eye shadow, liner and false lashes if worn, and lastly mascara. The variety of makeup textures available will alter this routine for high fashion effects, but the basic sequence remains a convenient guideline for general applications.

Types of Eye Makeup

Eyebrow Makeup   Pencils, crayons, and powders provide a good range of colours and textures for all colourings and age groups. Well-shaped brows can be tinted if necessary to reduce the task even further.

Eye Shadow   Creams, liquids, compact powders, powder cream, sticks and transparent tints provide an immense range of products for enhancing the eyes. Cream shadows are easy to apply but tend to crease, and so for mature skins powder creams offer the best solution, combining a soft appearance, with colour-retaining properties. The powder cream has the texture of a fine cream product and is applied in the same way, but it sets into a matt film, whilst retaining its soft fluid appearance.

Younger skins, free from lines and crêpiness, can combine all textures to achieve the desired effect, and can easily mingle irridescent and transparent items without creating an over-done appearance if the colours blend together harmoniously. Eye makeup can be the most flattering, or obvious item of the sequence, according to whether it suits the client's personality and age. High fashion effects, so attractive on young bright eyes, accentuate faults on the older client, and are out of place and unattractive. The therapist's skill in eye makeup applications will be to guide her older clients away from over-young effects, and devise flattering, but suitable colour combinations individually for her needs.

Eye Emphasis

Eye Liner   Lining the eyes is a fashion effect which swings in and out of favour, depending on the fashion scene at the time. Heavy eye accentuation is not used at present, but may revive if a swing back to harder, more elegant fashions occurs. The lashes can be emphasized by a fine line of deeper eye shadow colour, or dark liner, applied close to the roots. Use of liner can appear to open, lengthen or emphasize the eye, depending on the area of application and colour chosen. If false lashes are applied, they should be attached over a fine lash line, and then the finished effect can be balanced by additional use of liner and mascara.

Kohl   Accentuating the eyes with a soft black Kohl eye makeup is popular with younger clients, applied in a softly defined fashion right around the inner eye rim, and smudged through the lashes to create a romantic, rather Eastern effect. Similar in consistency to the traditional Kohl, worn by Indian women, it is applied in a similar manner, with a brush or blunt ended stick, a soft pencil version is also available. To apply the product the therapist must face the client, who has to keep her eyes open and steady during the procedure. A steady hand is needed to prevent the Kohl touching the eye-ball itself. Some clients may prefer to apply this final step of the eye makeup themselves, wearing it all the time as in the case of Indian women, they have a very exact idea of how they wish it to look.

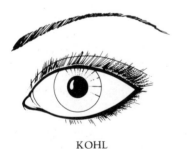

KOHL

Although very attractive and in keeping with Eastern features and costume, the use of Kohl in the European nationalities should be confined to younger clients with sufficient confidence to wear a makeup that will balance its dramatic effect. Large clear eyes, strong makeup tones, and defined lip colours are necessary to exploit the effect to the full.

Mascara   Block, spiral and liquid forms of mascara provide a large variety of products. Mascara wands offer the most convenient but expensive form of eye-lash emphasis and, due to their liquid formulation, use is restricted in the case of sensitive or allergy prone eye skin conditions. Both contact lens wearers and clients with sensitive eyes should be advised to use hypo-allergenic mascara, or tint their eyelashes to prevent the need for heavy mascara applications.

Eye Makeup Application

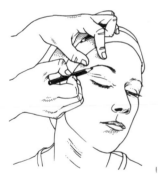

EYEBROW PENCIL

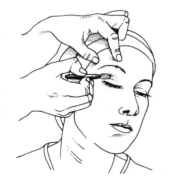

EYE SHADOW APPLICATION

The basic sequence for day makeup should be followed, with the eyebrows being formed into a natural shape with pencils or eyebrow powder using short light strokes in a mixture of tones to create a groomed appearance. Blunt ended pencils prevent a harsh finish, and even up the sparse areas of the brow. Application of the shadow items should be accomplished with a small brush or foam tipped stick, to transfer the preparation to the eye skin, where it may be blended with the fingers. The area of eye skin involved will depend on any corrective elements required in the makeup, but may include the middle and outer part of the lid, extending out towards the eyebrow arch.

This form of colour accentuation gives prominence to the eyes, and avoids the areas of worst skin texture in the mature client. Lightening the area under the brow to give the illusion of larger more brilliant eyes can be achieved with ivory-toned highlighters, which can also be reflected on the cheek bone area above the cheek shading or colour.

Application of socket emphasis, with deeper-toned products, is best confined to younger clients with large eyes and full smooth lids, and should not be applied on deep-set, small or crêpy skinned eyes.

If used, liner should not be apparent, but give emphasis to the lashes and eye generally, to present a more contrasting appearance between the eye and the shadow. Modern trends in makeup do not include the use of liners to a large extent, so their obvious appearance would give a dated look to the

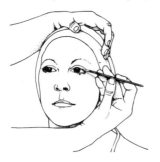

EYE LINER

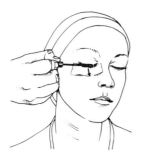

MASCARA DOWNWARD
APPLICATION

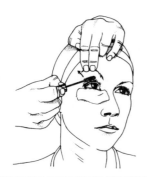

UPWARD SWEEPING STROKES

finished effect. However, subtle use can give eye emphasis, and can accentuate the most expressive feature of the face. The different makeup fashions worn throughout the world require that a makeup artist is competent in all facial effects, and eye liner is a standard eye makeup item for many overseas clients.

The line should be fine, but soft, and applied with a tapered brush close to the roots of the lashes, not extending beyond them. A coloured shadow line can be applied close to or instead of the dark line, to soften it and give additional colour brilliance.

Additional lash emphasis or careful fragmented liner application is usually required on the lower lashes to balance the effect and prevent a top-heavy appearance.

Mascara and false or individual lashes also have periods of popularity and decline, but the flattering effect of emphasizing and lengthening the natural lash retains mascara as a very popular client product, from which they will not be easily parted. The mascara should be applied first downwards over the upper lashes, coating them evenly, then lifting and sweeping them outwards and upwards to give an attractive curve. The procedure may then be repeated, until the desired effect is achieved, and then the lower lashes should be covered, taking care to keep the lashes separate, and avoiding touching and staining the skin.

Unsteady eyes should be made up with care and use of tissues to prevent under eye skin becoming coated with mascara when the client blinks. Insignificant, sparse, or very straight lashes should be tinted in preference to heavy mascara applications as a more natural effect will be achieved, and the mascara will only be needed to curl the lashes not to coat them.

Lipstick Choice and Application

Colour and texture have equal importance for mouth emphasis and improvement. Personal preference regarding texture will decide the range of possible lipstick applications, and the variety of colours and consistencies available provide products for all occasions, age groups and fashion effects. The lipstick is a very vital part of the entire makeup, as it gives the appearance of pulling the whole effect together, harmonizing eye, cheek, and facial tones, whilst giving vitality and life to the expression.

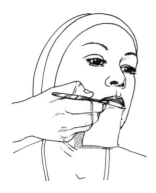

First the lip line should be evenly and clearly applied, and then the lips filled in with colour to achieve even coverage. The lips may be blotted, and fresh colour applied, to establish a long-lasting effect. In the case of transparent lip tints one application is sufficient, as the effect is designed to be superficial, and reapplication is unavoidable.

Full lips should be toned down with soft colours, with their natural shape used as sufficient emphasis. Irregular or narrow lips can be disguised with brighter or more pearlized lipsticks, which can be used in combination to fill out, diminish or bring out areas of the lips into prominence.

LIPSTICK APPLICATION

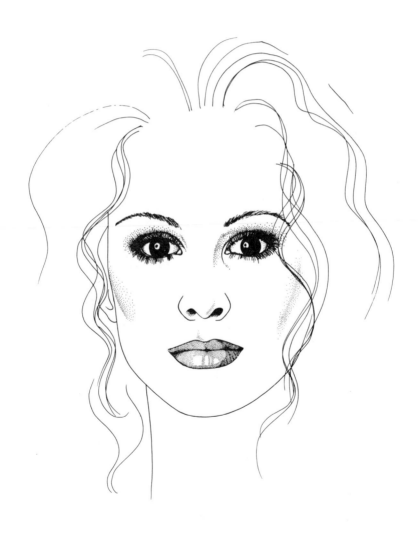

THE FINISHED EFFECT

Basic Makeup Conclusion

Makeup of the face must be approached as a total effect, rather than as a combination of the individual areas. An attractive facial expression can often bring beauty into a face comprised of few redeeming features, and this personality element should be fully developed by the makeup artist to create individual effects.

Examination of the finished effect will indicate any final touches, necessary to achieve the most flattering makeup. The need for additional colour on the eyes and cheeks, may be apparent, after the lipstick application, and should be accomplished prior to the client's inspection.

Completion of the makeup will include tidying the client's hair after removal of the head-band, robes etc., and it is important that the finished effect should be established before the client views the makeup, to avoid disappointment.

ANALYSIS OF THE FACE FOR PHOTOGRAPHIC, EVENING AND HIGH FASHION MAKEUP

Before the makeup is commenced, its purpose should be determined, so that the finished effect can reflect or create the required illusion. The lighting under which the makeup will be viewed will indicate the colour toning possibilities and suitable textures. Daytime high fashion effects require great subtlety of technique, as the makeup may have to be suitable for both close and distant viewing, i.e. demonstration and modelling applications. Evening or photographic effects permit more extreme contrasts of colour and texture due to the artificial lighting throwing the face into relief, an effect which can be emphasized by facial and reflective makeup contouring.

Analysis of the Face

The individuality of facial features can be developed by the makeup artist, who no longer has to attempt to fit her client's looks into an accepted mould. Interesting facial contours and attractive features should be noted and emphasized, to create an entirely individual look. Irregularly shaped eyes or lips can be made to appear less noticeable by drawing attention away from them to other more distinctive features.

The face should be viewed in profile and full face, and natural contouring requirements decided. Angular plains of the cheeks can be shaded and highlighted, and any faults such as a double chin or over-hanging lids minimized. The areas of shading should be definite, with the edges softened, and blended in to prevent harsh lines.

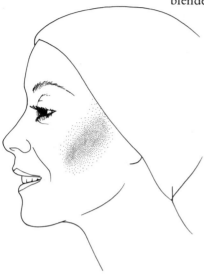

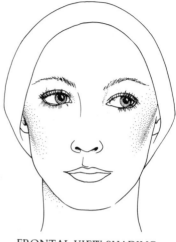

FRONTAL VIEW SHADING

FACIAL CONTOURING IN PROFILE

Facial Contouring and Correcting

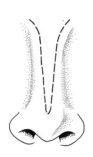

NOSE SHADING

The primary contouring and highlighting should be applied prior to the tinted foundation, so that its effect is softened by the overall colour, and it becomes fixed into position by it. The more obvious the contrast permissable, i.e. photographic makeup, the more evident can be the colours used for shading and highlighting.

Fleshy or irregularly shaped noses can be refined, straightened, or an illusion of a narrower nasal bridge created. The tip of the nose should not be shaded, as this always appears as a smudge. Jaw contouring, with light and dark foundations, can appear to firm the jaw line, minimize fleshy areas under the mandible, and be made to lengthen and slim an ageing neck.

Eyes may be emphasized, enlarged, and opened with cream or ivory coloured highlighter for evening or fashion effects, and white shader for photographic work. Overhead lighting throws the eyes into shadow, and so lifting and accentuating the area is usually beneficial.

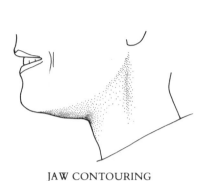

JAW CONTOURING   EYE ENLARGING WITH HIGHLIGHT

Corrective Eyebrow Shapes

The eyebrows can be used to create an angular or rounded appearance on different facial contours. A well-shaped brow is essential for all makeup work, but it can be made to change, refine, or improve a facial shape. Tinting can be used to emphasize, lengthen, or slightly change the eyebrow shape to accentuate a particular effect.

Angular Shape

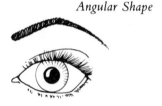

An angular shape can be used to give flat plains to a rounded face. The angle of the brow can be reflected in the shading and contouring to give the illusion of an elegant appearance. The angular eyebrow can be used to create many looks, and can reflect an appearance of harshness, elegance and sophistication.

Rounded Shape

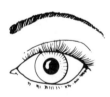

The more natural line of the rounded brow can give an innocent, fresh appearance, and blends well if a more general makeup is required. The line should follow the prominence of the frontal bone, and be shaped into a tapered end, encompassing the rounded shape of the eye itself. Clients with large eyes or very wide foreheads should be given a rounded eyebrow shape to show their eyes to the best advantage.

Sweeping Shape

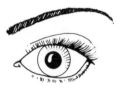

A sweeping eyebrow shape is very flattering to the majority of clients, giving width and expression to the eye area of the face. The sweeping eyebrow shape frees a large expanse of upper lid skin for eye makeup, and allows full artistic expression in this area. The sweeping line of the brow opens the eyes, gives interest to a narrow face, and can help to balance an over-large mouth or nose shape. This shape of brow can be used to create many different illusions, from the romantic, to the very natural look, depending on the rest of the makeup.

Facial Foundations for Fashion, Evening and Photographic Makeup

The texture of the foundation should be even, matt, and give good coverage without appearing heavy. For a natural texture a cosmetic sponge may be used to apply and settle the foundation. Different tones of tinted foundation may be used to reflect the underlying shading, but they must be well blended or will be obvious. The finish at this stage is important, as the face is being prepared for its final more flattering makeup elements, and poor preparations will prevent a long-lasting or perfect finished effect.

The foundation should cover the face and neck, and may also be applied over the eye and lip areas, depending on the subsequent makeup products to be used. Brighter tones than normally worn will be required for evening and photographic work, due to the draining effect of the artificial lighting.

Blushers and Additional Colour

Coloured blushers of the cream and stick compact type may be used to emphasize the shading at this stage, but care must be taken to avoid colour build-up, particularly for the day fashion makeup. The colour should not dominate the face, but give prominence to the eyes and vitality to the face.

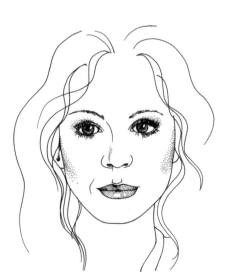

HIGH FASHION EFFECT

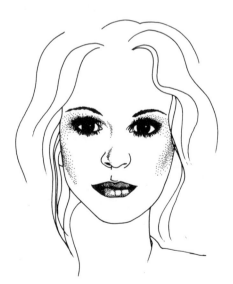

PHOTOGRAPHIC EFFECT

Face Powder   Use of loose powder has lost its popularity for basic day wear, but it is important for setting high fashion day effects and vital for evening and photographic work to merge together all the detailed layers of the makeup, and set the final result. The light reflection on the face from spot and background lighting in photographic work would spoil the effect if it were not diminished by thorough powdering. The powder should be chosen to harmonize, not change the foundation shade, and it should be applied carefully but liberally over all the face, neck, eyes, and lips with a rolling movement of the puff.

The residue can then be brushed from the face with a soft powder puff, following the natural vellus hair growth of the area. All parts of the face should be inspected, for loose powder, and the brows especially brushed and retouched.

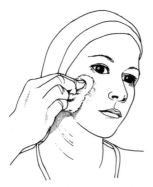

LOOSE POWDER APPLICATION

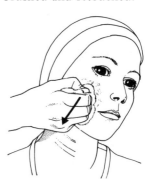

POWDER REMOVAL

Eye Makeup

As the underlying work has prepared an even-coloured, and highlighted matt base, only final colour touches and lash emphasis are required. Day fashion effects may include basic colour-toned shadows, socket emphasis (on the fuller eye), additional brow reflective highlighting, and liner, full or partial false lashes and mascara. Socket emphasis should be modified for evening and photographic work, otherwise the eye will appear deeply shadowed due to overhead lighting. The amount of makeup worn will depend on the effect or illusion to be created, and the direction of lighting used to illuminate the face in photographic work. The wishes of the photographer really decide the type of makeup that is required, and so the finished effect is a joint effort and cannot be accomplished in isolation.

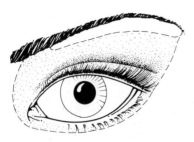

HIGH FASHION EYE MAKEUP

Corrective Eye Makeup

The principle of emphasizing, bringing forward into prominence, and diminishing or regressing, with light and dark tones, can be used to advantage in improvement of difficult or irregularly shaped eyes. Use of vibrant colours, tones of the shade picked, and contrasting textures enable the skilful makeup artist to correct or reflect interest away from the eye fault. No rules can apply to corrective makeup, as it is not only the feature that has to be considered but its relationship to the rest of the face. The profile and frontal view of the eye should always be considered, and difficult eyes not seen as a fault, rather as a challenge to present them to their best advantage.

False Lashes

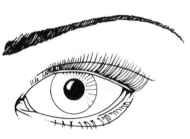

FINE LASHES: TOP

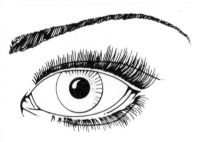

HEAVY LASHES: TOP AND BOTTOM

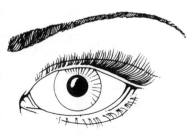

PARTIAL LASHES: OUTER EYES

The variety of false lashes available gives a wide range of possible effects for enhancing or correcting the eye. Very fine false lashes produce a natural appearance, emphasizing the density of the existing lash without seeming artificial. The heavier lashes attached to a more solid base require a more exaggerated makeup to complement them, and should be restricted to distance and photographic work. Partial lashes to extend width, give uplift, or general emphasis can be very useful in corrective eye makeup applications, as they can balance the eyes, improve the profile appearance, and disguise eye faults.

The decision to use false lashes will depend on the client's acceptance of artificial products around the eye, general eye sensitivity, and the sophistication of the client's normal makeup and personality. False lashes have to be integrated as part of the total makeup concept, and can give a very elegant and attractive appearance to the face, if chosen and applied with care. In the same way as eye liners, false lashes follow fashion trends, losing and regaining favour, but remaining popular at all times with the younger client. For photographic work false lashes form a standard part of the makeup, and are generally applied in all makeups designed to flatter the face rather than change it.

The lashes should be clean, naturally curled, and shaped to suit the client's eye. The variety of thicknesses and lengths should restrict the need for extensive individual trimming and reduce the application time. The eye makeup should be completed up to the eye-liner stage, and then the false lashes may be applied to the roots of the natural lashes to form a firm attachment. Adhesive may be applied directly onto the base strip of the lashes, or with an orange stick in the case of very light-weight

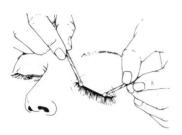

ATTACHMENT OF FALSE
EYE-LASHES

varieties. The client must remain with her eyes closed for a few seconds to permit the adhesive to set and prevent the preparation entering the eye and causing irritation. The lash should be firmly but gently pressed into position with the orange stick, and then the finished line can be inspected, and the inner and outer corners checked for firm attachment and appearance. An attractive shape should be attained with the false lashes blending and combining with the natural lashes to form a thicker, longer, more flattering effect. When the adhesive has set, and become transparent, the eye makeup may be finished by attachment of lower lashes if used, and retouching of eye-liner and shadow etc., to achieve a perfect finish. The lower lashes are attached with the eyes open, and emphasis should be placed on the outer area of the eye to prevent an artificial effect.

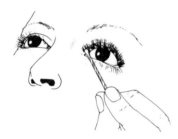

CHECKING LASH ATTACHMENT

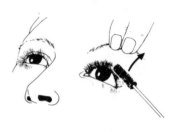

BLENDING FALSE & NATURAL LASHES

The completed lash attachment may be brushed into a natural shape with the minimum of mascara, or just a clean brush, to combine the false and natural lashes, and ensure separation of the top and bottom sets.

CORRECTION AND EMPHASIS OF EYE SHAPES
Deep-set Eyes

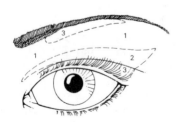

1 The eyes may be brought forward with pale irridescent colours, blended in an oval around the upper and lower lids.

2 The overhanging brow bone should be shaded as a fine line spreading out to wing along the crease.

3 The arch of the brow can be emphasized with a white or cream-coloured pearl shadow, also repeated in the centre of the lid.

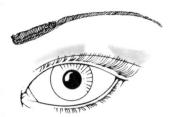

No eye-liner but fine pointed upper and lower lashes may be applied, for increased definition in the younger client.

Colour Suggestions

(1) Violet. (2) Pearl white. (3) Grape for shading.
(1) Pale pink. (2) Pearl pink/white. (3) Bergundy.
(1) Pale yellow. (2) Cream. (3) Gold/bronze.

Round Eyes

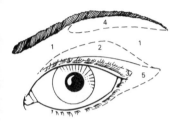

1   The entire upper lid may be highlighted with a pale tone.

2   In a full lid socket emphasis may be softly applied to form a sweeping curve, echoing the brow line.

3   A fine dark line, or a more brightly coloured shadow line, can be applied close to the lashes.

4   The arched line of the brow can be accentuated with an irridescent pearl white or ivory toned highlighter.

5   A medium tone of the general shade may be applied at the outer corner to lengthen the eye shape and give an attractive profile appearance.

Individual or false lashes to lengthen and thicken the lash line may be used, with the emphasis placed from the centre lids outwards.

Colour Suggestions

(1) Ivory. (2) Dark gold. (3) Gold/brown shadow or brown liner. (4) White or cream lightener. (5) Cream/gold.

(1) Pale pink. (2) Dark burgundy. (3) Grape shadow or liner. (4) White/pink irridescent highlight. (5) Medium grape.

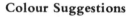

Small Eyes

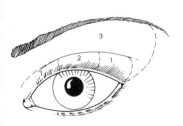

1   Colour the entire lid with a bright but soft tone to enlarge the eye.

2   Accentuate the centre lid area with a more definite and slightly contrasting shade, blending in to give fullness to the lid.

3   Echo the brow line with a soft sweep of colour in a deeper but harmonizing shade.

The outer lashes may be emphasized with mascara, and for the younger client individual false lashes may be applied at the outer corners.

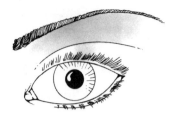

Colour Suggestions

(1) White/pale blue. (2) Violet. (3) Blue/dove grey.

(1) Soft yellow. (2) Lime green. (3) Greeny/bronze.

Overhanging Lids

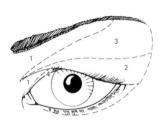

1   The inner eye corner may be highlighted with a soft light colour, which can be repeated under the lower lashes.

2   The overhanging lid area can be subtly shaded to diminish its prominence with a matt-textured, deeper-toned shadow.

3   The under brow area may be highlighted to deflect interest from the overhanging lid.

4   A stronger line of colour close to the roots of the lashes may be applied to add vitality and definition to the eye.

Lashes may be emphasized with mascara to form a natural appearance.

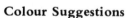

Colour Suggestions

(1) Beige. (2) Goldy/bronze. (3) Ivory. (4) Dark gold.

(1) Pale aquamarine. (2) Soft grey. (3) White/grey. (4) Aquamarine.

Close-set Eyes

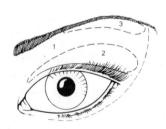

1   The entire orbital cavity area should be brought forward with a pale coloured, soft textured shadow, in a slightly oval shape.

2   A winging sweep of slightly darker, brighter shadow may be applied, commencing as a fine line, broadening into a wider curve.

3   The under arch area of the brow may be highlighted with a light, bright irridescent shadow to give a contrast of textures.

The sweeping brow line can be reinforced with fine, long, individual or partial false lashes applied to the outer third of the eye.

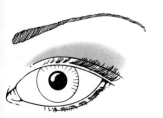

Colour Suggestions

(1) Pale cream. (2) Russet brown. (3) Ivory irridescent highlighter.

(1) Pale avocado green. (2) Brown/green. (3) Pale moss green highlighter.

Prominent or Heavy-lidded Eyes

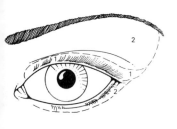

1 A sombre but rich shade of shadow should be applied to the upper lid to diminish the prominence of the eye

2 The shape of the eye may be redefined by illuminating the brow bone area to deflect interest from the protruding lids. This colour may be reflected under the lower lashes, depending on the overall fullness of the eye in profile.

Natural lash emphasis is sufficient definition, as over-heavy or curled lashes increase the rounded and prominent appearance of the eye.

Colour Suggestions

(1) Plum. (2) Medium pink.
(1) Green/bronze. (2) Pale creamy green.
(1) Grape/grey. (2) Pale grey.

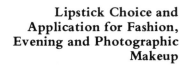

Lipstick Choice and Application for Fashion, Evening and Photographic Makeup

The intensity of lip colour must balance and be in harmony with the rest of the makeup. Artificial lighting tends to drain colour from the face, so sufficient brilliance is necessary to avoid an unfinished appearance. Working with soft but bright tones permits more improvement in mouth shape and gives definition to the lips.

The texture of the lipstick is important, and again can help to reduce or increase the apparent size of the mouth or improve the proportions of the lips to each other.

An Over-large Mouth   An over-large mouth should be made up with soft colours and a fairly matt lipstick consistency, otherwise it will tend to dominate the face. The lip line should be even, but not too hard, and kept well within the natural borders of the mouth. Every effort should be made to make up the face to deflect interest to the eyes or cheek-bones, diminishing the importance of the lips in the overall effect.

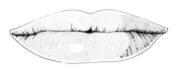

Uneven or Small Lips   Uneven or small lips can use matt and pearlized lipstick textures to give apparent fullness to central areas, or to regulate the different lip shapes. It is impossible to make a small mouth appear large by over painting the borders without it appearing obvious, but skilful use of colour can considerably improve the general appearance.

Lighter and darker tones, irridescent and matt textures, lip gloss, and outlining are all elements of technique available to the makeup artist to produce a more attractive lip appearance to complete the finished effect.

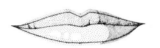

General Conclusion of Fashion, Evening and Photographic Makeup

All forms of cosmetic makeup can only be learnt by practice, experimentation, and development of a good eye for colour and texture. Working with skilled photographic and makeup artists is the finest way to increase personal makeup talents, by first watching their interpretation, and then developing personal techniques. Makeup application in general therapy is important, as otherwise the therapist's work will never be seen to its best advantage by the client. As the most immediate beneficial effect of a cosmetic facial is the improvement in appearance, noticed by the client, its importance should not be underestimated.

MAKEUP FOR THE DARK AND NON-EUROPEAN SKIN

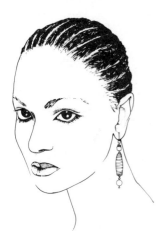

MAKEUP FOR DARK SKIN

Making up a dark skin does present a new challenge to the makeup artist, as many of the basic rules for the European skin either do not apply, or have to be altered drastically to be of use. More use has to be made of real artistic ability to devise attractive flattering makeup, using colour blending skills and working with primary colours to correct or enhance the darker skin tones. Working with a range of differing facial structures, skin colours and textures is also excellent practice for remedial camouflage work, as it throws the therapist back on her own resources and really stretches her makeup abilities. It makes her develop an eye for the correct colour or effect needed, which is invaluable, and is part of the true skill of the makeup artist.

The best approach is to rethink the normal manner in which makeup is chosen, and work from some basic points on facial shapes, shading and colour. These are obviously very different in the darker skin, whether the client is of African, Asian or Afro/Asian origin. The therapist can learn a lot by observing women of all nationalities, looking for points of beauty and how these are emphasized by the individual. Many of the aspects of facial adornment have a religious significance, particularly in the Asian women, and some knowledge of this should prove useful. Adornment of the face and body has a history in many cultures far more ancient than our own, so it is a very old art that is being practised.

Facial Shapes

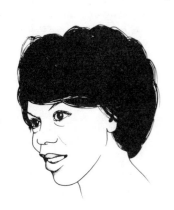

The diversity of facial shapes in the Afro/Asian races makes it impossible to record them as round, oval, square etc., as often the entire positioning of the facial bones is different from that of European women. The facial planes are differently positioned, and the jaw bones may be more prominent in the African face, emphasizing the larger mouth shape and giving a flatter nasal bridge. This can provide a beautiful cheek contour, tilted back to above the eyes, which gives excellent opportunities for emphasis of the upper cheek and eye areas.

The Asian face is more oval, but can sometimes be rather long and angular, requiring a makeup to soften the contours. Like all nationalities Asian beauty is very varied, but in all cases it is different from the stereo typed European view of beauty. The face has flatter planes across the cheek bones and more prominent and expressive features. The eyes are normally the dominant feature of the face, being emphasized with Kohl which adds an exotic appearance to the entire facial makeup. The attractiveness of the Asian beauty is to a large extent intrinsically linked with an elegance of movement, and calmness of manner which is seldom seen in Europeans.

It is important, rather than trying to fit the racial characteristics into the more familiar European mould, to devise a makeup effect that brings out individual ethnic beauty. Features such as a beautifully shaped head, attractive profile and large, brilliant eyes can then be emphasized.

Ethnic Characteristics

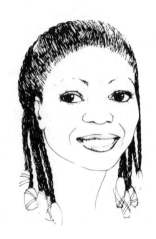

Devising a makeup which brings out the client's natural beauty will be to some extent be based on how the client sees herself, what her personal image of herself is. This can be drawn out of her through discussion prior to and during the makeup, whilst considering what are thought to be good and poor aspects of the appearance. In this way some idea of the different concepts of beauty valued within the client's own nationality can be gained. It is very hard not to view all facial makeups from the European standpoint, and a real effort has to be made to expand out the normal appreciation of beauty, to encompass all the differing nationalities.

A large number of differing ethnic characteristics exist, related not only to the colour of the skin and the bone structure, but also to the way the hair is worn and its physical appearance. Many Asian and Afro/Asian women have beautiful hair, which retains its sheen and colour well into middle age, and does not appear to go white as early as their European counterpart's. The extremely deep blue-black colouring of the hair forms a dense contrast to the face, and so has a bearing on the colours needed to complete the makeup. Far more rich tones can be used in the makeup without appearing brash or harsh, when such deep hair and skin tones exist.

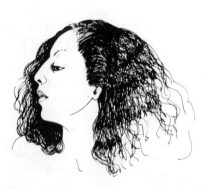

Even where the hair is tightly curled or frizzy as in the negro women, there is less inclination now to adopt European hair fashions by torturing the hair into smooth straightened styles. It is more normal now to either enhance the natural effect to show off an attractive head and neck profile, or emphasize the national characteristics with beading, plaiting of the hair etc. Now that young negro women have discovered that Black is Beautiful, there is a great upsurge in interest in making the most of personal assets, creating makeup effects which exploit the

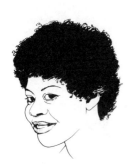

ethnic characteristics to the full: The popularity and attractiveness of these effects has even caused them to be copied by European women, often unfortunately without the natural grace and character they really possess on their natural owners.

In some cases the older woman will still strive to look European, and will attempt to make her complexion look paler, also using eye and lip colours more suited to a lighter colouring. It is up to the therapist to convince her client of the beauty of her own racial characteristics, and devise a makeup that combines all these elements to personal perfection. Many of the clients will have modelled their looks on the European idea of beauty for so long, that it may be impossible to get them to accept, or appreciate a different image, even if it is really their own rather than copied. So a compromise may be needed, to give the client the sophistication she desires, without making the makeup appear artificial or unnatural on her dark skin.

One of the major problems has been lack of suitable colours in makeup for the darker skin, particularly in high-quality cosmetics. This is slowly changing, and the cosmetics available are growing in colour choice and quality as the cosmetic companies realize the importance of this market. Even in parts of the world where a large proportion of the population are coloured, choice of makeup items is often limited to the lower-priced ranges, and women have experienced difficulty achieving a co-ordinated makeup range. So therapists will still have to use a bit of ingenuity to encompass all their coloured clients makeup needs, and will often find themselves advising clients how to make the best use of what is currently available for paler complexions.

Skin Colours

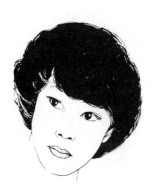

The colour range of African and Asian skins is vast and covers from pale olive, through to the darkest blue-black. The basic skin tones have as much variety as pale complexions, as is discovered when colour matching is attempted. It is wise to consider the primary tones of the skin, whether yellow, greeny olive, warm russet or grey brown, and use these to develop corrective or flattering makeup effects.

In many cases the deeper tone of the skin acts as a basic canvas and does not need to be covered as in a paler skin, but merely enhanced. Imperfections appear less obvious in the deeper skin, and evenness of skin tone is an asset many Afro/Asian clients

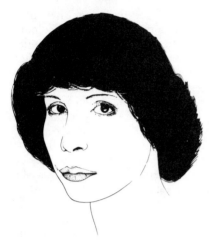

enjoy. Where variations of tone do exist, they appear as patches of pigmentation different in colour, and sometimes texture, from surrounding skin. Really dark African skins can suffer from very dark pigmentation patches of a satiny grey-black, even blue-black, appearance which is very obvious and disfiguring. Vitiligo or loss of pigment is also seen on coloured skins, which is very distressing to the individual, and needs to be treated with remedial camouflage methods, which produce excellent results.

These alterations in the skin colour relate to the presence of melanin forming (pigment) cells in the superficial skin tissues, and irregularities in their behaviour (see Chapter 3). The number of melanin-forming cells, the melanocytes, is not thought to be more abundant in the coloured skin; only their production of melanin for protection is increased. So there are not more cells, but they are more efficient in providing protection against the ageing effects of sunlight.

Coloured clients appear to have a higher skin temperature, and more oily skins which in youth can cause blemished complexions. In humid climates the condition seems worsened, through lack of the drying effects of the sun. The oiliness does appear to diminish in later life, and the skin then needs very careful deep cleansing to prevent a thickened sallow appearance developing. In very dark complexions this gives the face an ashen, dull look, as if the skin were coated.

If well cared for, the thicker skin of the coloured client can retain its youthful bloom and even colour longest, and seems to suffer less from lines and wrinkles in the middle years of life. This may be due to dietary factors keeping the skin supple and elastic, or may be associated with the increased weight many African and Asian clients carry as they advance in years.

Skin Sensitivity

As the minute changes of skin temperature are less obvious in the darker skin, it is easy to assume that it is less sensitive than a European skin, but this is not the case. As with all skins, variations exist, but on whole the skin is rather sensitive and liable to injury in treatment as it does not provide an instantaneous visual warning of its sensitivity through increased colour (dilated capillaries, etc). It does increase in temperature however, and this tactile warning of skin irritation should be heeded by therapists, using their hands to guide them on suitable treatment.

The darker skin has a higher skin temperature and seems to produce more fluid oils on its surface, but it is also subject to scarring and can suffer from Keloid scars after injury, deep-seated infection, etc. Grazing on a really dark skin can result in Keloid scarring, which forms slowly and becomes apparent some time after the injury has healed superficially. The Keloids can form sinewy cords of scar tissue around a damaged area, and are extremely disfiguring and difficult to disguise by camouflage methods. So all treatments that hasten the desquamation process (skin-shedding) should be applied with care, for example biological peeling, or abrasive masks designed to remove the dead and scarred surface tissue.

When one is acquainted with the darker skin, differences in colour can be recognized which relate to changes in temperature, oiliness, moisture levels, and behaviour. Erythema is apparent in the very dark skin, under magnification, as even darker more dense areas. Stretch marks or lines show as a change in texture and elasticity, and assume a silvery, pearlized appearance. The stretch marks may be more wide and soft, less defined than they would be on a paler skin. These may be visible on the breasts, and other areas of the body.

Makeup Choice

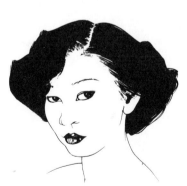

With such a wide range of skin colours, no range of cosmetics can hope to satisfy all the needs, but amongst the ranges will be colours able to enhance or correct most standard colour tones. Until recently many of the more unusual skin colours would have had to turn to theatrical makeup to find the depth and range of colour needed. Even now the Japanese and Chinese skin colours, an attractive creamy tone with just a hint of greeny yellow, are very difficult to match or enhance with available foundations. So also are the blue-black skins which really need colours of the plum and magenta type to show off their richness and beauty. These unusual skin colours will need makeup blended especially for them, often incorporating many different forms of makeup, eye and lip colours mixed into foundations to achieve the subtle tones needed.

Luckily many Afro/Asian skins need no tinted foundation or powder, as they have an even base tone which hides many small imperfections. Also in youth they often have a lovely bloom to the skin which would be a shame to hide with makeup. The skin might have yellow, red, russet, olive or grey undertones which the makeup artist may need to correct or blend in, to brighten the complexion and even out colour differences around the face.

The darker skin soon looks mask-like and cloudy, with the makeup appearing to stand away from the skin if it is the least bit too pale, or too thickly applied. With the base skin tone as the basis for the makeup, more covering is not really needed, and this stage of the European makeup, which is like putting on the base coat of a painting, may be omitted if desired on the coloured skin. The colour depth and evenness is already there and can be built onto, with translucent shaders, shapers, and highlighters to emphasize the beauty of the bone structure.

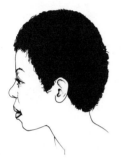

Unevenness of skin colour around the face, darker or lighter patches, and shadowing around the eyes can be camouflaged at the primary stage of the makeup. However even this must be achieved with a light touch, otherwise attention is drawn to the fault rather than away from it. Older Asian women particularly suffer from darkening around the eyes, the skin taking on a reddish purple tone. This is probably concealed more effectively by deflecting interest away from the skin around the eyes, to the attractiveness of the eyes themselves, their fineness and expression, rather than through straightforward cosmetic concealment which might appear obvious.

The basic principles of light shades bringing a feature forward, and darker tones making it appear less obvious, still apply on a dark skin, though different colours have to be employed to achieve the effects. More emphasis has to be placed on highlighting to shape features and bring areas of the face into prominence, rather than shading to diminish weak areas, as the dark shading may not be visible on a really dark toned skin.

Cosmetic Items

Foundations

Transparent products are ideal on the darker complexion if it is clear and free from scars. These show off the colour and enhance it rather than hide it. Foundation should not be oily, and should be heat resistant to cope with the higher skin temperature, and increased sweating that is associated with this condition.

Designed for the European complexion, many of the warmer-toned tinted foundations have a strong orange-red tone to them, which really does not correspond to the darker complexion. If the skin naturally has yellow undertones then a base with

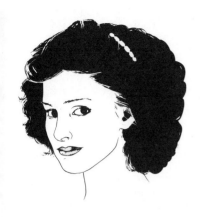

warm peachy orange tones will make the skin appear even more orange, like a technicolour red Indian. So to enhance the yellow undertones, and subdue the red or warm tones, a beige tinted foundation can be used to accomplish both. The very grey ashen skin with a purplish sheen to it can make an individual look very drained and older than they are, so colour lift and brightness should be added to correct the grey tones. This may be achieved with warm beige tones, or use of a tinted moisture base in apricot or peach tones to cancel out the ashen shade of the skin. It is necessary to try out the colour combinations on the skin and learn from experience. If colours are worked out from basic colour blending knowledge, as learnt in related art lessons, it will be possible to achieve some improvement on even the most difficult skin colours.

All colours need to be tried on the client before purchase, as the product looks quite different when in the bottle or jar compared to its appearance on the skin. This is due to the intensity of background colour the darker skin presents behind the cosmetic when on the skin. Even transparent products do not always produce the expected results, being primarily designed to be applied over a pale base. Some translucent products disappear into the skin leaving no trace, others look very obvious and unattractive. Glittery or shimmery products can look very attractive on the right personality, but are best reserved for the younger women.

Face powder tends to flatten the look of any foundation used and if chosen should be neutral in tone. If used heavily it gives a dull, lifeless grey look to the skin. If to be used, loose powder is the best, fluffed on very lightly to finish off the foundation effect without spoiling it.

Blushers   Many of the textures of the blushers available are suitable for the darker skin, but the apricot, peach and pink colours most widely available are not really of use on the darker or olive complexion. The blusher needs to be non-greasy, a creamy gel or fluid, and should be fine in texture. Wine-coloured shades are effective on really dark skins, and where not available as blushers may be utilized from ranges of facial colour crayons. These are designed for painting the eyes, or creating body makeup designs for fantasy or party effects. Lip colours, eye makeup products, or stage makeup items may all need to be used until the specialized ranges of products for coloured skins, available on the Continent, are more freely available world wide.

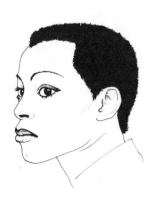

Greater awareness of cosmetic products and a greater sense of their potential beauty among coloured women, may force these products to become more widely distributed. As the demand increases so will the quality and range of products available.

Lip Colours

The deep tones of the lips, sometimes almost purple, need to be corrected on the negro mouth, and clear yellow-toned shades picked to minimize the density of the mouth colour. A compromise is normally necessary, between correction and enhancement, to make the mouth appear less large and dark-lipped. Transparent lip tints are very useful, but shouldn't be over glossy and liquid, otherwise the mouth seems to attract attention and is too prominent in the face. Discovering the most flattering lip colours for darker skinned clients is a matter of experience, but harsh or over-vivid colours should be avoided if a natural effect is to be achieved. The more subtle rose reds, dusky pinks, and muted red golds are all delightful in contrast with the darker skin tone. If the mouth colour and shape is attractive as it is, then lip gloss may be all that is required.

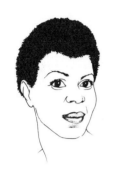

Eye Makeup

All the normal crayons, eye pencils, pressed shadows and eye-gloss can be used to shade the eye area and give it prominence. The deeper the skin is, the richer can be the eye makeup worn, but intense deep glowing colours rather than light vivid ones should be chosen. Often the eye is prominent enough without a lot of added colour, but needs definition and lash emphasis to exaggerate the contrast of the eyes against the dark skin. Ivory and creamy gold are useful neutral colours which show up well on the darker client. Translucent tints of pink and plum are also effective, apart from where the eye skin tends towards this colour naturally, then it should be avoided. Young coloured girls, particularly young negro women, can wear primary eye colours in a kaleidescope effect around the eyes without it looking overdone. This obviously is only for the very confident, and has to be balanced by a fashion makeup on the rest of the face. Eye emphasis around the lashes can be from kohl, or a liner dark enough to show against the skin colour. Lashes can be emphasized in the normal way, and are often a feature of the face.

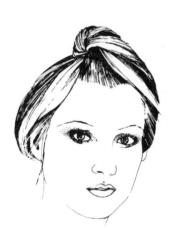

Corrective Elements

Corrective elements in the makeup follow the same pattern as for the European skin, apart from altering the colours used. Deflecting interest to attractive features of the face seems more successful

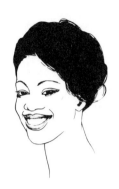

than attempting to shade away or disguise faults. Slimming the nose is useful in the negro face, with contouring cream or darker foundation applied down the sides of the nose, and a paler shade used to straighten and slim the centre of the nose. This gives it elegance and diminishes the broadness of the nostrils. On a really dark skin, where shading would not show, the straightness of the bridge of the nose should be carefully modelled with light makeup or highlighter, so that it catches the eye and draws attention away from the broadness of the nose generally. For day time makeup work, correction of the features is rather limited, as much of the correction would be obvious on close scrutiny. For photographic makeup or distance work as for modelling, a lot of correction is possible, and effective.

Slimming the round or heavy jawed face requires darker contouring creams applied down the sides of the lower cheek and jawline, and highlighting emphasis of the upper cheek bone area.

General points in Makeup Choice

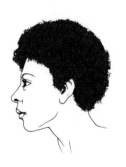

Making up the coloured or non-European woman with whom one has less experience is a challenge and a delight, and some of the ideas gained of how they maximize their own beauty can be transferred to their European counterparts. By observation it is possible to become aware of the special advantages the coloured client possesses, and build on to these to create an individual effect.

It is perhaps even more important when devising a makeup for a non-European client, to realize that their own traditions, life-style, religion etc. can have a strong bearing on what they feel is acceptable in their own personal appearance. So time spent in discussion, before and during the makeup application will insure that the client feels correct and not ill at ease with her new appearance. Much of the traditional ornamentation and makeup of the Asian women is an inherent part of their life, and even when they come for advice, it is of more value to improve on their appearance, than to attempt to change it drastically. It is part of the therapist's rôle to guide and help her clients to greater awareness and fulfilment of their personal beauty, rather than make them feel that their way is wrong and must be changed to conform with European fashions.

Luckily these days all nationalities are considered to have women of equal beauty, and it is really only a question of the therapist's skill to be able to develop it to perfection.

COSMETIC CAMOUFLAGE

Special cosmetics are now available for making up the face for remedial purposes, and these can be used by a skilled beauty therapist trained in cosmetic camouflage to make a new face. Faces can be changed, moles, birthmarks and pigmentation abnormalities disguised, and scarring from acne and skin grafts improved with camouflage. Badly damaged faces can be restored after accidents, burns or surgical treatment by the skilful work of a cosmetic camouflage expert. Blemishes on all parts of the body that cause distress, split capillaries, naevi, etc. can be treated in the same way to good effect.

The cosmetic camouflage expert is a beauty therapist who has had special training and experience in the art of masking skin blemishes of all kinds. She should have a sound knowledge of the skin and the ranges of available cosmetics from which she will have to work. The price and value of the items will be important as, although remedial in effect, the cosmetic masking products may have to be purchased by the patients. They are available on the NHS through prescription, but availability depends on individual Hospital Authorities.

Special training is necessary within the hospital situation to develop the techniques of camouflage procedures, using the minimum of ordinary makeup, combined with masking products, to achieve a natural skin colour and texture, completely disguising the imperfection. The effect of the blemish on the patient may also have resulted in a condition of severe psychological stress, making instruction and co-operation difficult.

The camouflage technique depends basically on the application of a number of opaque covering creams which are non-irritant and have a matt finish. Their durability and capacity to allow the skin to perspire normally, permit extended periods of wear, without ill-effect. These masking agents are blended onto the skin to achieve a perfect match with the surrounding area, and then set with a special untinted, unperfumed finishing powder. A standard range of colours can be mixed to achieve perfect colour results, and even men can match their complexions, changing the blend as the natural tone deepens in the sun. Natural shadows, freckles, beard growth can be balanced, and the patient taught the sequence, once the correct blend of preparations has been determined by the camouflage expert. One application should last all day as the majority of products are waterproof, and the masking sequence once learnt should not exceed 15 minutes application time a day.

A successful change in appearance can sometimes be a starting point for a new approach to life for many patients, and the psychological benefit to the individual is very apparent.

COSMETIC SELLING AND DEMONSTRATING
Reasons for Selling

The facial specialist has a duty both to her client and her profession to sell the required preparations and cosmetics needed for successful treatment. Her obligation to selling has advantages for the therapist in that a more beneficial result is accomplished, and additional profit is obtained from the treatments. The client's advantage is that she gains the fullest attention and application of skill from the therapist if all her cosmetic needs are diagnosed and their use explained during the facial treatment. The efforts of the therapist within treatment must be reinforced and extended by home use of suitable cosmetics, which will not only increase results but encourage the client to persevere with salon visits. A client coming for professional help realizes that she has a part to play in her improvement, and she has a need to be involved in the process to contribute towards the finished result.

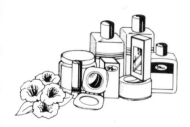

If treatment sales are neglected the client will feel disappointed in the therapist's disinterest in her overall progress, and may well obtain her products and her treatment elsewhere, where her full needs are understood and fulfilled. Part of the responsibility of the beauty specialist is to sell what is needed, to who needs it, and not decide for clients what they should spend, or how much they can afford, otherwise she is robbing the client of the pleasure of purchase. Completion of a facial treatment should permit discussion of necessary home care items and their application, and then the therapist will have done her job well and satisfaction will result. It is necessary to sell seriously, technically and systematically after treatment, or during a facial consultation for general advice. The client must gain the impression that the therapist is the ideal person to consult regarding her needs, and that she has the ability to advise the correct preparations and treatment which will obtain results.

Selling Itself

Selling is revealing an unconscious need to the client. The ability to handle a sale naturally will be increased if a genuine interest is present in the client and her needs. Natural client conversation will reveal areas of treatment or skin care neglected or unknown to the client, and the therapist's care for her client will demand that satisfactory treatment and home care is advised. New products or treatments should be introduced to keep the client aware of fashion trends and abreast of current developments in the beauty industry. If she is made to feel up to date and knowledgeable, it is more likely that she will avail herself of the new concepts available in the establishment rather than in more neutral or commercial surroundings where she is not known.

A skin chart should be prepared listing all the necessary preparations which the client should be given for her personal reference. The products should be offered to the client in order of importance, stressing the priorities, and in this way the client can decide her financial commitment and plan her sequence of purchases.

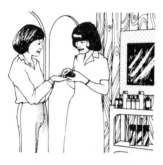

COUNTER SALES

High pressure sales methods are unnecessary, unethical and create a bad image for the salon, which often results in a loss of regular business on which the salon relies. Specialized treatment products should be advised where possible, so that items recommended can only be purchased at the salon, thus assuring repeat sales and avoiding the client seeking unknowledgeable cosmetic advice from a chemist or store.

Casual sales inquiries should be dealt with sympathetically, as they may conceal a more serious need for skin care or treatment advice, which could result in increased business for the salon. Honest and unbiased advice is desirable in general therapy applications, but in particular the younger therapist should not make the mistake of underestimating her client's need to believe in the products and have enjoyment from their use. The luxurious appeal of personal attention and beautifully presented goods and services to the mature or depressed client is difficult for the younger therapist to appreciate, as she will not normally have personally felt the need for such props to morale.

The operator's ability to give ungrudgingly of her interest is part of both successful salesmanship and technical therapy applications, and it is essential to achieve personal fulfilment in therapy practice. The technical ability and ethical behaviour of the therapist will help her in her sales duties, as clients are impressed by a confident, competent manner, and feel they can benefit personally from such knowledge and experience. Advice on home care and salon treatment requirements and cosmetic needs will be gladly accepted, willingly followed, and should prove to be mutually beneficial.

Demonstration Techniques

One of the most popular methods of selling is through demonstration, which combines entertainment and education of the audience as to the value and efficiency of the products used. Demonstrations are not always sales-linked, but may be designed to show the audience a technique or procedure, rather than sell them a range of cosmetic products. The link to sales is so strong however within demonstrating, that even if products are not being sold directly, the audience will demand to know where items used may be purchased, or treatments obtained. So to demonstrate and not to sell does seem a waste of an opportunity.

Initially when one is planning a demonstration it is necessary to know its purpose, whether informative, or sales orientated, and the audience it will attract. The numbers expected and general age of the audience are also important considerations, so that the talk can be planned to be either of a wide appeal or specifically related to one age group and its problems.

The topic of the demonstration should be considered beforehand, whether to be concentrated on one aspect of beauty, or be widespread in appeal giving greater scope for audience questions. Product-linked talks and demonstrations exert some guidelines on the speaker, there being a certain amount of information that has to be transferred in the course of the available time. This leaves less scope for personal views, but is good discipline for the demonstrator.

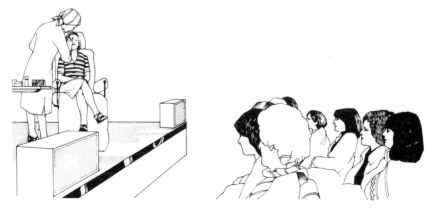

A TYPICAL DEMONSTRATION

Once the topic, venue and audience are known, the real plan of the demonstration can be considered. First it is important to know your subject, particularly if speaking to a knowledgeable audience. Then check that all the facts are available for reference, either on cards for easy scanning and prompting, and that you are familiar with the subject, in case of questions. If promoting a new range of items, make sure you are totally familiar with the items in the range, their prices, sizes available, etc., and the advantages the products have over rival products. Then you will be able to do them justice, and make them appear superior to comparable products, when the individual client is making a choice.

If models are to be picked out of the audience for makeup demonstrations, make sure that they are of a type to benefit from the preparations you are showing. Nondescript faces obviously showing a greater before, and after difference, than a previously well made up face. Where the emphasis is to be on makeup, a good-looking young face clearly shows the products to greater advantage than a middle age face, but again if you use your own judgement on which age group the audience would prefer to see made up, this will be the most successful. It may be appreciated by the audience when you are able to bring about a subtle transformation on one of their own age group, rather than on a model who has all the advantages of youth, looks, etc. to start with.

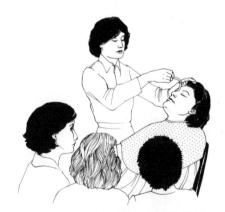

DEMONSTRATION OF EYE-BROW WAXING

In some cases providing a model for the demonstration is preferable, so that no unknown factors emerge during the practical application. There are usually quite enough things to cope with whilst demonstrating and talking, without having to cope with model problems such as hyper-sensitive skin, eyes that twitch etc. Once experience grows, the skilled demonstrator can over-ride any difficulties without her audience realizing the problem, but initially it is better to verve on the safe side and pick an easy model.

Actually working practically, and talking to the audience at the same time is difficult, but it can be practised during training in front of other members of a class. They will be quick to tell you when they can't hear, or can't see because you are blocking your own work. All the comments (constructive or otherwise!) will act as good preparation for live demonstrating, where coping with the behaviour of the audience is all part of the art. A demonstrator who can hold the audiences attention, and divert unwanted questions, whilst performing an excellent practical application, is skilled indeed.

Skill can be built up initially during training, by working in teams, so that the task is split. One pair of students can be working and talking, whilst a third is the model. Each student gives the others moral support, and working together to do a demonstration for a real audience then seems less traumatic. Working as one of a pair with an experienced lecturer is also very valuable, and builds confidence. As the total responsibility for the demonstration is lifted from the student, the experience can then freely develop skills of participation with the audience, answering questions, etc.

Once over the initial anxiety and embarrassment of giving a talk, most young therapists find their confidence boosted by the audience's obvious enjoyment and interest in what she, as the therapist, has to say. It can also confirm that much more knowledge and expertise had been acquired during training than had been imagined!

Essentials of Demonstrating

Whether demonstrating on a one to one basis, as in a makeup lesson, or to a large static audience, or to a general free-moving audience as in a store situation, several things are essentially the same.

Communication

First is the need to be able to communicate to the audience, be it one or many, and to hold their attention and make them interested in what you have to say. That is not too difficult in the beauty field, as looking good is of tremendous importance to people of all ages. Whether for reasons of self-esteem, or to appear attractive to the opposite sex, everyone is interested in making the most of what they have got, so therapists have a committed audience and should make use of it.

Timing

The next aspect is to cover the subject as fully as time permits, and endeavour to complete the practical application to match the talk. Depending on the audience, a cleanse and makeup for example could take anything from 20 minutes to one hour. This being dependant on whether questions were answered as the talk progressed, or whether they were kept to the end, in a general question period. A good demonstrator will judge which is the best method at the time, and it is not always the most efficient talk that is the one most enjoyed and appreciated by the audience. Questions do keep interest alive, and if voiced by one member of the audience, may speak for many others watching. Where timing is important, as in a planned programme of talks, demonstrations, etc., as at a conference, then it is worthwhile doing a trial run to make sure the demonstration can be accomplished in the allocated time. Talks likewise can be taped to see how they sound, and how long they actually take to say.

Where audience turn-over is fast, as in the In-store cosmetic promotion demonstration, one therapist will complete the practical effects while another or a compère will describe what is happening and answer questions. In this way timing is very slick, and a large volume of people can participate in some way with the demonstration.

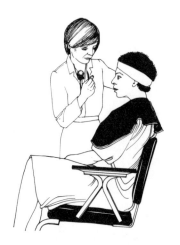

MAKEUP DEMONSTRATION

Organization and Preparation

Good organization of a demonstration can make or mar the whole event, so it is worth checking carefully before setting out that everything is prepared. Think your way through the routine, physically checking that all the items needed are packed conveniently in light-weight containers that will not seep or spill. Touring with a demonstration sales team in a hot country presents special problems of keeping the products in first-class order, as some tend to liquify at high temperatures. Special packing and the use of cold retaining bags, such as used for freezer food, can help in this instance.

Product houses normally provide attractive display cases for demonstration purposes, with all the items in moulded trays to avoid spillage or breakage. Tops should be checked carefully after use to see they are firmly screwed up, as the movement of being carried about, especially in a car, tends to shake them loose, and contents spill causing a terrible mess in a short time. The moulded trays of the product houses can be copied by anyone who demonstrates, by preparing a makeup case which permits items to stand upright, or be firmly packed

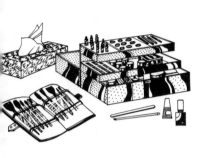

into it to avoid breakage. If glass containers have to be carried to display branded preparations they can be separated by foam sponge pieces to prevent them shattering. Placing each individual bottle in a polythene bag also ensures other items in a case do not get soiled, if one item does get broken by accident. Many cosmetic items are packaged in plastic these days, and this has lessened the problems of travelling and demonstrating.

Pull-out makeup trays, in cases such as those used for stage makeup, can be purchased to house the selection of makeup items; or tool or fishing tackle boxes utilized to provide convenient storage for the makeup items.

Tool kits or makeup boxes which fold back on themselves to form a steady stand are ideal for demonstrating, as they save time in preparation, and setting up the actual practical sequence. They provide everything close to hand, and allow the therapist to work quickly and efficiently.

If water is not going to be readily available close to the demonstration position, cotton wool tissues can be prepared beforehand and stored in light-weight plastic containers, which can also double as waste bins. Disposable tissues can be used for head-bands, or washable gowns and capes used with tissues placed to prevent soiling. The choice depends largely on the nature of the demonstration, whether it is constantly repeating as in a store, or is a single performance, where more luxury would be appropriate.

When the demonstration commences it is desirable that all the preparation is complete, with the table laid out invitingly, leaflets to hand, samples available, and all the items needed for the actual application ready for use. This preparation avoids too much movement slowing the work, and causing interruptions which spoil the quality of the demonstration. This is particularly important if a static pedestal microphone is used, as used in a large hall, or on a dias in a perfumery hall of a store, where a large audience has to be reached. Even when using a neck microphone, one should avoid unnecessary movement, as this picks up on the sound system.

The model for the practical demonstration may be positioned beforehand in a semi-upright chair or couch, or she may be brought to it quickly at the start of the talk, and settled with the minimum of fuss.

Audience Contact   Try to pause when explaining some point in the application, so that the audience have visual contact, and they are drawn to look at what is being done on the face of the model. Speak clearly and decisively, so that it appears that you know what you are doing, and why. Remember also that many of the spectators will be unfamiliar with some of the items used, so give their purpose briefly. This saves unnecessary questions, and may answer the question someone is too timid to ask.

Lastly don't intimidate the audience if you hope to sell a lot of cosmetics or wish simply to have increased their knowledge and regard of the beauty industry. The secret is to build interest and enthusiasm for both the possibilities of treatment and self-improvement. From this springs naturally the wish to become involved with this beautifying process through the purchase of cosmetic products or undertaking treatment.

For demonstration is a wonderful way to promote the beauty therapy business, revealing to the audience what is possible, talking casually about problems and faults so that the audience feels their particular problem is not unusual and can be readily solved. It reveals possibilities of resolving personal worries which may have nagged for years. Also a technically qualified beauty therapist with a full knowledge of her business at her finger tips can make the audience believe that almost anything is possible. This feeling can then be converted into real salon or cosmetic sales revenue if the opportunity is grasped.

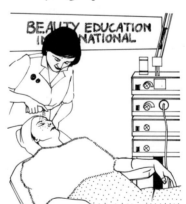

DEMONSTRATING THERAPY TREATMENT TECHNIQUES

Specialized Electrical Treatment: Choice and Application for the Dry, Delicate and Dehydrated Skins

INDICATIONS FOR ELECTRICAL TREATMENT

The addition of electrical applications in the facial sequence will be decided on the basis of:

1 The existing skin condition.

2 The effect of the specific electrical treatment.

3 The skin's response to previous manual or electrical treatment.

4 The temperament and wishes of the client.

Electrical applications can add beneficial elements of a stimulating, toning, or germicidal nature to a facial treatment programme, increasing the improvement or correction of existing skin conditions. The treatment may be applied at any convenient stage of the routine, according to the action desired. Apparatus which increases the cleansing and stimulation aspects of the routine should be applied prior to the mask, combined with or replacing the manual massage. Toning, refining, drying or germicidal effects are most beneficial after, or instead of, a mask application, when the skin is deep cleansed, free from adhesions, and has regained its normal temperature. Certain apparatus has a twofold action, i.e. cleansing and germicidal, and then, convenience of application, and the skin's reaction to the treatment, will decide its most suitable location within the facial routine.

Choice of Electrical Treatment

The varied effects of electrical treatment allow a large range of possible applications on differing skin conditions and age groups. The client's natural temperament and nervous disposition will be a decisive factor in the choice of application, limiting the range of beneficial actions possible. Contra-indications to certain treatments (reasons why the application is not suitable) differ with each specific piece of equipment, but must be visually and verbally investigated prior to treatment. Physical and temperamental contra-indications to electrical therapy prohibit all but the most superficial applications, and manual and cosmetic treatment methods are preferable.

General Contra-indications to Electrical Facial Therapy

1 Hyper-sensitive skin, prone to allergic reaction.

2 Diabetic clients, due to the unstable nature and poor healing abilities of the skin. With medical approval, adapted treatment may be possible to balance and maintain skin texture.

3 Skin infection, sepsis, and inflammation. Certain adolescent skin conditions may be treated with medical approval, i.e. acne, see Chapter 9.

4 Sinus conditions, where treatment could cause discomfort.

5 A large number of fillings in the teeth or bridge-work in dentures could cause discomfort in certain treatments, i.e. muscle contraction around the mouth.

6 Extremely vascular skin conditions, where the capillaries have dilated and ruptured to form a wide-spread varicose appearance, are contra-indicated to most forms of electrical treatment.

7 When the client is undergoing medical treatment for a general condition, approval must be sought prior to therapy applications, e.g. high blood pressure, asthmatic conditions.

8 Later stages of pregnancy.

9 Epileptics. Mild controlled forms, Petit Mal, may have superficial forms of treatment, i.e. vibrators, wax masks etc, but are contra-indicated for treatments involving current flowing through the skin's surface, or where discomfort is present, as this could precipitate an attack.

Beneficial results wil be obtained with electrical treatments if the skin diagnosis is accurate, the effects of the equipment are known, and the treatment is applied safely, with regard for the client's comfort.

SAFETY POINTS IN THE APPLICATION OF ELECTRICAL TREATMENT

The protection and safety of the client is the primary concern of the facial therapist, and observation of correct safety precautions will eliminate accidents and assure greater client satisfaction.

Location of Equipment

1 Equipment should be conveniently placed for safe application on the right or left side of the therapist, according to her natural dexterity.

2 The therapist should be able to perform the treatment satisfactorily with an adequate range of movement and support to ensure client safety and achieve results.

3 Lead connections to the mains supply must be positioned so that they do not become over-stretched or disconnected from the sockets. Long trailing leads must be avoided to prevent accidents resulting from clients or therapists tripping.

4 Leads from electrical treatment machines should not be allowed to trail along metal parts of couches etc. An unexpected current passing through the client or operator could result in discomfort, an unpleasant experience, or even a serious accident occurring.

Choice, Maintenance and Use of Apparatus

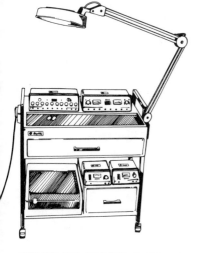

COMBINED TREATMENT UNIT

1 Well-made, sturdy equipment should be chosen, as the therapist is very dependent on the constant performance of her equipment, and the sophisticated nature of the apparatus makes repair a specialist task.

2 The performance required from the equipment should be considered prior to purchase, to avoid overheating, or strain being placed on motors unsuited to the task. Constant or heavy usage of steamers, vibrators, muscle contraction machines etc., calls for heavy duty clinic models if performance is to be maintained.

3 The equipment should be well maintained, correctly wired, with proper earth connection or, alternatively, double insulation, symbolized by ☐ on the rating plate. The apparatus should be ready for use before commencement of the

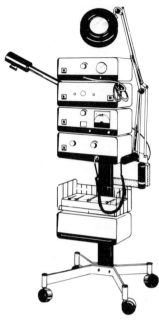

COMBINED FACIAL UNIT

facial routine, and tested for intermittent performance prior to the client's arrival. Continental apparatus may have different wiring from British models, and so it should be checked by a qualified electrician if there is any doubt as to its safety, or its performance regarding interference to other electrical fittings in the proximity, i.e. display lights etc.

4   The therapist must be familiar with the treatment application, the safety routine, and special points relating to the specific method to be applied.

5   The machine should be left ready for the next treatment after the conclusion of the routine, with controls at zero and mains connections off, unless immediately required.

6   The machines should be moved as little as possible to prolong their working life and prevent intermittent performance due to loose connections. Home visiting or mobile beauty specialists should obtain apparatus especially designed for the additional stresses it will have to endure during transit.

ELECTRICAL TREATMENT FOR THE DELICATE SKIN

Indications for Electrical Therapy

Delicate or sensitive skin conditions, where manual manipulations would be contra-indicated due to overstimulation, may benefit from gentle forms of electrical treatment designed to improve the cellular function of the skin's basal layers, without surface irritation, dilation of capillaries, skin distension, or a change in the pH value.

The degree of sensitivity observed at the skin inspection or occurring during treatment will determine the most advantageous routine of therapy, and may call for adaptation or exclusion of elements of the sequence planned.

Recognition

Several points of diagnosis, see Chapter 2, will be evident on the delicate or sensitive skin, including increased colour, fine texture, and a fast response to stimulation. On the younger client, the cheeks and prominent areas may be thin in appearance, with an apparent vascular network close to the surface. In the more mature client, or where premature capillary damage has occurred through neglect, dilated blood vessels will be evident, with extreme sensitivity and reaction to stimulation being observed.

Care must be taken to prevent further dilation and rupture of the surface vessels into skin tissue. Caution should be exercised in all applications on the sensitive skin, and tolerance to the treatment should be permitted to develop over a period to prevent over-reaction or irritation forming. Neutral treatment products should be combined with electrical therapy to prevent additional reactions being created, which could prove too active in effect for the sensitive or delicate complexion.

Delicate or Sensitive Skin Treatment Suggestions

1 Basic facial routine, including manual cleansing, massage, setting mask (calamine based), toning, and makeup with hypo-allergenic cosmetics.

2 Vibratory facial, comprising manual cleansing, audio-sonic vibratory massage, biological mask, spray toning and makeup.

Home Care Suggestions for the Sensitive or Delicate Skin

The purpose of a home care sequence for the sensitive skin is to maintain an adequate oil and moisture balance, whilst preventing irritation, dryness or sensitivity forming from over-exposure or incorrect care. Mild action or non-allergic preparations should be advised, with adequate day protection with moisturizers, and elimination of drying elements in daily care such as washing the face. Very few delicate or sensitive skins can survive facial washing without premature lining, dehydration, flaking etc., and clients must be persuaded out of the habit if at all possible.

Daily Skin Care

Cleanse

A semi-liquid cleansing emulsion should be applied to remove cellular matter and secretions produced during the night. Removal can then be gently accomplished with damp cotton-wool tissues, which are used at all times on this skin condition.

Tone

Complementary toning lotion may then be used to refine and refresh the skin, and prepare it for the pre-makeup base. The lotion should be smoothed, not patted, onto the surface to prevent over-stimulation.

Protect

A moisture emulsion or light-textured cream should be sparingly applied over the neck and face. Special protective creams for the exposed capillaries may be applied prior to the moisture base to prevent further damage and hold the condition in check.

Makeup

Oil or moisture-based tinted or transparent foundations may be applied to give additional protection and enhance the complexion. Loose powder application may be necessary to settle the foundation and avoid an over-shiny appearance. A very small amount should be used, and compact powders avoided due to their drying properties.

Nightly Skin Care

Cleanse

Application of a light textured cream cleanser, thoroughly covering the face and the neck to ensure complete removal of tinted foundation, grime and natural secretions. Thorough cleansing is very important for the sensitive skin in order that it may benefit from subsequent cosmetic applications.

Tone

Gentle toning to refresh the skin, remove remaining cleanser, and refine the pores. Exposed capillary areas should be toned with a rolling motion of the tissue only, but should not be excluded from the toning aspect of the routine, as gentle stimulation can prevent stagnation of the blood in the tiny vessels and encourage improved elimination of the area.

Nourish

Application of an active but fine textured cream over the entire neck, face and eye areas will maintain skin texture and increase the skin's ability to function and protect itself more efficiently. The consistency of the product should be fine enough for the under-eye skin, and will then be ideal for the rest of the face. Elaborate patterns of nightly skin care are unnecessary and confusing to the client, and should be avoided. Skin distension and over-reaction to certain product ingredients will confine the choice of suitable preparations to hypo-allergenic and unperfumed creams and products. The texture should be light, and the consistency easy to apply, with fast absorption properties, precluding the need for massage movements in its application. In this way damage from the client's

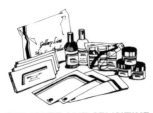

DELICATE AND SENSITIVE
TREATMENT PRODUCTS

unskilled techniques will be avoided, and the professional work will be reinforced not hindered by the client's home care activities.

Night or nourishing creams may be recommended, but more active hormone or cellular-based creams avoided.

VIBRATORY TREATMENT

Facial vibrators produce a succession of mechanical manipulations or vibrations which emulate or replace the effects of manual massage. Vibratory massage has a stimulating effect on vascular and lymphatic circulation, increases cellular activity and has a relaxing general effect if correctly applied.

General Characteristics

1 Low penetration power, with a superficial effect on subcutaneous tissues (percussion).

2 Activates local vascular and lymphatic circulation.

3 Increases local skin temperature, and colour (erythema.)

4 Does not excite muscle fibres.

5 No chemical formation on the skin's surface.

Percussion and Audio-sonic Vibrators

There are two types of vibratory treatment, basic percussion, which produces simple mechanical vibrations of low penetration, and audio-sonic, which produces vibrations, on the soft tissue of the body.

Comparison of Vibratory Methods

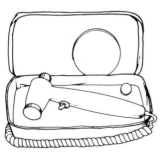

AUDIO-SONIC VIBRATOR

Audio-sonic vibrators do have some advantages over percussion methods in certain skin conditions. The vibrations have a deeper effect on the tissues, without causing surface discomfort or irritation. This gives them the ability to be used on delicate skin conditions, without overdilation of surface blood vessels and client discomfort. The reduced surface sensation, with increased cellular stimulation, extends the application to the mature client, where skin distension and overstimulation of surface vessels have previously contra-indicated the use of percussion vibrators.

Applications for Percussion and Audio-sonic Vibrators

Percussion Vibrators

1 Dry, dehydrated skin conditions requiring general stimulation.

2 Normal skin conditions, to maintain biological function and skin texture.

3 Mature, even-textured skin, with firm contours, and sufficient subcutaneous adipose tissue, to regenerate and stimulate basal layer activity.

4 General relaxation purposes, on the face, shoulders, upper back and extremities of the limbs. Increased vascular activity and warmth produce a relaxation of tense muscle fibres, and help prevent the formation of fibrous thickenings in the muscles, particularly the trapezius.

Audio-sonic Vibrators

1 Delicate, sensitive skin conditions, to stimulate the skin to function more efficiently, without creating surface irritation or discomfort.

2 Mature skin conditions, with loose skin tissue, associated with a delicate, or vascular surface appearance. Stimulation of the deeper basal layers increase mitotic activity (cell division), and encourages desquamation and improved skin texture.

3 Normal, dry and dehydrated skin conditions, to increase cellular function, improve sebaceous secretion, and stabilize the fluid balance.

4 In any condition where manual manipulations cause discomfort, audio-sonic may be used to advantage, due to reduced surface reaction, and slight impairment of sensation. Stiffness in the upper back and shoulder areas may be treated to relax tense muscle fibres, and prevent reoccurrance of the condition. Any condition of pain or inflammation however must be directed for medical attention, and permission gained prior to treatment.

Contra-indications to Vibratory Treatment

1 Extremely vascular skin conditions.
2 Inflammation, sepsis, and skin irritation.
3 Recent scar tissue.
4 Skin infection.
5 Sinus blockage (which causes discomfort).
6 Extremely bony facial areas should be avoided, particularly with audio-sonic vibrations, due to the possible depth of the sound waves.

Equipment   Both types of vibrators have a range of applicator heads for specific conditions and variable intensity controls to permit their application on both soft tissue and muscular areas.

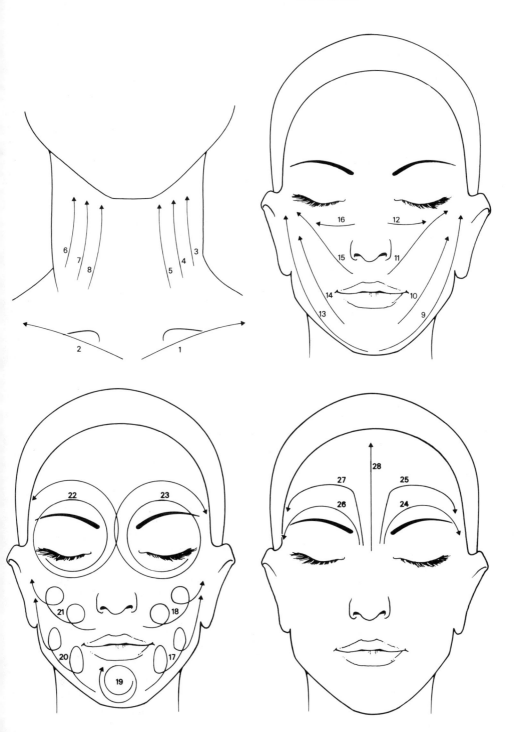

Applicator Heads   Sponge (percussion) and flat disc (audio-sonic) heads are used for general facial and neck massage, producing a gentle effect which can be applied directly or indirectly over the back of the therapist's hand.

Hard surface discs (percussion) and round hard applicators (audio-sonic) are used where an intensified action is required, e.g. fibrous infiltrations in the trapezius muscle or around joints.

Hedgehog-type applicator heads (percussion and audio-sonic) are used mainly for scalp massage, or where an extreme desquamation effect on skin tissue is required, e.g. rough skin texture on the upper arms, or post-acne scarring on the back. The vibration should be applied lightly, and regenerating cosmetic preparations used in combination to encourage improved skin growth.

Care of Apparatus   The motor-driven vibrators should not be applied for more than 20 minutes continuously, otherwise overheating will result and the life of the apparatus will be reduced. The applicator heads should be cleaned and sterilized after use with cold water methods (Savlon Concentrate, diluted to suitable proportions), and then kept in a sterile container until required. The sponge applicators must be dried thoroughly, and can be lightly powdered to keep them in good condition. All preparations must be removed from the rubber applicators or they will perish and also be a source of cross-infection in the salon.

Vibratory Treatment Application   As the treatment has only a superficial action on the tissues, the direction or pattern of strokes is devised to follow natural facial contours, avoiding bony areas, and be generally upward in direction. The main effect of the treatment is the local increase in vascular circulation. Areas poorly covered with subcutaneous tissue may be treated indirectly, with the vibrator placed over the back of the therapist's hand, with only the reduced vibrations passing to the client. The additional contact this method produces can reduce the jarring effect of vibratory massage experienced by some clients. The initial contact and release of the vibrator onto the skin's surface must be accomplished smoothly, and even rhythmical strokes used throughout. The established speed of movement for manual massage is a good guide for vibratory strokes. Straight and circular patterns may be alternated to vary the routine and add client interest. Skin reaction, erythema (reddening), local warmth and a generally stimulated appearance will determine the duration of the

VIBRATORY TREATMENT.
DIRECT APPLICATION

application, and should be used as a future guide. The skin reaction may vary slightly on each occasion due to internal and external influences, and so the immediate observed reaction is the deciding factor in concluding the sequence.

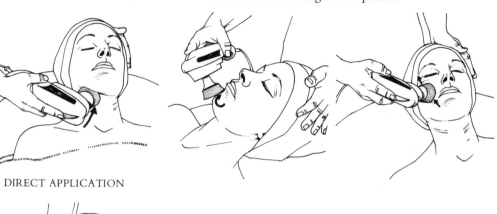

DIRECT APPLICATION

Normal application time may vary from 5-15 minutes due to the variation in reaction, which at all times occurs more swiftly than with manual methods, and should be noted immediately to avoid over-treatment. A choice of cosmetic medium, cream for dry skin, and talc for normal to oily skin will increase the smoothness of the application and prevent skin distension.

Repetitions of individual strokes may be increased or decreased according to skin reaction, sensitivity or loose skin texture in any area. When the required reaction is achieved the treatment should be smoothly concluded, the cream or talc removed, and the remainder of the facial routine completed.

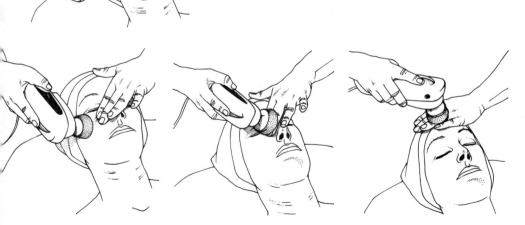

INDIRECT APPLICATION

BLOOD CIRCULATION OF THE HEAD AND NECK

All superficial applications increase the blood circulation of the face and neck, causing a rise in local skin temperature and increased colour (erythema). The superficial capillaries dilate to regulate the temperature, and the interchange of tissue fluids increases nutrition to the skin's surface layers.

Arteries of the Head and Neck

The arch of the aorta gives off three large branches that supply the head, neck and upper limb: these are the inominate artery, the left common carotid, and the left subclavian artery.

The External Carotid Artery gives branches:
Thyroid artery.
Facial artery.
Temporal artery.
Lingual artery.
Occipital artery.
Maxillary artery.

The Internal Carotid Artery gives branches:
Ophthalmic artery.
Middle cerebral artery.
Anterior cerebral artery.
Posterior communicating artery.

Venous Return from the Head and Neck

Superficial veins
Thyroid vein ⎫
Facial vein ⎬ empty into the external jugular
Occipital vein ⎭ vein.

Deep sinuses
Superior sagittal sinus ⎫
Inferior sagittal sinus ⎬ empty into the internal
Straight sagittal sinus ⎪ jugular vein.
Transverse sagittal sinus ⎭

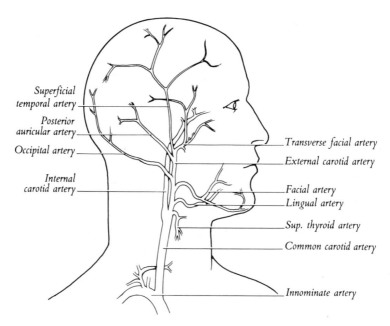

Superficial temporal artery

Posterior auricular artery

Occipital artery

Internal carotid artery

Transverse facial artery

External carotid artery

Facial artery

Lingual artery

Sup. thyroid artery

Common carotid artery

Innominate artery

ARTERIES OF THE HEAD AND NECK

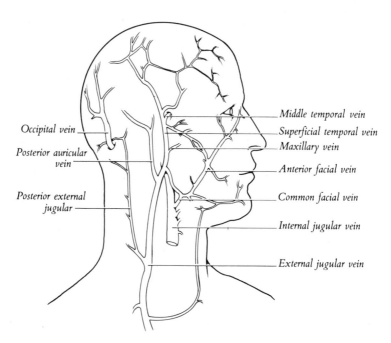

Occipital vein

Posterior auricular vein

Posterior external jugular

Middle temporal vein

Superficial temporal vein

Maxillary vein

Anterior facial vein

Common facial vein

Internal jugular vein

External jugular vein

PRINCIPAL VEINS OF THE HEAD AND NECK

ELECTRICAL TREATMENT FOR DRY AND DEHYDRATED SKIN

Indications for Treatment

Electrical treatment may be applied as an alternative, or in addition to manual methods, to increase the effectiveness of the sequence, or to accomplish a specific effect impossible to achieve manually. Neglected, over-exposed, or dehydrated skin conditions may be corrected and discomfort alleviated more promptly with a skilful choice of combined manual and electrical techniques.

Electrical treatment can increase cellular activity and maintain a firm fibrous skin condition, so delaying the formation of fine lines and ageing tendencies. Premature wrinkling, crêpy skin, and softening of facial contours can be arrested and corrected with an extensive programme of linked cosmetic treatment and electrical stimulation, i.e. paraffin wax or hot oil mask treatments, which increase the skin's nutrition, without distension of surface tissues.

Recognition of Dry and Dry/Dehydrated Skin Conditions
Dry Skin

Many important points of diagnosis will give guidance as to the most beneficial and suitable treatment programme (see Chapter 2, Diagnosis). The dry skin is recognized by a fine texture with no apparent pores, and often has areas of sensitivity and dilated capillaries. The decreased rate of sebaceous secretion and cellular function produce a softening of skin tissue and fine wrinkles around the eyes and on the neck. A loss of subcutaneous adipose tissue further aggravates the condition, and can give a crêpy loose appearance. Reduced mitotic activity of the basal layer can cause improper functioning of the skin's protective mechanisms, and minor imperfections may be present, i.e. fibrous malformations, split capillaries, and milia.

The normal oil and acid/alkaline balance of the skin may have been altered by external and internal factors, including dieting, over-exposure to sun, or simply incorrect skin care. Attention should be given to revising the home care cosmetic routines to reinforce the beneficial effects of professional treatment.

Dry/Dehydrated Skin

This skin has an additional problem of moisture loss, and needs an adapted programme of dry skin treatment, including highly hydrating elements, i.e. facial steaming, paraffin wax mask, and galvanic iontophoresis. Moisturizing preparations should be used throughout the sequence to increase the skin's hydric balance.

The client's age and general disposition will limit the intensity of the routine, and will determine the rate of progress in skin texture improvement. Client co-operation is vital if results are to be obtained.

Dry and Dehydrated Skin Treatment Suggestions

1 Continental facial routine, comprising manual cleansing, massage, setting or non-setting mask, toning and makeup.

2 Viennese facial, including brush cleansing, spray toning, indirect high frequency massage, biological mask, toning and makeup, if desired.

3 Paraffin wax mask treatment, comprising manual cleansing, massage (if not contra-indicated), paraffin wax mask, and moisture protection only.

4 Iontophoresis treatment, comprising manual cleansing, vapour steaming, short duration massage, and galvanic iontophoresis (to pass active substances through the skin's surface, for hydrating and regenerating purposes). See Chapter 9, Galvanic Treatments.

Home Care Suggestions
Daily Skin Care

Cleanse

Use of a light textured cleansing cream or emulsion, with a high oil to water proportion, to offset the detergent action on the skin's surface, whilst achieving a thorough cleansing action.

Tone

A skin tonic preparation to tighten the skin tissues, without causing dryness or irritation, may be applied with light tapping movements.

Nourish/Protect

1 Specialized products may be applied prior to the general moisture preparations to prevent further capillary damage or loss of moisture, and to add nutrient elements to the daily protective programme.

2   Moisturizing cream may be generally applied as a pre-makeup base, and to protect the skin from external elements.

Makeup

An oil-based, or cream-textured tinted foundation should be worn to give additional protection. Scant use of loose powder may be applied. All cream preparations are more suitable in texture and appearance for the dry and dehydrated skin. Compacted and compressed powder preparations should be avoided, due to their drying effect on skin tissue and the artificial appearance created.

Nightly Skin Care

Cleanse

A cream cleanser should be used to remove the tinted foundation and surface grime, and the procedure repeated until the skin is free from all external matter.

Tone

A more active tonic preparation may be applied to activate cellular function, refine the skin and prevent further loss of skin tone. A tissue-bracing lotion can be used, applied briskly over all but the most sensitive areas of the face and throat.

Nourish

Extremely light-textured but active creams should be applied, with gentle upward massage movements, to increase the blood circulation, and so improve biological function. Tissue creams may be alternated with nourishing or astringent creams to firm the skin tissue and add nutrient elements to the dermal layer. Regenerating active ingredients may be included if the skin is neglected, out of condition, or suffering from premature ageing. Regular application is more important than the choice of preparation, as the skin benefits more from the circulation improvement, than from the lubricant effect of the cosmetic applied.

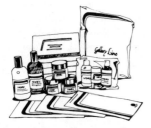

TREATMENT PRODUCTS FOR
DRY AND DEHYDRATED
SKIN

HIGH FREQUENCY TREATMENT

The high-frequency current may be applied indirectly (Viennese massage) and directly (for germicidal effect). The high-frequency current alternates so rapidly that it does not stimulate motor or sensory nerves. It has a frequency of 200 000 Hz (cycles per second) or more, and is termed an oscillating current. Indirect HF passes through the surface of the body and produces a stimulating, anti-congestive effect, with no chemical formation on

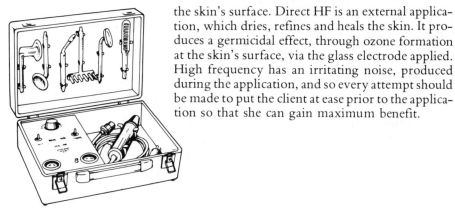

HIGH FREQUENCY UNIT

the skin's surface. Direct HF is an external application, which dries, refines and heals the skin. It produces a germicidal effect, through ozone formation at the skin's surface, via the glass electrode applied. High frequency has an irritating noise, produced during the application, and so every attempt should be made to put the client at ease prior to the application so that she can gain maximum benefit.

General Characteristics

Stimulation of Surface Tissue

HF can penetrate to the subcutaneous tissues and generates heat there which increases the interchange of blood and tissue fluids. Improved nutrition and elimination produce an improved skin texture and oil and moisture balance.

Relaxation

The generated warmth within the scalp and facial tissues produces a sedative effect, increasing relaxation and relief from tension. The current flows through the surface of the body (indirect method), but due to the speed of the oscillations it does not excite muscle fibres.

Germicidal, Drying Effect
(direct method only)

Directly applied the HF current produces a germicidal, anti-bacterial effect, limiting the sebaceous secretion, and drying and healing pustular infection.

Destructive
(fulguration, direct method only)

Incorrectly applied, direct HF could have a destructive effect on skin tissue and sebaceous glands, so adhering to the correct sequence of application for therapy purposes is essential.

Contra-indications to High Frequency Treatment

1   Highly strung clients of a nervous disposition.
2   Epileptics.
3   Asthmatics.
4   Extremely vascular skin conditions.
5   Skin infection. Adolescent acne may be treated directly with medical approval.

6 An excessive number of fillings in the teeth.
7 Clients undergoing treatment for defective circulation. Oedema (swelling), high blood pressure, etc.
8 Later stages of pregnancy.
9 Sinus blockage.

Indirect High-frequency Treatment (Viennese massage)

Preparation

The client should be prepared for general massage, and cream or talc applied to permit free movement of the hands over the area. The cream medium is chosen if a more soothing, relaxing effect is desired, and talc used if a more superficial but stimulating action is required. All jewellery should be removed from both the client and the therapist to prevent induced electricity causing discomfort and possible loss of contact.

The apparatus should be prepared, placed conveniently, and the glass saturator electrode attached to the holder to form a firm connection. Plugs, switches, and leads should be checked, with the intensity dial at zero and the machine switched off for safety.

Application

The client is given the saturator to hold, and advised to maintain contact throughout the treatment in order to complete the circuit and facilitate an even flow of HF current through the superficial tissues. A brief explanation of the sensation to be experienced will dispel nervousness and increase the client's enjoyment and benefit from the application. The therapist places one hand in contact with the client's forehead and commences the massage, whilst the second hand turns on the machine, and gradually increases the intensity, until the client's immediate tolerance level is reached. Verbal contact gives guidance as to general effect, and may indicate a possible increase in intensity level when the client has relaxed and become accustomed to the HF current. The second hand (nearest to the HF machine) is then placed in facial contact, and both hands perform rhythmical massage movements over the neck and face. The movements may be superficial (stimulating) or deep (relaxing) to achieve the desired effect. Facial contact must be retained by at least one hand throughout the routine to prevent a break in the current flow and subsequent prickling and discomfort to both client and therapist. This discomfort is due to the transient nature of the HF current, accompanying the sudden change in the electrical circuit when loss of hand contact occurs.

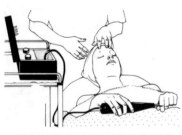

COMMENCING AN INDIRECT
HF TREATMENT

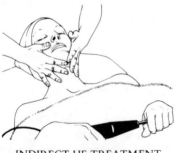

INDIRECT HF TREATMENT
IN PROCESS

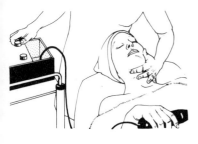

ADJUSTING THE INTENSITY

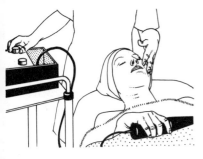

Areas of increased subcutaneous tissue may have the intensity increased, according to the client's tolerance, to achieve a more stimulating, regenerating action. With both hands in contact the current is evenly spread, but if one hand is removed the effect is intensified, and care should be taken to avoid creating a feeling of pressure and discomfort, particularly on the forehead.

When the necessary reaction is achieved, the skin will appear stimulated, with increased local warmth and colour and an improvement in texture. Normal application time varies from 8-20 minutes, with no area of the face receiving excessive attention. The treatment may be concluded by releasing one hand from the face, reducing the current intensity to zero, and switching off the machine. The second hand may then be released, and the saturator removed from the client, prior to further treatment.

The HF machine and electrode should be left placed safely out of the way, and the facial treatment progressed by removal of the cream or talcum preparation and application of a suitable mask. The glass saturator should be cleansed and sterilized after use, and retained in a sterile container until required.

Direct High-frequency Treatment (germicidal and drying effect)

Direct HF may be applied prior to the mask, replacing the massage, or concluding the facial routine, depending on the degree of action required. Directly applied HF has an extremely stimulating effect on the surface blood circulation and, due to the production of ozone as a by-product, its action is also germicidal, anti-bacterial and drying to the skin stratum corneum. Its main application is within the treatment of seborrhoea and acne conditions (see Chapter 9, Control Treatments), but it may be used in moderation to give a tonic effect to the dry, dehydrated and mature complexion.

Preparation

The facial area is prepared with talcum powder to permit a smooth passage of the electrode over the contours, and to absorb the natural secretions formed during treatment. A glass bulb-shaped electrode replaces the saturator, and the client is not connected into the HF circuit as an indirect HF. The current is applied to the skin by contact with the externally applied bulb electrode.

Application

The application commences at the forehead, the apparatus is switched on, and the intensity

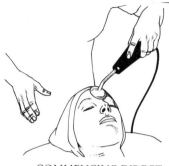

COMMENCING DIRECT
HF TREATMENT

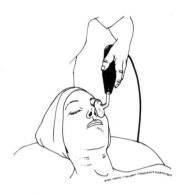

DIRECT HF IN PROCESS

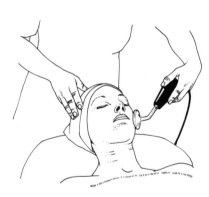

increased slowly to the client's maximum tolerance. Circular movements cover the face and neck, with the current intensity and pressure regulated to the skin's sensitivity and degree of subcutaneous tissue. The more superficial movements create the greatest stimulation, as the HF current ionizes the air when a slight gap exists between the electrode and the skin. This is seen as a small spark, which activates the sensory nerve endings.

The high frequency output terminates in the low pressure gas-filled glass electrode, which offers protection to the client and operator from the risks of electric shock. In normal use the gas becomes ionized and gives a blue/violet glow in the tube of the chosen electrode. Ozone is produced as a by-product and causes a chemical reaction on the skin's surface. The spark created by providing an air gap should not exceed ¼ inch (or 6mm) in general therapy practice, as its effect becomes destructive to skin tissue beyond this length. This technique of 'sparking' can be used to advantage on scar tissue, or to activate a sluggish complexion, by improving lymphatic circulation and achieving an anti-congestive effect. Sparking must be applied with care by an experienced therapist to prevent client discomfort and subsequent skin irritation and flaking.

Erythema, increased warmth, and a generally stimulated appearance will indicate when the desired effect has been achieved. The treatment may then be concluded by reducing the current to zero, switching off the machine, and releasing the electrode from facial contact. The talcum should be removed with damp tissues, and the skin left free from tonic preparations in order to maintain the refining, drying and germicidal effects of the HF.

SPARKING
METHOD

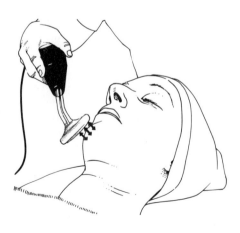

Application time varies according to skin texture, sensitivity, and the individual client's tolerance to the treatment. Dry, dehydrated and mature skins require a short duration, low intensity application of 3-5 minutes, to achieve the necessary dilation of superficial blood vessels and subsequent interchange of tissue fluids. Oily, blemished and scarred complexions require longer applications to fully benefit from the controlling elements of the HF, on sebaceous secretion and bacterial growth. Applications of 10-15 minutes may be given, according to the individual reaction.

Long-term benefits of direct HF include refined skin texture, increased cellular activity of the skin's basal layer, and an improvement in the skin's defence against bacteria.

BRUSH CLEANSING AND MASSAGE.

Brush Cleansing

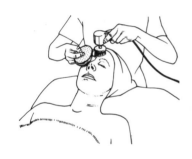

BRUSH CLEANSING

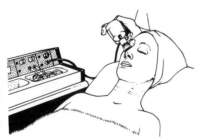

Electrical brush cleansing may be used as an alternative to manual methods to give variety to the facial routine and maintain client interest. The equipment for brush cleansing and massage applications may form part of a combined facial treatment unit, in association with any combination of High Frequency, Galvanism and Vapour applications, or it may be an independent treatment unit, usually free-standing.

The action of brush cleansing is gently stimulating whilst it affects a thorough and fast skin cleansing. Water-based preparations are applied on the chest, cheek, and forehead areas, and the brush cleanser is applied in a pattern over the entire area to spread the preparations and cleanse the skin. A range of brushes for varying skin conditions is available, from soft tapered bristles for cleansing to firm bristle brushed in different shapes for activating and abrasive massage. The brushes are powered by a variable speed motor positioned within the equipment, which through a flexible drive system rotates and gently vibrates the chosen applicator. A slightly damp brush applicator is attached and applied with light pressure over the area to deep cleanse the skin, remove cellular blockage and free surface adhesions.

The equipment head should be contoured to the area under treatment, and bony and sensitive sections treated with reduced pressure and speed and the minimum number of strokes possible to accomplish complete removal. The client should be advised to keep her eyes closed throughout the routine to prevent preparations entering them.

The range of brushes and speed variations permits all but the most sensitive of skin conditions to be treated by this method.

Damp sponges may be utilized to remove the cleansing products, with the procedure repeated until the skin is thoroughly clean.

Brush Massage

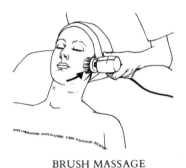

BRUSH MASSAGE

Brush massage is a more stimulating form of treatment than manual methods, producing faster vascular response from the skin's dermal layers. It is not a relaxing form of massage, but applied to accomplish a specific task, i.e. improvement of skin texture, through desquamation on a rough skin surface. The shaped brushes are designed for general face and back applications, abrasive massage and general toning purposes. The pumice block applicators are included for abrasive mask removal purposes on the scarred and pigmented complexion. Brush massage is a useful alternative to manual techniques for the younger client, where hand contact is not always accepted and electrical applications preferred, and for male skin treatments due to its increased stimulatory action.

Cream or talcum may be used for the application, according to skin type. Brushes should be cleaned in mild detergent products prior to cold water sterilization to remove all the cleansing and tinted makeup preparations accumulated and to keep the bristles soft.

PRESSURE SPRAY TONING (VAPORIZERS)

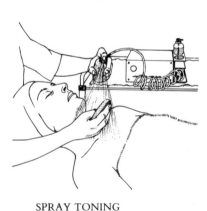

SPRAY TONING

The use of vaporizers for tonic and liquid applications during the facial treatment is becoming established, due to the fineness of the spray produced and the convenience of application. The spray is directed onto the face under pressure, and forms a fine penetrating film which is readily absorbed into the tissues. The motor-powered apparatus must be kept in good condition to prevent blockage in the connection tubes and intermittent performance resulting. A variety of toning and astringent lotions may be prepared according to the size of the equipment, all of which require dilution to prevent blocking the outlets and due to the increased stimulatory effect of the product when applied under pressure. Vaporizers are often combined with other small facial equipment, i.e. vacuum suction, for convenience and economy of space.

The application should be directed onto the neck and face at a distance of 9-12 inches, with the spray produced by placing the index finger over the air outlet. The controlled film should be applied in broad sweeping movements, with the surplus moisture forming and being removed by the second hand which follows. The client's eyes should remain closed, and care should be taken to prevent droplets of moisture forming in the inner eye, nose and mouth areas. Sponges can be used to capture the residue of liquid not accepted by the skin.

The larger vaporizers are also equipped for mask removal having spray jets which produce a continuous stream of high-powered water for removal of setting type masks. The client is placed upright, and a plastic receptacle (a curvette) is placed in close contact under the chin. The surrounding area is protected with towels, and the mask sprayed off, with the water jet directing the mask fragments downwards into the bowl. The client's eyes must remain closed, and care in the application is necessary to prevent soiling the gowns, blankets, etc.

This technique of mask removal is particularly useful in removal of acne setting-type masks as it speeds the removal and tones and refreshes the skin in one operation.

PARAFFIN WAX MASK TREATMENT

Paraffin wax treatment functions on the principle of heat penetration to produce a local increase in skin temperature. Natural perspiration is gently produced and the skin's capacity to absorb cosmetic preparations, oils, creams, etc., is increased, due to dilation of the superficial vascular network. Respiration of the skin is improved, surface adhesions are freed, and the skin shows an immediate difference, and a sustained reaction in the period following treatment. Increased elasticity, smoothness and softness of texture and improved colour and tone become evident over a course of wax therapy treatments.

The cleansing action of paraffin wax removes surface cellular and bacterial build-up, increases desquamation, and controls the pH balance. Surface horny cells are released, and regeneration from the dermal layers produces a younger fine skin texture.

Indications for
Paraffin Wax Therapy

1　Dry, dehydrated skin, requiring stimulation and correction of oil and moisture balance.

2　Mature skins, where regeneration of the basal layer is desired, without over-stimulation, or distension of surface tissues, through manual methods.

3　Crêpy, finely lined skin, where stimulation and absorption of nutrient products is desirable.

4　Uneven textured skin (unstable pH) to deep cleanse and free the skin, promoting desquamation and a refined skin texture.

5　Seborrhoea conditions, to remove surface adhesions, oily skin blockage, and promote desquamation.

Contra-indications
to Paraffin Wax Therapy

1　Highly nervous, tense clients, due to the need for immobility during the application.
2　Extremely vascular complexions.
3　Sepsis, skin infection and irritation.

Preparation　　A small quantity of clean, sterilized paraffin wax should be prepared in a thermostatically controlled wax heater, with an outer casing, by bringing it to a moderate working temperature of 49° C. The wax unit prepares the wax quickly and hygienically, and maintains it at a constant temperature, ready for use.

The client is prepared in the normal way for facial treatment, with adequate protection of gowns etc., to prevent damage from the preparations to be used. Disposable paper may be placed over the normal towels etc., to prevent wax adhering to the fabric in the case of an accident. A semi-reclining chair position is ideal and creates a safe application angle for wax treatment, whilst preventing the client feeling claustrophobic during the application. The cleansing sequence should be thorough, but endeavour to avoid over-stimulation of the skin, as this will alter the skin's tolerance to the heat application and reduce the effect of the treatment. Skin inspection should follow to determine sensitivity and any imperfections which would alter the intensity or duration of the application.

Application

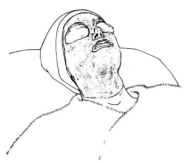

PARAFFIN WAX
MASK

Appropriate creams are applied to the neck and face to ease removal and enhance the effectiveness of the treatment through absorption into the epidermis. Eye pads must be applied for safety reasons, and to aid relaxation. The wax should be applied as warm as can be comfortably tolerated by the client on to a clean skin (after massage if indicated), to form a fine layer over the neck and face. The wax is applied swiftly, with the therapist working in such a way that at no time can warm wax fall on the client. A firm layer of wax is built up, over first the entire throat, then the cheeks, chin, nose and forehead, to form a complete mask avoiding the lips, nostrils, eyebrows and hairlines. A small brush is the ideal applicator, and permits swift and neat work to be achieved, without the problems of the wax setting before it can be applied to the area.

First, heat will build up within the mask, and features will be immobilized as the mask sets and cools. The client should be aware of the therapist's presence, but encouraged to relax, until all the therapeutic effects of the heat are gone, but the mask is still pliable and just warm to the touch. The length of application time will depend on the natural skin temperature, its tolerance to heat, and the reaction to the paraffin wax. The normal duration varies from 10-20 minutes, and fits within the 1-hour facial sequence, as a setting mask is not applied and makeup is not indicated, since the skin is unsettled for a time after the routine.

Removal

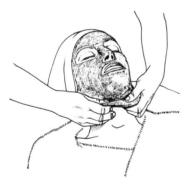

Removal is completed by easing the edge of the wax, all round the mask and internal spaces, removing eye pads, and lifting the mask off gently in one piece. This is accomplished by placing the hands under the mask at the throat, and bringing it away from the face, a little at a time. An attempt should be made to keep all the wax fragments attached to the bulk of the mask to avoid unnecessary cleaning up after the removal. The remainder of the cream, wax, etc., can then be removed with the protective disposable paper, and the treatment can proceed. Gentle pressure toning, with water only, can be applied to freshen the skin, and finally moisture protection to complete the routine.

Conclusion

Natural perspiration is produced, the skin appears softer, finer in texture, and clean and fresh in appearance. Fine lines are eased, and ageing tendencies controlled. Clients should be encouraged to look upon paraffin waxing treatments as a preventative measure against skin ageing.

Chapter 9

Control Treatments for Seborrhoea and Blemished Skin Conditions

Control of greasy skin may be accomplished with reasonable success if the underlying factors behind the condition are understood, and the treatment planned to control the malfunction, not to aspire to its cure. Over-secretion of the sebaceous glands during adolescence and early maturity is a natural physical occurrence, affecting a large proportion of the population. Without correct skin hygiene and general good health, however, the condition can develop into an excessive oil secretion, seborrhoea, which can progress into a pustular infection of the follicle, acne vulgaris. (See Chapter 5, Skin Disorders.) It is characterized by the appearance of blackheads, papules, and pustules, which may occur on the face, neck, shoulders and back.

Juvenile acne unfortunately is often regarded as a trivial complaint which will be grown out of in time. Apart from the demoralizing effect it has on its young sufferers, the condition can cause serious disfiguring and permanent scarring. The frequency of its occurrence in adolescence, with an incidence of as high as 50 per cent, and the reluctance of sufferers to seek medical aid, brings it constantly into the realm of the beauty specialist. The responsibility of the beautician is to see that medical attention is obtained if necessary, and that her treatment and cosmetic guidance will minimize the severity of the complaint and avoid aggravating the existing condition. The primary cause of an infected acne condition should be diagnosed medically to determine the extent and nature of the infection and to assess whether medical or therapy treatment would prove the most beneficial in the circumstances.

There are a number of factors which cause acne. It has been known and accepted for many years that the condition is associated with the physiological changes which accompany puberty. In recent years medical research has shown that the administration of androgens (male hormones) increase's activity of the sebaceous glands, whereas oestrogens (female hormones) decrease the secretion, and that a sufficient quantity of oestrogens administered would control acne in both sexes. Thus correcting the hormone balance offers a radical treatment for many cases of acne, but this of course is correctly and clearly in the province of the medical profession. Changes in skin texture, a regression in skin infection and a generally improved skin appearance during pregnancy and whilst taking the female contraceptive pill seem to confirm the beneficial effects of increased oestrogen levels in the body. As these methods are obviously not applicable to young men, their treatment presents greater difficulties and an increased need for local antiseptic and antibacterial methods to control the skin eruptions.

Whilst treatment of clinical acne is a medical reponsibility, minor forms of adolescent acne may be controlled and improved by the beauty specialist, if agreement is given by the client's own doctor. Oily skin, seborrhoea, and discoloured or scarred complexions are well within the province of the beauty specialist, and excellent results are possible. As young men and women are at a time of their life when appearance is of paramount importance, if the skin condition is not professionally controlled by salon and home care measures further aggravation will be caused by desperate camouflage and incorrect treatment methods.

As the skin is over-productive, a rational therapeutic and cosmetic treatment programme should be designed to reduce skin oiliness, and control bacterial growth by electrical and cosmetic methods. Improved skin hygiene and efficient cleansing routines form the basis of effective home care sequences, as the oily skin is one of the few conditions that benefit from regular soap and water applications. Specialized antiseptic products for controlling and camouflaging the condition have an important part to play in the improvement of the psychological state of the client. Bactericidal and bacteriostatic agents can be incorporated into cover creams, which are primarily used to cover rather than cure the blemishes. The presence of the active ingredient, whilst not necessarily improving the skin condition, ensures that the risk of secondary infection is minimized.

Client co-operation is vital for successful control of seborrhoea or acne vulgaris conditions, and personal encouragement and a sympathetic understanding of the embarrassment suffered will help to maintain progress and lift client morale. A flexible attitude towards camouflaging the skin during its programme of treatment is essential, if progress is to be made and client co-operation sustained.

Recognition of Oily, Blemished, and Scarred Skin Conditions

Establishing the degree of the condition is important both for deciding whether medical permission is required, or for planning the sequence of salon and home treatment.

Oily Skin

The most evident points of diagnosis for the oily skin are the age of the client, the general sheen and coarse texture of the complexion, and its unstable pH value. In younger clients the condition may be widespread, and affect the entire facial area, whilst in post-adolescence it may be confined to the central area of the face giving a 'combination' skin condition. The pH balance of the skin becomes unstable, and an over-acid condition exists, which causes a patchy complexion, and subsequent colour change in tinted foundation applications.

Seborrhoea

The sallow colour, heavy compacted appearance, and excessive oiliness of the seborrhoea skin makes recognition obvious. Comedones affecting the mouths of the follicles may also be present, particularly in the centre of the face, where sebaceous glands are most numerous. (See Chapter 5, Skin Disorders.)

Acne Vulgaris

A condition combining all stages of the oily skin, with associated pustular infection of the follicle. Excessive oil secretion (sebum), blackheads, papules, and secondary infection are present, and medical approval is required prior to treatment. If the client is undergoing medical treatment for the acne condition, therapy applications must be postponed until its conclusion. (See Chapter 5, Skin Disorders.)

Scarred Pigmented Conditions

The increased keratinization, and scar tissue formation after acne vulgaris, appear as discoloured patches, with rough skin texture, and indentations due to the damage of the basal layer. The thickened appearance of the skin and its discoloration can be considerably improved with treatment, but no cosmetic treatment as yet exists for the pock marks and indentations caused by acne scarring. Peeling methods however lessen the uneven texture of the skin.

Treatment Suggestions

Seborrhoea

1 Pore treatment, comprising manual cleansing vapour, herbal or ozone steaming, vacuum and manual massage, setting mask, and corrective toning.

2   Base cleansing treatment, comprising brush cleansing (with normal and biological soap preparations), ozone steaming (vaporzone), biological or setting mask and toning (vegetable extract).

3   Lymphatic drainage treatment, based on manual cleansing, lymphatic drainage massage, with galvanic desincrustation for removal of sebum.

Acne Vulgaris and Blemished Skin Areas

Based on forms of ozone therapy:

1   Ozone steaming treatment, comprising manual cleansing, with neutral products, prolonged ozone steaming, setting acne mask, and pressure spray toning with antiseptic lotions.

2   Direct high-frequency treatment, comprising brush cleansing (with normal and biological 'soap' preparations), setting mask application, and direct high-frequency treatment, using stimulatory and sparking techniques.

3   Ultraviolet exposure. Progressive or constant U/V exposure to control the blemished condition and improve skin texture.

Post-acne Scarring and Discoloured Skin Conditions

Based on increasing the skin's natural desquamation:

1   Biological peeling, normally comprising manual cleansing, the biological peeling process, and application of protective products only.

2   Progressive or chemical peeling, applied in a similar manner.

3   Abrasive mask treatment, comprising manual or light brush cleansing, massage if indicated, abrasive mask treatment, and application of hydrating or nourishing mask or cream preparations to conclude.

HOME CARE SUGGESTIONS FOR OILY AND BLEMISHED SKIN CONDITIONS

Skin hygiene is the most important factor in caring for the skin between salon visits. Removal of surface oiliness, bacteria and dirt, reinforce the drying and healing effects of salon treatment, and prevent aggravation of the condition and subsequent lack of improvement. Younger clients may be encouraged to steam their faces, and apply clay masks between visits, if this would appear to help the drying process, and involve them in the improvement programme. All clients with oily or blemished skins should have impressed upon them the importance of thorough cleansing and the use of the correct preparations for their skin conditions. General health factors such as a balanced diet, avoidance of constipation, and the importance of sufficient sleep and exercise, should be discussed, as these factors are often abused in adolescence, and may have a part to play in the overall improvement.

Daily Skin Care

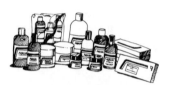

TREATMENT PRODUCTS
FOR OILY AND
SEBORRHOEA SKIN

Cleanse

Use of liquid, 'soapless', or biological soap products will remove natural sebum formed during the night. The product may either be wiped over the face in the case of the liquid cleanser, or applied to a damp skin in the case of the soap substitutes, and worked up to a thin lather with a complexion brush. The product may then be rinsed off, leaving no trace, and the brush washed and placed in antiseptic solution.

Correct

A corrective or acne lotion may be applied, diluted according to skin sensitivity, to protect and dry the skin, whilst continuing the healing process. Initially the lotion may worsen the condition, and the client must be prepared for this occurrence.

Protect

A greaseless lubricant (for extremely oily or acne conditions) or a hydro–emulsion (for centre panel oiliness only) may be applied over the entire face and neck to act as a protective film if no makeup is worn, or as a pre-makeup base. If this protective step of the sequence appears to aggravate the oily condition, it may be suspended until further skin texture improvement is achieved.

Makeup

Medicated block, semi-liquid, or covering-type foundations may be applied if necessary to maintain client morale. Clients should be encouraged to leave the skin free from tinted preparations whenever possible. Disposable cotton-wool or a clean sponge should be used to apply the block foundations to prevent reinfection of the skin.

Nightly Skin Care

Cleanse

Thorough removal of tinted preparations is necessary, and should be accomplished by first application and removal of a light-textured cleansing milk, using tissues or cotton-wool pads, and secondly by a repetition of the morning 'soapless' routine.

Tone

Corrective or acne lotion, as in the morning.

Protect and Heal

On the oily skin a medicated cream may be sparingly applied and massaged in to promote healing and refine the texture. Blemished skins may benefit more from re-application of the acne lotion, to bring sepsis to the skin's surface and prevent the spread of the condition. If the surface appears flaky due to treatment, the nightly procedure should be to soothe and protect the epidermis by application of a non-greasy emulsion or lubricant to re-establish the skin texture.

General Points

It is necessary for the client to keep in close contact with the beauty specialist so that the effects of the home care sequences advised may be seen, and the routine moderated or revised as the skin condition alters. As the blemished and seborrhoeic skins often become worse before they improve, the client must understand and be encouraged through these regressive periods by sympathetic handling. The correct home care sequence is vital for the younger client, who will find it financially more difficult to maintain regular salon treatment, than the slightly older working and independent individual. Treatments may be adapted to suit the needs of the individual, without reducing the profitability of the routine, by careful assessment and application of the most effective element of the sequence.

The cosmetic needs of the client must be completely fulfilled by the beautician to avoid the purchase and use of incorrect products during the improvement programme, which could aggravate the existing condition.

REGIONAL LYMPH NODES AND VESSELS OF THE HEAD AND NECK

The Lymphatic System

Composition of Lymph Fluid

Lymphatic fluid closely resembles blood plasma in its composition, but it has a much lower concentration of protein. There are also a large number of lymphocytes (the only living cells in the fluid) which come from the lymphatic glands.

Lymphatic Capillaries and Vessels

The lymphatic capillaries commence in the tissue spaces of the body as minute blind end tubes. These minute capillaries join with one another to form a close network of very fine vessels, which drain away the fluid that has passed through the walls of the capillaries into the spaces of the tissues. All lymphatic vessels open into lymphatic nodes which have a nodular appearance and are placed in strategic positions throughout the body. The lymph from the vessels drains through at least one lymphatic node before it passes eventually into one of two main ducts, the thoracic duct and the right lymphatic duct.

Lymphatic Nodes

The nodes are almond or bean–shaped structures situated at strategic points in the course of the lymph vessels, the lymph nodes perform several important functions, including acting as filters of the lymph in its course from the various organs and tissues, to the point where it is returned to the blood. If the body was without lymphatic nodes, general infection of the blood by pathogenic bacteria would be inevitable.

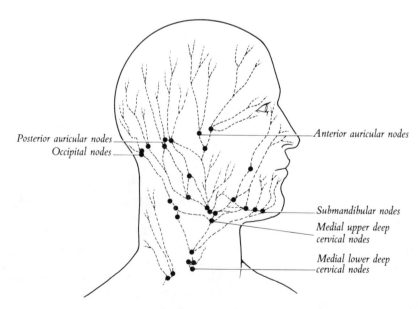

Posterior auricular nodes
Occipital nodes

Anterior auricular nodes

Submandibular nodes

Medial upper deep cervical nodes

Medial lower deep cervical nodes

Functions of the Lymphatic System

The lymphatic system offers a second line of defence against bacterial invasion, the first being the presence of leucocytes at the site of injury or infection. The lymphatic system is also responsible for the production of lymphocytes, and blood plasma protein, to some degree, with the lymphocytes being formed in the lymph nodes, and the plasma protein being formed by disintegration of these same cells into plasma globulin. The manufacture of plasma globulin and of lymphocytes are functions of lymphoid tissue in general.

Facial Vacuum Treatment for Cleansing and Massage Purposes

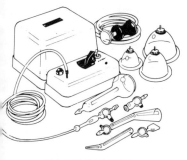

VACUUM UNIT

The vacuum massage is a mechanical method of draining lymphatic vessels. The treatment may be applied after manual cleansing or steaming, to reinforce the cleansing effect and increase removal of skin blockage, blackheads and oily matter. Vacuum and galvanic desincrustation treatments are often combined to achieve removal of established blackheads without skin injury. The direction of the lymphatic vessels is followed, with straight strokes, applied in a light upward lifting manner. The fluid in the minute lymph spaces drains quickly, because the small ducts are emptied under pressure and blockages are released. This evokes a vigorous response from the circulation, fresh lymph and blood with nutrient elements replace the loss and degenerated matter and deposits are eliminated.

Indications for Treatment

1 General skin cleansing purposes, for removal of tinted facial preparations and skin blockage caused by incorrect cleaning etc., on the normal dry and combination skins.

2 Specialized cleansing on the seborrhoea skin for removal of oily and cellular matter, follicle blockage, and dead keratinized skin cells. Small aperture cups and applicators are required in different shapes for specific areas. The treatment is most effective after vapour, herbal or ozone steaming applications, when the skin is softened, or after galvanic desincrustation.

3 For stimulation purposes on the dry, dehydrated skin conditions, to promote cellular function, and biological activity, and to increase the elimination process via the lymphatic vessels of the neck and face.

Contra-indications to Treatment

1   Delicate, sensitive skins due to over stimulation and possible capillary damage.

2   Crêpy loose skin condition, where skin distension is contra-indicated.

3   Infected acne conditions, where secondary infection of the follicle is present, due both to the discomfort caused and the risks of increasing the infected area.

4   Very fine areas of skin texture, or dilated capillaries, around the eyes, and on the upper cheek in dry or sensitive skin conditions.

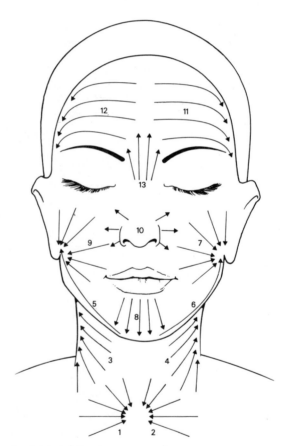

PATTERN OF FACIAL VACUUM STROKES

Application

The vacuum or suction massage is applied on a clean skin, previously prepared with a fine oil to facilitate an easy flowing stroke over the surface. A

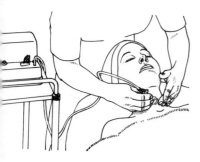

GENERAL SKIN TREATMENT

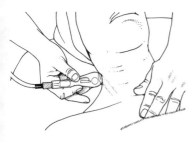

reduced pressure is formed within the cups, which lifts and stimulates the skin tissue throughout the stroke. The intensity must be adjusted to the skin's reaction and resistance, and the lift into the applicator should not exceed 20 per cent, otherwise skin distension and capillary dilation will result. The skin's natural elasticity alters the degree of skin resistance present.

The pattern commences at the neck, with the speed and vacuum adjusted to the skin reaction observed and the client's tolerance. The routine progresses up the face, concluding between the eyebrows on the corrugator muscle. The size and shape of the applicators used depends on the sensitivity of the skin and the effect desired, i.e. general cleansing, toning, or removal of skin blockage.

The duration of treatment may vary from 3–5 minutes for general cleansing purposes to 10–12 minutes for massage and drainage of lymphatic vessels. Specialized cleansing routines for the younger skin commence with the general cleansing pattern, and then with specific cups, treatment of the blackheads, scarred areas and uneven texture, progresses until the desired effect is achieved.

The oil is removed and the treatment proceeds, either with a cleansing mask or further manual applications, according to the routine chosen.

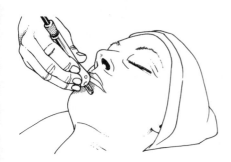

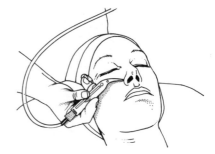

CONCENTRATED CLEANSING ON THE CENTRE PANEL

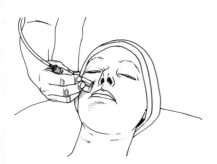

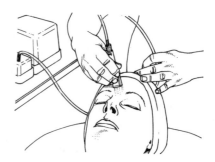

LIFTING VACUUM MASSAGE ON WRINKLES

Pulsed Air/Tapping Massage

The pulsed air system of lymphatic drainage treatment operates on a principle of applying intermittent suction to provide a tapping or patting effect on the skin. The skin is gently stimulated by the action of the pulsed air. Lymphatic drainage is increased, and vascular circulation improved, by the faster interchange of tissue fluids.

Glass applicators called ventouses are applied in unison, following a pattern which increases lymphatic drainage. The vascular response from the skin is achieved without excessive stretching or pulling of the skin so the more delicate or mature skin conditions can be treated successfully. The rhythm of the pressure and suction air impulses can be infinitely varied. Consequently it is possible to start with vigorous tapping massage, with a rhythm of 4–5 impulses per second on skin needing a stimulating and toning effect, and then change gradually to a delicate vibratory massage on the delicate skin areas such as the cheeks.

Application

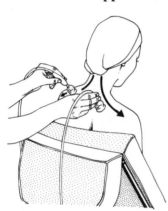

BACK TREATMENT

The treatment should ideally commence on the upper back, working in a *downwards* direction, from the occipital cavity at the base of the skull to the shoulder areas. Strokes are applied using the large ventouses, following the fibres of the trapezius muscle in the upper back area. Smooth unbroken strokes are used, alternated with circular strokes following the same path. The whole area is treated until a skin reaction is achieved, then the client rests back into the chair and the treatment progresses to the decolletage and neck areas. It may not always be possible to include the upper back area into the treatment, if chair positioning will not permit access to this part of the body, without inconveniencing the client. Wherever it is possible to commence on the upper back, the results of the treatment will be seen to be enhanced, with improved lymphatic drainage and general relaxation of tension in the area, due to the vascular stimulation.

Changing to a lower intensity (reducing the pressure) the area over the upper fibres of the Pectoral muscles is then treated, with the movements working up to the bones of the clavicle, with alternating smooth and circular strokes. The area of the sterno-mastoid muscle is treated next using a smaller pair of ventouses, and regulating the pressure as necessary. The movements work *downwards* from behind the ears, towards the natural indentation at

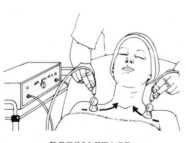

DECOLLETAGE

the base of the throat. Care must be taken not to exert pressure over the area of the trachea (windpipe), the main emphasis of treatment being the sternomastoid muscle area. In fact because of the unique action of pulsed air massage, the therapist has only to guide the applicators along, and keep them in rhythm to ensure a successful treatment, and pressure as such is never needed.

Treatment of the area under the mandible follows, either applied with the hands working in unison or alternately. The movement works from the point of the mandible bone, to behind the ear and then down to the clavicle following the previous pattern on the neck. This is often easier to accomplish one hand at a time initially, until skill develops in keeping the applicators working together to maintain contact and rhythm in the strokes. The applicator not in use may be prevented from altering the effect of the working applicator's pressure, by blocking its opening with a thumb or finger for the few minutes needed.

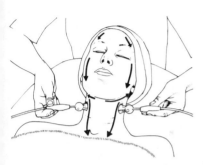

GENERAL LYMPHATIC DRAINAGE
METHOD

The treatment progresses to treat the borders of the face, starting at the temples, passing in front of the ears, and down to the clavicle as before. A slight alteration in the strokes encompasses the cheeks at this stage, avoiding any dilated capillaries in the area. The size of the ventouses and the air pressure used may need altering at this stage, depending on the size of the clients features and her skin condition.

Forehead strokes then commence, and again follow the pattern of lymphatic drainage previously established, down to the clavicle. With the broad surfaces of the skin completed the ventouses are again altered to treat the chin, upper lip, laughter lines and under-eye skin areas, more specifically if required. Forehead wrinkles and blocked pores can also benefit from this more concentrated approach. The intensity of the pulsed air or suction is increased, depending on the effect desired, and the treatment applied in a localized manner until the desired result is achieved. For cleansing effects more suction may be necessary, and for gentle stimulation (such as the eye areas) less suction is needed and more pressure is useful to give a vibratory sensation. So the system can be tailored to fit the needs of the skin. As the ventouses used for this aspect of the treatment have such small openings (apertures), it is possible to use a fairly high level of suction without causing unwanted skin reactions. However, if the skin reaction to pulsed air massage is not known, or the skin appears to react excessively, it is wise to use caution.

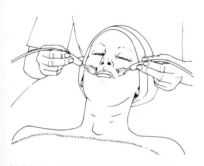

SPECIAL TREATMENT OF WRINKLES AND FLEXURE LINES

On a first treatment it is always wise to moderate the duration of the application, both in the general and more concentrated aspects, to avoid skin damage. For it is possible to cause a wheal on the skin, or a blood spot formation, with the skin appearing raised and covered with dilated capillaries in the treatment area. This is simply the skin's natural response to injury in action, and normally it will recede in time. On older clients any dilation of capillaries can cause permanent damage so it should be avoided at all cost. In all cases of skin damage or excessive reaction to pulsed air massage, it is the therapist's negligence to blame. Attention to skin reaction, caution in initial treatments and a vigilant approach to changes in the skin will prevent bad reactions occurring. Pulsed air massage is a skilled application to become proficient with, as it relies on attention to the skin's reactions, control of the equipment, and very good co-ordination of the hands with the mind. As with all specialized routines, practice makes perfect.

LYMPHATIC DRAINAGE MANUAL MASSAGE

Massage for increasing lymphatic drainage is applied in a downward direction in the facial and neck areas towards the subclavial vein. The special massage techniques employed empties the ducts, accelerates the lymph flow, and increases elimination of waste products. Rotary movements are used to lift the tissues whilst moving fluid downwards, in an even but light manner. To achieve successful lymphatic massage a highly developed sense of touch is necessary, to feel by palpation the condition of the lymph nodes, and the pressure needed to progress the drainage. Special training is necessary for this form of massage to achieve the beneficial effects and promote the full range of applications.

Indications for Treatment

1   Poor local circulation, causing dry skin, atrophy of the subcutaneous tissues, and superficial lines and wrinkles.

2   Scar tissue, due to the regenerative effect of lymphatic massage on the circulation.

3   Lymphatic stagnation, infiltration, oedema (swelling), particularly around the eyes.

4   Blocked pores, acne vulgaris, seborrhoea, and general poor skin texture.

5   Skin congestion, vascular complexions, areas of dilated capillaries (working around the affected area), and general skin tension.

6   For general relaxation purposes, on clients suffering from fatigue, nervous tension or depression.

Application

Treatment commences at the pectoralis muscle area, and progresses to drain the lymph nodes of the neck (sterno-mastoid and upper fibres of the trapezius muscles), working from the occipital cavity downwards and forwards towards the sternum area. The lymph nodes under the mandible are treated next, and all the following strokes then follow the same path, from the central area to the outer borders of the face, firmly along under the jaw, and downwards over the neck to the sternum and clavicle bone areas. In this way the lymphatic system of the face and neck is drained, by first freeing the larger vessels, and subsequently draining the superficial system.

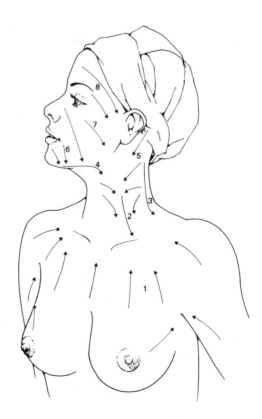

LYMPHATIC MASSAGE DIRECTIONS

General Points   Lymphatic drainage is not a massage of the muscles but a treatment which cleanses and regenerates the skin, improves the blood circulation and promotes elimination of waste products. The massage relaxes tense muscle fibres, soothes sensory nerves and achieves a rested facial appearance.

OZONE THERAPY TREATMENTS

Drying, healing, anti-bacterial and stimulatory treatments for the seborrhoea or acne conditions may be classified as ozone therapy treatments, if they are based on either a wet or dry form of ozone application. Ozone formation in minute quantities can be extremely beneficial to the disturbed and blemished skin, and is available to the therapist via the following mediums:
Ozone steaming (Vapozone or Infrazone)
Direct high-frequency treatment
Ultraviolet exposure (ray lamp treatment).

As ozone is also a destructive element, its use must be carefully controlled in skin treatments, otherwise destruction of skin tissue could result from over exposure.

Ozone Steaming

Ozone steaming is a natural means of activating the circulation of the subcutaneous vessels and providing them with oxygen. The Vapozone application has a disinfecting, anti-bacterial action on skin tissue, which normalizes the pH and promotes healing on blemished skins. Ozone is produced in the head of the equipment by means of a quartz tube high-pressure mercury lamp, over which the water vapour passes and becomes ionized.

The physiological actions include:
(a) the heating action of the ionized water vapour,
(b) the action of the ozone and its derivatives,
(c) the action of the ultraviolet radiation arising from decomposition of the ozone.

Slight perspiration is induced, the stratum corneum becomes hydrated and softened, and desquamation is increased. Ozone and the active oxygen produced by its decomposition destroy organic substances and bacteria, The increased blood circulation caused permits the effects of the ozone to act not only on the surface of the epidermis but also in the cutaneous tissues.

Indications for Treatment

1 Normal skin conditions, to maintain skin texture (application 10 minutes at approx. 12 inches (30cm)).

2 Seborrhoea and blemished skin conditions, to heal and disinfect the skin (application 15–25 minutes at 10 inches approx. (25cm)).

3 Mature skin conditions for regenerating purposes (application 3–6 minutes at approx. 15 inches (38cm)).

Contra-indications Treatment

1 Hyper-sensitive skins.
2 Extremely vascular complexions.
3 Acne rosacea.
4 Sunburn or previous ultraviolet exposure.
5 Skin irritation, abrasions, etc.

Method of Application

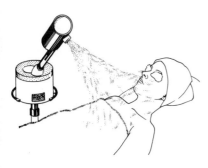

OZONE STEAMING

The equipment should be checked for a sufficient supply of purified water in the reservoir tank, and switched on 5–10 minutes before it is required to permit water heating to commence. The vapour switch only is required at this stage. When vapour starts discharging from the head of the equipment, the production of ozone may be added to the process by switching on the ozone control. The steam then changes its consistency, becomes ionized, cloud-like and very fine in appearance. Crackling is heard from the vicinity of the Quartz tube, positioned within the equipment head.

The client may be prepared for facial treatment, and the skin cleansed, whilst the steamer is heating the water source. Explanation of the treatment and its effects will alleviate client anxiety, and prepare her for the unusual smell and noise of the apparatus. The eyes must be covered with damp cotton-wool pads to avoid irritation, and any areas of sensitivity, e.g. upper cheeks, protected with dry cotton-wool. The client should be placed in a semi-upright position, and the fully operating steamer applied so that an even distribution of ionized vapour is achieved. The client should be prepared for the application to avoid surprise.

The length of application time depends on the state of the skin, and only approximate durations can be given:

1 General cleansing and toning purposes: 5 minutes on the lower neck, 5 minutes on the lower face, and 4–5 minutes on the full face area.

2 Disinfecting and anti-bacterial effect on the oily and blemished skin: 10 minutes on the lower face and jaw, 10 minutes on the upper face, followed by vacuum massage or pore treatment massage, and re-exposure of ozone steaming for 5 minutes, generally applied.

3 Regenerating effect on dry, dehydrated or mature skins: 2–3 minutes on the neck, and 1–3 minutes on the face, to achieve erythema, and increase cellular function. The treatment is used in combination with nourishing and hydrating preparations to prevent skin irritation.

When the desired effect has been achieved, the steamer should be removed and the routine progressed. Surface moisture should be removed and the appropriate cream or mask applied, according to the sequence being undertaken.

Younger clients may have ozone steaming at frequent intervals, to control and heal blemished areas of the face and back. The possible range of application positions permits the ionized vapour to be directed at an angle on to the face and back, without danger arising from moisture formation and scalding.

The use of ozone apparatus is restricted in some countries and therapists in practice should consult their local Public Health Authorities so as to safeguard their position.

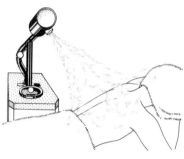

STEAMING ON THE BACK

DIRECT HIGH-FREQUENCY TREATMENT

The direct form of HF application, as explained in Chapter 8, has a very beneficial effect on oily and blemished skins. The convenient and hygienic method of application via the glass bulb electrode makes treatment of infected skin possible, due to the elimination of hand contact and the subsequent risk of increasing the extent of the condition. The response to treatment is swift, with the skin showing an immediate improvement in texture, decreased sebaceous secretion and brighter colour.

There are several methods of treatment combination, which may prove to be the most effective on the different stages of the oily or blemished skin. The beauty specialist must use her own judgement to decide the most suitable routine.

Treatment Applications and Suggestions

1 Cleanse (biological soap or 'soapless' cleanser), mask (acne), and direct high-frequency (10–15 minutes over the face and neck).

2 Within the normal pore treatment, concluding the routine after the mask, for refining and drying purposes.

3   Cleanse, direct high-frequency (short dura-tion), mask, and re-application of HF direct, for the seborrhoea condition, to activate the circu-lation and improve elimination.

4   On post-acne scar tissue, particularly around the chin area, to increase skin desquamation, using the sparking technique, to produce flak-ing and a dry condition. Moderate durations and intensities should be used, according to the client's tolerance, and the irritation caused to the sensory nerves. The treatment must be combined in a regenerating programme of cosmetic applications to promote new skin growth, and avoid an unpleasant facial appear-ance due to the peeling effect.

5   On blemished back and shoulder areas, to dry and heal the skin. The pore treatment routine may basically be followed, with direct HF replacing or following the mask application. For severe conditions, soapless cleansing and direct HF only may prove the most suitable treatment, applied several times a week. The direct HF may be applied with equal benefit to young men and women.

ULTRAVIOLET TREATMENT (RAY LAMP)

Ultraviolet rays are electromagnetic waves with wave-lengths of between 3 900 and 136Å, those within the range 3 900 and 1 849 Å being available for treatment purposes (Å stands for angström unit; 10 Å = 1nm or nanometre). Ultraviolet rays are absorbed in the skin, and it is there that the reactions occur which cause the beneficial effects. The effects of ultraviolet rays on the body may have a local reaction, or a more widespread effect depending on the degree of the irradiation (output and general exposure to the rays).

Local Effects

Erythema Reaction

A mild dose causes slight reddening of the skin, which is accompanied by no other symptoms, and soon fades. The reaction usually appears within 12 hours of the irradiation. There are four degrees of erythema; only the first reaction is a permissible application for the beauty specialist, but she should be aware of the consequences of over-exposure and its effect on the skin.

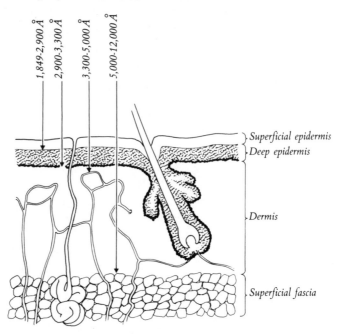

PENETRATION OF RAYS INTO THE SKIN

A first degree erythema is a slight reddening of the skin, with no irritation or soreness, which fades within 24 hours.

A second degree erythema is a more marked reddening of the skin, with slight irritation. It fades within two to three days.

A third degree erythema is a marked reaction, which causes the skin to become red, sore, hot and swollen. The reaction lasts about a week and is very painful.

A fourth degree erythema is similar to the third degree reaction, with the addition of blister formation.

Desquamation

Ultraviolet exposure accelerates the skin's normal shedding process. The amount of peeling varies with the strength of the erythema reaction.

Pigmentation

Rays with wave-lengths between 2 800 and 3 300 Å (280 to 330 nm) are absorbed in the deep epidermis, and initiate a chemical reaction which results in the conversion of the amino-acid tyrosine into the pigment melanin. The degree of pigmentation found depends on the client's natural colouring and the method of application. Constant duration treatments for germicidal purposes do not alter the skin's colour greatly, whilst progressive applications for cosmetic tanning and tonic purposes affect a considerable colour change over a period of time. The local applications appear to increase the skin's resistance to infection.

General Effects

Sufficient UV exposure:

1 Increases the body's general resistance to infection.

2 Gives a general tonic effect.

3 Enables vitamin D to be produced, if of sufficient intensity and duration, produces pigmentation, and an improved skin condition.

Indications for Treatment

1 Sluggish complexion, with uneven texture and pH value.

2 Seborrhoea, for improvement of skin texture and to regulate secretions.

3 Acne vulgaris, to promote healing by its antibacterial and peeling effects.

4 To provide additional protection against natural sunlight and heat effects in the delicate or sensitive skin conditions, and permit a tan to form without discomfort.

5 For cosmetic tanning purposes, to produce or maintain a tanned complexion.

Contra-indications to Treatment

1 A very sensitive skin.

2 UV should not be used in combination with certain other treatments, which alter the skin temperature, i.e. prolonged vapour steaming.

3 When a client is taking medically prescribed drugs classed as sensitive to UV: gold, the sulphonamides, insulin, thyroid extract, and quinine.

4 Acute eczema or dermatitis or any unknown skin complaint.

5 An unnatural rise in temperature from any source.

APPLICATION OF
ULTRAVIOLET
IRRADIATION

Assessment of Exposure Required

The most satisfactory method of assessing the dosage required is by observation of the erythema reaction created by a patch test or short primary exposure. The following factors determine the intensity of the reaction:
the output of the lamp,
the duration of the exposure,
the distance between the lamp and the client,
the sensitivity of the client to the treatment.

Equipment   Ultraviolet lamps vary in their output, according to the type of lamp, its size, and the source of UV rays within the lamp. The bulb-shaped UV lamp contains a hot quartz tube (high pressure mercury vapour, HPMV) and is most commonly used in facial applications. Also for general skin effects and cosmetic tanning. Quartz tubes are also used, either in single or multiple form, to cover small or widespread areas. The hot quartz lamp produces a mixture of short and long rays, and is suitable for tanning, tonic, cosmetic and germicidal purposes.

The lamp chosen should be of sturdy construction, with a stable base, and sufficient reflector span to permit general exposure of larger areas, i.e. the back. The cross arm section should permit a free range of heights and angles, to accommodate the need for variation in the distance between the client and the bulb during the complete sequence of the treatment programme. The reflector must be free from dents, otherwise hot spots will result, which intensify the reaction and could cause burns.

Application

The effect of the UV rays on a client may be tested to determine sensitivity by giving an extremely short-duration irradiation at a distance of 3 ft, and requesting the client to remember the effect (if any) apparent after 4–8 hours. The distance and duration of subsequent treatment may then be determined, using the principle of inverse squares, for bulb type lamps.

The intensity of rays varies inversely with the square of the distance from the lamp. Thus the intensity of the radiation at 1 foot is 4 times that at 2 feet, and 9 times that at 3 feet. This law applies to infrared, visible and ultraviolet rays, so when a lamp obeys the law of inverse squares, four minutes at 2 feet, and nine minutes at 3 feet, are required to produce the same effect as 1 minute at 1 foot.

Both bulb and tube lamps require 1–2 minutes to reach maximum output or intensity, so they must be switched on in preparation for the treatment, and placed in such a way that the rays do not fall on unprepared individuals. A curtained area or individual cubicle is required for UV treatments. The lamp should be moved as little as possible prior to, or after, the irradiation, until it has cooled, otherwise its life is reduced. There is also a risk of spontaneous implosion of the bulb, if it is moved or knocked whilst hot.

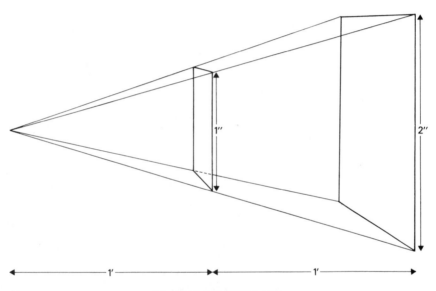

INVERSE SQUARE LAW

Preparation of the Client

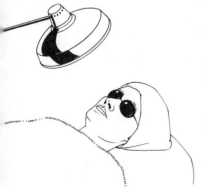

The skin should be cleansed and all oily preparations removed. Tonic lotions should not be applied, but the skin left free and clean. The eyes of the client and operator should be covered with close-fitting goggles, and the client placed in a comfortable position, either upright facing the lamp, or in a semi-reclining posture. The rays must strike the skin at a right angle, so the alignment and distance of the lamp from the client must be measured accurately. The therapist must ensure the client does not alter position during the exposure. When the lamp is in position over the client, it must be checked to ensure that it cannot fall on the individual. The cross-arm should be over the leg or section of the base that lies under the couch, to prevent over balancing, and all screws on the movable arm should be firmly tightened.

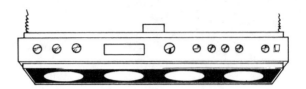

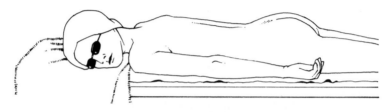

MULTIPLE LAMP APPLICATION

Records of Treatment

A record must be kept of the date, the lamp used, the area exposed, and the time of exposure and distance from the lamp. The general effects, erythema reaction, and any related information should be noted. Progressive cosmetic tanning treatments may be applied in rapid succession, as soon as the erythema reaction has faded, possibly every other day until a tan is established. The progression should be planned according to the client's general colouring and skin reaction. Fair skinned clients may take 8–10 treatments to progress from a ½ minute exposure to a full 10 minutes, with the application for the face being in the form of (1) ½ minute, (2) 1 minute, (3) 1½ minutes, (4) 2 minutes, (5) 3 minutes, (6) 4 minutes, (7) 6 minutes, (8) 8 minutes, (9) 10 minutes. Darker skinned or previously tanned clients may commence on a 1 or 2 minute exposure, and progress quickly, (1) 2 minutes, (2) 4 minutes, (3) 6 minutes, (4) 8 minutes, (5) 10 minutes, and then the tan can be maintained by regular but spaced exposures. If the skin appears irritated for any reason, treatment should be suspended, otherwise severe desquamation will result and the skin will peel and be sore.

Treatments to restrict bacterial growth, improve skin texture, and heal infected areas should be applied on a constant basis to avoid pigmentation.

Areas of scar tissue can become very apparent under the influence of UV, so a moderate exposure programme is the most suitable. A ½ or 1 minute irradiation repeated at regular intervals to the face or back should control the condition, and achieve a skin improvement. Ultraviolet is a very acceptable treatment for blemished skins, as it produces a fast response, which is encouraging, and it is hygienic in its application.

Over-exposure

The skin becomes hot, red, extremely sore and there may be blister formation. In the event of an over-exposure, the client must be advised to consult her own physician. The effect of over-treatment would not be evident immediately after the exposure, taking up to several hours to develop, so the possibility of its formation should not be ignored but discussed with the client to avoid anxiety. The precautions against an overdose lie in careful technique and attention to all the points mentioned previously. A strong reaction can occur if the client interferes with the exposure programme and undertakes excessive natural sun tanning at the same time. Wind exposure can also increase the skin's erythema reaction, and so verbal and visual investigation are necessary prior to treatment.

Sun Beds

Lie-on sun beds, which permit a natural tan to develop slowly without all the associated hazards of natural sun-bathing, have revolutionized tanning as a clinic treatment. By eliminating most of the procedures associated with traditional artificial tanning, the sun bed system has become immensely popular with clients. This has been to the advantage of clinic owners with the space to install such a system and thus fulfil the public demand, the high initial cost of a sun bed unit soon being returned through the increased salon revenue.

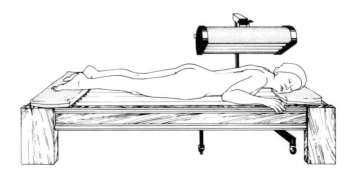

The sun bed system operates by screening out the burning elements of the ultraviolet spectrum, leaving only tanning elements to produce a natural and comfortable treatment. The ultraviolet spectrum is made up of ultraviolet A (UVA) ultraviolet B (UVB) and ultraviolet C (UVC), and it is the UVB and UVC rays which do all the damage. These cause sunburn, degrees of erythema and other side effects.

The risk of burning, which was difficult to assess, made it necessary to control the dosages of ultraviolet very carefully with ray lamps, and to progress the treatment cautiously to avoid painful skin inflammation and irritation, It also made the wearing of goggles to protect the eyes a necessity.

With the screening out of the UVB and UVC rays, goggles are no longer necessary, and clients can undertake longer tanning sessions on the sun beds, with no fear of sunburn. The spectrum of the solarium sun bed is similar to that of the natural sun, but with the special mercury vapour low pressure radiators used, a 10 m W/Cm^2 radiation intensity is normally attained in the UVA range. While UVB rays are only 0.04% of the specified total radiation. *So the tanning radiation content is improved and the burning components drastically reduced.*

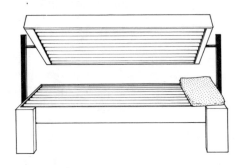

The sun beds need very little maintenance, and the ten 80 Watt mercury (Hg) low-pressure lamps typically used, can be replaced easily at the end of their life. Aluminium-plated reflectors provide for a uniform radiation field up to the edge of the bed surface ensuring that the sides of the body tan as evenly as the back and front. By using an overhead solarium 'sun-roof' unit at the same time, treatment time is cut by half, as all surfaces of the body are treated simultaneously. This saves the client turning over half way through her treatment period. It also increases the potential profitability of the sun bed for the clinic, as the same area of space can cope with twice the number of treatment bookings over the same period. This is an important point, as apart from high initial purchase costs, the sun bed area cannot be utilized for any other treatment (as could an overhead solarium unit over a treatment couch) so it must justify the space it takes up.

The sun bed unit should be enclosed as a treatment position, both for reasons of modesty for those who tan in the nude, and also to extend the working life of the equipment. When in almost continual use it should be left switched on, rather than turned off between consecutive treatments.

The power requirement is only 800 watts, which means little current consumption, and a normal mains power supply. The life span of the lamps is 1600–2000 hours without noticeable output loss. However, this will be reduced if the unit is continually being switched on or off in treatment. With the sun bed system, although timing procedures are not so critical, there is still the need to ensure that the client is suitable for tanning treatments. Contra-indications include those individuals unable to form pigment molecules in the skin, and those on drugs likely to act as sensitizers to ultraviolet.

Sensitive-skinned or very pale-skinned clients should also commence their treatment in a progressive fashion, starting with a total treatment period of 30–40 mins. This would mean 15–20 minutes front and back or with a 'sun roof' solarium 15–20 minutes, where the client is 'sandwiched' between the two UV units. For lightly tanned skins this can be increased to a total time of 60 minutes (30 minutes each side). For heavily tanned clients trying to maintain a tan, in a winter climate perhaps with no chance of natural sun bathing, up to 120 minutes total tanning time can be undertaken (60 minutes each side).

Normally a one-hour period is sufficiently long for most clients, and it is normally booked on a half-hour or one-hour basis, to maximize treatment use. The client normally can only spare this amount of time for treatment, when it has to be undertaken on a regular basis, to build up the tan in a progressive fashion. The advantage of having the sun roof unit is obvious, as cutting down the treatment time, provides results in half the time for busy clients (and reduces boredom).

Treatment plans are usually sold on a course basis of 10 to 12 treatments of an hour's duration. Initially clients can take treatment in ½ hour sessions till their tolerance for the treatment develops. Sessions must be progressively undertaken, particularly when attempting to produce a tan on a

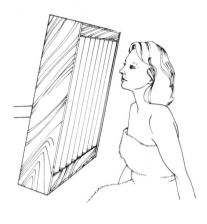

pale skin, and two or three sessions can be undertaken the first week. As the effects of the application are to tan rather than dry or irritate the skin, sun bed session's can be taken every day, by clients who find it easy to achieve and maintain a tan naturally.

Most sun beds available make it possible to exclude the face from the tanning effects, which is an advantage in many cases, such as dry, dehydrated or mature skins. For though attractive in itself, a tanned skin becomes tougher in the process, and it is wise to avoid this on facial skin.

For skins where tanning can be used to dry and heal the skin, such as the young blemished skin, mini solarium units are available. These operate on the same principles, but are portable, and can be moved into position more easily to treat the face, back and shoulder areas.

GALVANIC SKIN TREATMENT FOR DESINCRUSTATION AND IONTOPHORESIS

Galvanic Current

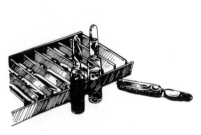

GALVANIC AMPOULES

Equipment

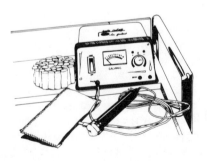

Generation of a steady direct galvanic current can be utilized in facial therapy to introduce water soluble substances through the skin (iontophoresis), and to remove surface oiliness, blockage, and regulate secretions (desincrustation). The polarity of the active ingredients to be introduced into the skin varies, i.e. there are those effective at the cathode (negative pole), and others effective at the anode (positive pole). Positive (+) ions (cations) progress from anode to cathode; negative (−) ions (anions) progress from cathode to anode. The efficiency of the introduction process depends on the time, concentration of ions, the current, and electrode area, the latter two of which have a certain influence on each other.

Whether part of a combined treatment unit, or as an independent galvanic unit, the effects of galvanic applications are similar in action. Therapists should become familiar with the particular application method of the unit they have available, as techniques do vary slightly from one system to another.

However, the galvanic equipment operates on direct current, and will normally incorporate a pilot light, an intensity control, a polarity changer, and an indicator by means of which the minutely dosed amperages can be determined. The equipment has

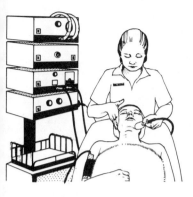

COMBINED FACIAL UNITS
WITH GALVANISM

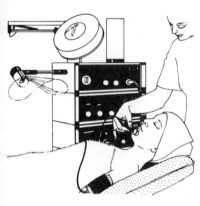

active (differential) electrodes, by which the application is made, and indifferent (passive) electrodes, normally of a plate form, which are attached to the client's upper arm to complete the circuit. Both active working electrodes, and the indifferent electrodes are attached to the equipment by leads.

The active electrodes may be in the form of wand, tweezer, rod, roller-type or face mask applicators, according to the system chosen. These allow for treatment on large areas, and concentrated effects on inaccessible parts of the face, such as the nostril area and chin cleft.

The indifferent plate electrode is of metal or conductive rubber, and is covered with a thick layer of moistened viscose sponge material to protect the skin, and to allow a good connection to be formed for the galvanic current. This is strapped firmly to the client to allow a perfect flow transmission to be established between the current generating unit, and the body itself. Hand-held indifferent rod electrodes are also widely used with galvanic apparatus available, but these do not allow for such efficient connection of the body to the galvanic current, and could cause more discomfort so plates are preferable wherever possible.

A full face mask may be used for both penetration of nourishing substances, and desincrustation purposes, which permits an even penetration of the active substances and increases the effect achieved. The mask electrode is also attached to the active connection. Clients do not always happily accept this method of galvanic treatment, finding it rather claustrophobic, so its use should be considered carefully by the therapist.

General Effects

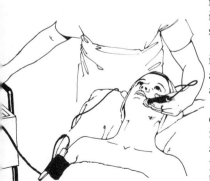

The application of direct current in galvanic applications can be used for iontophoresis (on-toe-for-resis) and desincrustation (des-incrustation). In cosmetic practice galvanic current (direct current) is utilized for increasing blood circulation, activating metabolic processes and infiltrating active substances through the intact skin (iontophoresis).

The introduction of active substances through iontophoresis is quicker, more intensive in effect, and results in deeper penetration than by manual applications.

Inorganic and some organic salts have the property that they dissociate when dissolved in water, i.e. they separate into positively charged cations and negatively charged anions. If a direct current is passed through such a solution of ions, the positively charged cations are attracted to the negative pole of the source of current, the cathode, while the negatively charged anions are attracted to the positive pole, the anode.

Iontophoresis consists of infiltrating such dissociable solutions through the skin by means of electrodes connected to a source of direct current. The polarity of the electrode to be used for introducing the substance is usually given by the manufacturer of the preparation containing this substance.

Application and Effect of Desincrustation

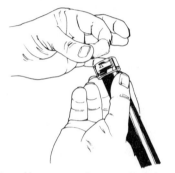

Disposable cotton wads are moistened and folded

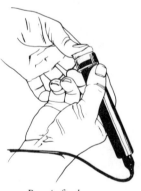

Press in firmly

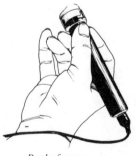

Ready for use

After cleansing and ozone steaming (if indicated), the desincrustation fluid may be applied on a negative charge, via the wand or tweezer electrode upon affected areas of the face. The wand applicator is prepared with its disposable cotton-wool wads being wetted and well squeezed out, and fitted firmly into the top collar of the applicator. The client is prepared by placing the indifferent pad in place in its damp envelope, and connecting the circuit via leads. The face is moistened and the active ampoule solution applied, and treatment commences.

After setting the correct polarity, the unit is switched on and application starts on the check, with the moistened wad being gently but firmly applied to the skin. The applicator is moved slowly over the affected areas, with stroking or circling movements, keeping the moistened wad firmly in contact with the skin. The skin must remain moist throughout the application, if it becomes dry, treatment must return to zero for remoistening of the skin. As the skin's resistance drops, and the lotion starts to be effective, the client will become aware of the galvanic current, and its intensity may need adjusting to avoid discomfort. Sebaceous blockage is dissolved, and oily matter removed, eliminating the need for forceful expulsion of blackheads. Ingrained skin blockage due to insufficient cleaning on the normal or combination skin may be dissolved over a period of time, and removed with vacuum massage without leaving enlarged pores. The cleansing effects of desincrustation are beneficial on all but the hypersensitive, extremely dry or mature complexions. Desincrustation may be followed by penetration of hydrating and nourishing substances on the normal and combination skins, using iontophoresis methods. Desincrustation may be applied for 4–5 minutes for general cleansing purposes and 8–12 minutes for oily skin treatment, depending on skin reaction.

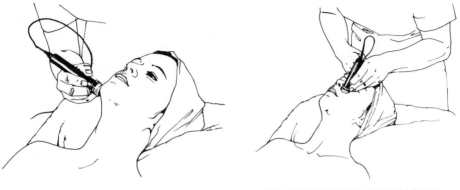

GENERAL FACIAL WORK CONCENTRATED APPLICATION
ON BLOCKED CENTRE PANEL

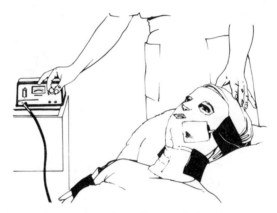

FULL FACE DESINCRUSTATION
OR IONTOPHORESIS

Application and Effect of Iontophoresis

Thorough cleansing should be carried out to remove all preparations, oils etc., from the skin. The treatment method is the same as for desincrustation, with the substance applied to a wet skin, and a wand or tweezer, roller, or face mask electrode used. Treatment on one part of the face should not exceed 3–5 minutes, whilst the whole face and neck may require 10–12 minutes to achieve the necessary circulation increase, and allow full penetration of the active substance. More sensitive skins may require shorter application times, or a longer treatment on a lower intensity, to avoid skin irritation. Nourishing, moisturizing, or normalizing ampoules may be applied, normally on a *negative charge*, this being the most penetrating pole. Certain treatment ampoules may contain substances, some of which travel to the cathode, and some to the anode. In this case the application time is divided, and the polarity

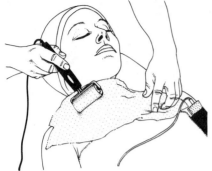

TREATMENT OF LARGER AREAS

reversed half way through the treatment, after reducing the intensity to zero. Some of the ampoules for normalizing the skin fall into this category, as they contain acidic amino acids, and organic acids which travel to the cathode, and basic amino acids which travel to the anode. Through the reversal of the polarity, all the substances of the natural treatment complex are transported into the deeper layers of the skin. The polarity of the ampoules will be clearly indicated, either on the sealed ampoule itself, or on the container pack in which it arrives. If no indication of polarity is apparent, the manufacturer's guidance must be sought to determine treatment application, for successful results.

Most ampoules are penetrated using the negative pole, with the positive pole being applied if needed for skin toning effects, right at the end of the application. If its more tightening effects are not needed, or are likely to cause skin irritation, the positive pole is not used, and the entire routine completed on the negative polarity

General Points

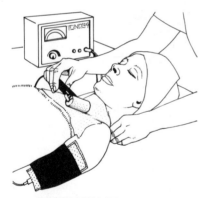

DECOLLETAGE

Active substances are available in sealed glass containers (ampoules), which should not be opened until required. They are sufficient for one application of the face and neck, and the treatment should endeavour to penetrate the maximum amount through the skin, as their effectiveness is lost after being opened, and they cannot be applied to advantage at a later stage.

Deincrustation is always applied on negative polarity and is rinsed away very thoroughly after application. Iontophoresis is normally applied on a negative charge, but may use both polarities (negative always applied first). Iontophoresis penetrates active products which are left to work in the skin – not rinsed away.

Conclusion of Treatment

The skin should be protected from exposure by moisturizing preparations of a bland nature, but left free of facial makeup items, apart from eye and lip colour. In this way the skin can gain full benefit from the treatment and should show an immediate improvement.

Readers who require further information on galvanism are advised to consult my book *Beauty Guide 3 – Galvanic Treatments*, also published by Stanley Thornes (Publishers) Ltd.

GALVANIC/HIGH FREQUENCY TREATMENTS

Combined galvanic and high frequency treatment routines have become increasingly popular over recent years, providing an efficient and effective method of deep and thorough skin cleansing, and gentle peeling. These effects are beneficial in nearly all skin 'types', as they help to rejuvenate the skin, whilst freeing it from surface blockage. The deep cleansing actions of galvanic desincrustation, when combined with the germicidal, toning and refining effects of direct high frequency, provide for an immediate improvement in skin appearance and texture.

There are several systems of treatment available, which though they all function on similar principles, can differ considerably in their product applications. So therapists should follow the manufacturer's instructions closely as to the routine of the electrical work and the application of associated treatment products without which the treatment is ineffective. Use of the ion action products (gels, emulsion, etc.), when covering the skin evenly, make cotton wool protection of the working electrodes (rods, and rollers) unnecessary with this system of treatment. However, care must be taken to ensure even coverage does exist, otherwise the galvanic treatment would be uneven in effect, and apart from being less effective, could be uncomfortable for the client.

Most combined galvanic/high frequency routines achieve their effects in a two-fold way: cleansing and then refining and regenerating the skin. The gels which are used to cleanse the face contain cations, which are activated by a low intensity of galvanic current (usually below a detectable level). This opens the pores and encourages a slight natural perspiration, which helps the skin to eject ingrained dirt, and clear clogged pores. The horny nature of the skin, stratum corneum, is gently broken down, and becomes easier to remove by subsequent treatment. This also helps remove scar tissue and pigmented skin, making the skin appear clearer and with a better colour.

The rejuvenation aspect of the treatment involves application of an emulsion, which releases oxygen when it comes into contact with the residue of gel, left on the skin from the desincrustation procedure. Application of direct high frequency converts this into ozone, which in turn has an oxidizing and purifying action on the tissues. It also encourages cellular growth of skin tissue, increasing the proliferation rate (desquamation), and hence avoiding skin keratinization effects. So the skin is helped towards improved functioning in a natural manner, by first freeing it, and then allowing it to bring itself back into the correct balance of oil, fluid, and pH levels.

Application

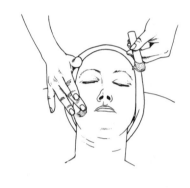

A typical treatment would commence with cleansing and toning of the skin, using products appropriate for the clients skin 'type'. The toning must be thorough and remove all traces of cream, grease etc. from the skin. The skin is then blotted dry with a tissue, in preparation for the actual treatment.

A generous coating of specially formulated gel containing cations is applied. These will be activated by the galvanic current, and bring about an effect of opening the pores, and deep-cleansing the skin.

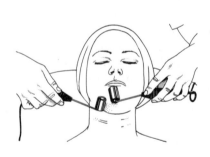

The neutral electrode of the galvanic unit is attached to the client, ideally in the form of a sponge-covered metal plate or conductive rubber plate, strapped firmly to the upper arm. A hand-held electrode may also be used if a plate electrode is not available, but this does reduce the contact area of the neutral electrode, which does not make for such effective connection of the client into the galvanic circuit. A larger neutral plate, well protected with sponge layers, makes for an improved flow transmission of current, and is always preferable to a hand held rod electrode. The machine is switched on, and treatment commences, first with rollers, working from the throat upwards, covering the area, with even rhythmical rolling movements, both hands working together. The rollers should remain in skin contact throughout the application. A timer may be used to guide the therapist as to application time, with 5–7 minutes being average, depending on the condition of the skin, and the amount of treatment it requires.

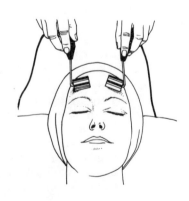

The rollers are slowly and evenly passed over the face, to activate a slight and natural perspiration which will help to bring out impurities and deep cleanse the pores. The client should not really be aware of the current, as it functions perfectly effectively with this system of treatment at a level below that at which the client can discern it. This also avoids the metallic taste in the mouth experienced with some galvanic applications, which clients can find unpleasant.

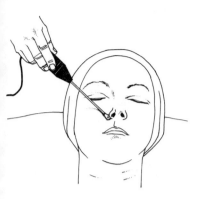

The treatment changes after the initial roller application, to use of a single-electrode applicator, for a further five minutes of concentrated work. The equipment should be switched off whilst changing over to the single-rod electrode. The client remains attached to the neutral electrode during the change over. The skin should also be checked to see that sufficient gel is still present, evenly covering the surface. The rod-like electrode allows more concentrated work on the inaccessible areas of the face, around the nostrils and sides of the nose, and the cleft of the chin. These being areas where the concentration of sebaceous glands is highest, and skin problems, blemishes, open and blocked pores are more likely to occur. So attention to these areas is especially beneficial.

The galvanic part of the treatment is then concluded, and the current switched off, and the neutral electrode removed from the client. The skin can be then examined under a magnifier, and dead surface skin gently removed with the side of a sterile probe. Any blocked pores which have had their contents loosened by the dissolving action of the treatment, may be *gently* scraped clear, but on no account must pressure be used to extract blackheads. Apart from being a pointless procedure as the blocked pores will simply reform, the skin damage that could be caused could result in permanent scarring. This occurs as a result of the skin trauma caused by the pressure on the surface and subcutaneous tissues, a natural result of which is scar tissue formation.

The pores may only be blocked with superficial debris, old makeup etc. from poor daily cleansing procedures, and then the dead surface skin and waste matter will come away without pressure or trauma to the skin. So therapists must use their judgement, and knowledge of the client's skin, to decide whether extraction of blackheads is advantageous, and at what stage of the course of treatments it is useful. Only when the skin is becoming refined naturally, will it be of any benefit to the established seborrhoea skin condition. The pores will then close naturally, preventing any repeat formation of keratinized matter. Use of vacuum treatment within the routine may also be of advantage in helping this pore cleaning process.

On skins which have a simple build up of old skin, the removal of dead horny skin is easy to accomplish after the desincrustation, as it has been softened by the application. So the horny layers and blockage may be removed immediately on a dry or

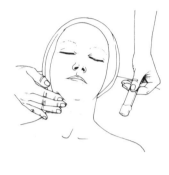

normal skin, usually on the first or second treatment application. With an oily, blocked skin this may not occur until ten or twelve treatments have been completed, as if the established blockage is to be dispersed without skin injury, the keratinized matter has to be dissolved slowly and gently, allowing the pores to be refined at the same time.

A generous coating of treatment emulsion is applied to the face and throat. When it comes into contact with the remaining gel from the galvanic application, a chemical change occurs and oxygen is produced on the skin surface. The products must be carefully stored, and be in a fresh condition for this to occur however. Their effectiveness decreases if the items have been left open, or been subjected to extremes of temperature.

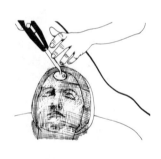

The face and throat are covered with a square of dry gauze, and direct high frequency applied. The gauze provides an even spark gap for the direct HF, and prevents the bulb electrode sticking to the skin, and perhaps causing a loss of contact. The HF application is used in the normal way, commencing on the forehead, to prevent the current becoming uncomfortable later in the application. Finger contact should be used to transfer the active bulb electrode to the client's skin, to avoid causing any initial prickling which might surprise the client, and cause anxiety. This could spoil the treatment enjoyment for the client, and might prevent her accepting the following HF application, so is worth taking care over. The treatment is applied for five minutes approximately over the face and neck, concentrating on areas of particular need. The treatment need not be given at a high intensity to be effective, but must be able to produce the germicidal effects which are the particular benefit of this form of treatment. The high frequency application causes ozone to be produced, both as a result of the combination of the gas with the atmosphere, and from the effects of the products on the skin's surface, which intensify the action. These effects have a rejuvenating and purifying action on the skin surface, and cause a change in skin texture, which is immediately apparent to the client.

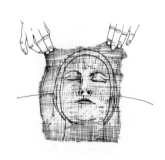

All traces of gel and emulsion are removed with a toning lotion. Next a gauze square soaked with a toning or soothing lotion is applied over the client's face and neck, and acts as a relaxing compress to settle the skin tissues. This compress is left for five minutes, and allows the skin to continue working from the effects of the HF, whilst regaining its normal temperature and colour in preparation for the mask.

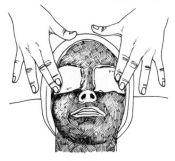

The gauze is removed, and the skin blotted dry with a tissue. A mask is then applied to complete the treatment. This is chosen to suit the skin condition at that time, and must take into account the stimulatory effects of the preceding treatment application. The eyes are covered with moistened pads of cotton wool to soothe the eyes.

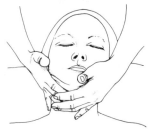

The mask is removed after 10–15 minutes and a moisturizer applied to protect the skin, chosen to suit the skin 'type'. The client should be advised not to wear makeup for the next 6–12 hours if possible, as the skin will still be active from the effects of the treatment. Also the effect of clearing the pores, and refining the skin should be given the maximum opportunity to be effective, a point most clients appreciate.

SKIN PEELING BY BIO-LOGICAL, CHEMICAL AND ABRASIVE METHODS

Skin peeling is a treatment that improves the quality and tone of the complexion. The process removes dead cells from the surface of the skin, increasing the skin's natural desquamation, and leaving a fresh clean appearance. It is a cosmetic process, based on biological (vegetable) or chemical products, which only removes dead surface cells and the products of keratinization in the horny stratum corneum of the epidermis.

Biological Peeling

This cosmetic method is achieved by application of a solution which softens the unwanted keratnized dead cells, without affecting the living skin tissue. The sequence is completed by application of a mask-like cream, which progresses the action initiated by the solution and eliminates the dead cells.

The skill in all forms of peeling is in diagnosis and recognition of the existing skin condition, rather than in the actual application of the cosmetic preparations. Observation of sensitivity, skin irregularities or irritation, produced by the first mild skin-peeling application, will give guidance as to future treatment possibilities, and should prevent over-treatment.

Indications for Treatment

1   Young problem skins, with blocked pores, blackheads and over secretion of sebaceous glands.

2   Sallow complexions, which require toning and stimulating.

3   Scarred, post-acne complexions, to refine the skin, and slowly remove the discoloured scar tissue.

4   General cleansing and refining purposes on normal and combination skin conditions.

Contra-indications to Treatment

With careful choice and application of biological products, very few skins are completely contra-indicated, but the following conditions might suffer irritation from the sequence.

1   Hyper-sensitive skins.

2   Extremely dry or dehydrated complexions.

3   Mature crêpy skin.

The manufacturer's instructions should be followed carefully as variations of application sequence exist. Basic principles, diagnosis, and the need for vigilant awareness of skin reaction, however, stay constant.

Application

1   General cleansing and toning should be completed. The skin should not be steamed as this pre-softens the surface and is disadvantageous.

2   The skin is thoroughly wiped over with the softening lotion, to remove surface dirt, and natural sebum, and prepare it for the peeling.

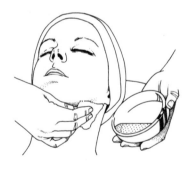

PREPARATION OF THE SKIN

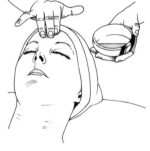

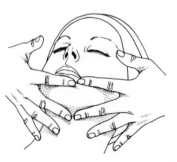

3   The entire area is moistened with the special lotion, which has a lysing action which helps to dissolve the dead skin cells. The liquid is gently worked into the face and neck until it is all absorbed. Any tingling or itching felt at this stage can be relieved by a few minutes light massage to alleviate the sensation and reassure the client.

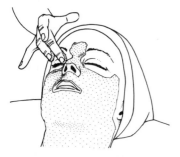

APPLICATION OF CREAM

4 The solution is left for 3–5 minutes, then the cream is applied in the same manner as a mask avoiding eyes, nostrils, etc. Eye pads are applied and the client rests for 15–20 minutes to enable the peeling process to develop.

5 When the cream is ready for removal, small cracks appear in the surface, and the texture becomes dry. The product is removed with light circular movements of the finger tips, commencing at the neck. A cuvette bowl may be placed at the neck to catch the dried mask fragments, as they are removed. The dead cells are removed with the dried cream, and on completion the skin will appear fresh and vibrant.

6 When the neck and face are completely clean, nourishing cream and a gauze compress soaked in mildly antiseptic hydrating lotion may be applied. The skin requires protection and rehydration at this stage, so it may be left until the skin appears calm and has regained its normal temperature.

7 Moisturizer may be applied to complete the treatment, and protect the newly-peeled complexion. Only lipstick and eye makeup should be applied after any form of peeling process.

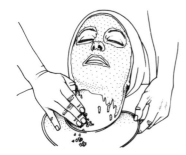

REMOVAL OF CREAM

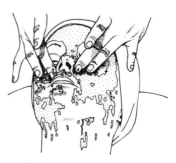

REMOVAL OF CREAM PELLETS AROUND NOSE

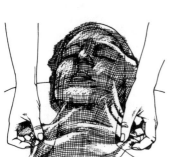

GAUZE MASK

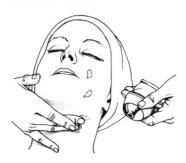

MOISTURE CREAM APPLICATION

Chemical (Progressive) Peeling

The chemical method of skin peeling has a progressive effect, becoming increasingly stronger as the treatment extends over a lengthening period. Unlike the biological peeling which has a fairly constant action, the progressive method is capable of causing skin irritation if incorrectly chosen for the skin condition. Previous knowledge of the skin, its reaction to treatment, and general sensitivity to chemical substances is vital prior to chemical peeling.

Indications for Treatment

1 Post-acne scarring.

2 Discoloured skin areas (mild peeling at spaced intervals only).

3 Sallow, thickened skin conditions.

Contra-indications to Treatment

1 Sensitive, dry dehydrated skins.

2 Mature skins.

3 Skin infection, irritation, abrasions etc.

Application

The treatment is composed of an active lotion which is combined with progressively more active powders to form a mask paste. The paste is applied like a mask, avoiding the eye areas, and left for 5–10 minutes according to the client's reaction. The mask should be removed immediately if, after the initial tingling sensation passes, irritation is felt strongly on any area. The mask powders are used in sequence, always combined with the activating lotion, to produce increasingly evident peeling effects. The mask is removed with tepid water, and nourishing or hydrating preparation applied to soothe the skin.

Progressive peeling forms part of a sequence of skin improvement treatments for the post-acne scarred, or discoloured complexion. It may be alternated with regenerating treatment for the more mature discoloured skin, or with antiseptic electrical routines for the adolescent skin. No infection should be present at the time of peeling otherwise irritation and soreness will result. The treatment may be applied at moderate intervals according to skin sensitivity and the effect desired. The skin should never be permitted to become over-exposed, otherwise capillary damage will result.

Abrasive Peeling Treatment

Abrasive brush treatment is accomplished by application of the brush massage equipment, with special attachments for abrasive effects (see Chapter 8, Brush Cleansing). Foam pads and an abrasive stone applicator are used to remove the abrasive mask paste from areas of hardened, scarred or pigmented skin tissue. The treatment may be varied to include all but the most sensitive complexions.

Indications for Treatment

1 Uneven skin texture on the face, back, and upper arms.

2 Discoloured skin areas.

3 Scar tissue.

4 Sallow, blocked complexions, with over-secretion of sebaceous glands.

Contra-indications to Treatment

1 Sensitive skins.

2 Dehydrated skin.

3 Mature skin.

4 Skin infection.

Application

After the cleansing stage, the abrasive powder is mixed into a fine paste with water, and applied as a mask over the entire face or to the affected areas only. For normal skins the paste should be thin in consistency and removed whilst still slightly damp with the moistened sponge applicator applied via the brush massage unit. For thickened greasy skins, the mask should be permitted to dry, and removal completed in the same manner. Scar tissue may require more extensive treatment, which may be applied on the second or third application by replacing the sponge applicator with the abrasive block for the mask removal.

Skin reaction will vary according to the mask consistency, the skin's sensitivity, and the method of removal. No pressure should be used during the removal, as the rotating heads accomplish the grinding effect unaided. Caution in the method of treatment will avoid soreness or over-exposure caused by the abrasive application.

The skin may then be cleansed with moistened sponges, and hydrating or nourishing preparations applied in the form of masks or creams. Wheat germ or royal jelly products may be applied over a gauze compress to soothe, normalize and protect the skin. No makeup should be worn after the abrasive mask treatment.

Chapter 10

The Ageing Process. Treatments for the Mature Skin

The treatment approach to the mature client differ both in general attitude and in its cosmeti emphasis from all other methods and application of facial therapy. The importance of regular an correct cosmetic care must be stressed, if the clien is to retain a youthful supple skin and prevent pre mature ageing and wrinkling. The actual age an apparent skin age of the client should be considere in planning the treatment to determine whether th ageing process is an inevitable or premature condi tion. Hereditary and physical factors exert an influ ence upon the skin throughout its life, and provid varying capacities to deal with the effects of exter nal forces, such as extremes of heat, sunlight, col and humidity. The neglect or care a skin ha received, the general health of the individual, an dietary factors will all have played a part in th maintenance or loss of skin texture and elasticity.

THE AGEING PROCESS

Ageing commences as maturity is reached bu because of the slow changes occurring, the condi tion may not become a cosmetic problem until we established and more difficult to reverse.

In the early thirties small expression line become a permanent feature, the skin starts to los its firmness, and minor imperfections may becom established. At this stage of life treatment results ar very satisfactory, and the ageing process can b considerably delayed.

Approaching the menopause age group or earlie if the skin has been neglected, fine lines form int wrinkles, the skin tone becomes crêpy, atrophied t a slight degree, and the thickness of the skin and it capacity for fluid retention decreases. Prematur ageing is seen more frequently in this age grou than any other, and may be associated with th lowered amounts of oestrogen present in the body An improvement in tone and vigour of the skin i clients taking oral contraceptives in this age rang would appear to confirm the delaying effects o oestrogen in relation to skin ageing.

The mature client in the post-menopause grou suffers from the inevitable characteristics of ski ageing: loss of elasticity, changes in the water reten tion properties of the dermis, and pigmentation an fibrous abnormalities. The progressive loss of resilience in the collagen fibres, appears to be part of the physiological process of ageing, and is thought to be accelerated by exposure to sunlight and drying elements. Although the effects of ageing can be delayed considerably, the process itself is inevitable, and may be associated with hormone changes occurring through alterations in the internal endocrine secretions, causing regressions of oestrogen levels and subsequent loss of youthful and vibrant appearance.

Ageing does not appear to be associated with a decrease in the skin's vascular supply, or with a change in its protective capacity. Mature clients do however appear to have a lowered tolerance for heat, light etc., possibly due to a decreasing function of the skin's thermostatic abilities (control of body temperature).

Causes of Premature Ageing

1 Over-exposure to sunlight and heat, which causes the skin to become leathery, with evident lines. This is a direct result of the skin's attempt to protect itself from injury, by a thickening of the corneous layer itself, and pigmentation formation (sun-tan).

2 Incorrect skin care routines, with use of harsh preparations, drying makeup applications, and insufficient cleansing and nourishing elements.

3 Lack of protective skin care, or general neglect.

4 Poor health, lowered resistance to infection, and lack of regular sleeping patterns.

5 Bad work environment, dirty, smoky, or over-heated surroundings.

6 Incorrect dietary balance, or an extreme loss of weight, causing loose skin texture, and loss of supporting subcutaneous adipose tissue. Low fat diet plans, which affect the skin's protective capacities and suppleness, may be balanced by a revision of the skin care programme (for the whole body) and the addition of more nutrient elements.

7 General depression, fatigue, stress and anxiety all have an ageing effect on the body and skin appearance. The attitude to the client in this instance may be even more important than the actual treatment in accomplishing beneficial results and an improvement in vitality.

Recognition of the Mature Skin

The skin may be thought of as mature when the signs of ageing mentioned previously are evident, regardless of the client's true age. Often the actual and apparent age of the client tally, and give important guidance to the therapist regarding treatment. Points of diagnosis (see Chapter 2) which will be evident in varying degrees, are decreased activity of sebaceous glands, lowered capacity for fluid retention, and imperfections of a fibrous and vascular nature. The degree or stage of the mature skin condition will determine the course of possible treatment, and may be sub-divided for convenience into:

(1) Preventative and Delaying Treatments

Performed on a dehydrated skin with fine lines, slight evidence of atrophy, but sufficient muscle tone and little or no evidence of vascular imperfections or fibrous malformations. This skin type is usually found in the 30–40 age group.

(2) Maintenance and Relaxation Treatments

Performed on the mature skin with etched facial lines and wrinkles, severe loss of muscle skin and tone, and a diminished thickness of skin tissue. Vascular and fibrous imperfections, and the damaging effects of skin distension, limit the electrical applications, and emphasize manual and cosmetic care for this skin condition. Ageing becomes progressively more marked from post-menopause onwards, and care must be taken to prevent aggravation of existing imperfections, i.e. dilated capillaries or milia.

Treatment of Ageing Skin

Elimination or correction of some of the causes of premature ageing brings immediate improvement in a large proportion of the pre-menopause clients. Simple neglect of the skin is the most common cause of 'dryness', dilated capillary formation, and fine wrinkling, and once a skin care programme has been established the effect of the salon treatment will quickly become evident. Unfortunately many clients seek advice for established conditions, where the possibility of regression is decreased, but much can now be achieved, due to recent cosmetological advances in development of substances which greatly improve the appearance of an ageing skin.

The general health and mental condition of the mature client is of significance, and a positive attitude to both professional and home care measures should be adopted by the therapist to foster harmony of interest in the mind and body of the client. Client involvement in her general health and appearance, through revised diet and skin care routines, should be reflected in a more youthful and vital attitude to life.

Salon Treatment Suggestions

Preventative and Delaying Treatments

1 Continental facial treatment, comprising cleansing, vacuum massage if indicated, manual massage of the shoulders, neck and face, non-setting mask, toning and makeup.

2 Warm oil mask treatment, comprising cleansing, oil mask application with infrared irradiation, and protection.

3 Paraffin wax facial treatment, comprising cleansing, manual massage if indicated, paraffin wax application, and neutral toning and protection only.

4 Viennese facial, comprising cleansing, massage with indirect HF, non-setting mask, toning and makeup if required.

5 Passive muscle contraction treatment, which may be applied in combination with manual techniques, concluding the facial sequence, or given as an independent short duration routine, applied at regular intervals.

6 Iontophoresis treatment (galvanic), using hydrating and nourishing ampoules.

7 Regenerating treatment, comprising brush cleansing, ozone steaming, brush method stimulatory massage, wheat germ mask and protection only.

Maintenance and Relaxation Treatments for the Post-menopause Client

1 Modified continental facial treatment, with adjustments in manual massage technique to avoid skin distension, and the addition of audio-sonic vibratory massage to conclude the sequence.

2 Viennese facial for relaxation and sedative effects.

3 Modified warm oil mask treatment, with protection of dilated capillaries, and decreased heat intensities.

4   Paraffin wax treatment, with modified heat intensities.

5   Lymphatic drainage massage treatment.

6   Iontophoresis treatment (galvanic), using regenerative and tissue building ampoules.

Cosmetic Care of the Mature Skin

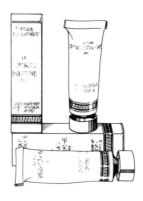

Differences of opinion exist as to whether the skin can actually be 'fed' by cosmetic creams, oils, etc. One important factor for the therapist to consider is that if the skin is kept supple, by the emollient and moisturizing products applied, skin chapping, flaking and soreness will be prevented, bacterial infection will be restrained, and premature ageing controlled. Nothing at present exists to prevent the ultimate wrinkling of the skin, but recent advances in cosmetological science have developed substances which considerably delay the process, amongst them the soluble collagen, hormone products and tissue extracts.

Soluble collagen

The connective tissue of the dermis changes as the body ages, from its flexible unlinked form with a high elasticity and capacity to absorb water. The skin loses its full soft appearances as the soluble collagen diminishes and becomes cross-linked and rigid. It changes to inflexible collagen (inelastic connective tissue), which is unable to swell and retain fluid, so that it cannot benefit from moisturizing elements around it or locally applied. Soluble collagen products are now available, which appear to increase the skin's capacity to retain fluid, improve its elasticity and provide a more youthful appearance. Combined moisturizing/collagen products, creams, and emulsions are available to fulfil all aspects of mature skin care, and delay the formation of wrinkles and the effects of premature ageing. The beneficial effects of soluble collagen will be fully acknowledged by physicians and cosmetic chemists only when long-term results are assessed, and the skin improvement seen to be accomplished without side effects. The results available to date would appear to show soluble collagen as a very useful medium for therapy applications in the treatment of the ageing skin. The popularity of collagen products with clients would seem to reinforce the view that they provide the effects claimed, as a visible difference in the skin's texture, smoothness, and firmness is quickly apparent.

Hormone Creams

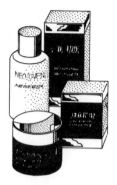

Hormone creams satisfy the skin's need for oestrogen on clients of post-menopause age, where the natural oestrogen level has decreased, and has a more vital general rôle to accomplish in the mature woman. The hormone content of the cream is too small to cause any general or systemic body effects, but it does improve the skin condition, and provide a more youthful appearance in the area of application. Hormone products are permitted to contain only 7 500 to 10 000 I.U. (International Units) of oestrogen per 1 oz. (28 grammes approx), which would provide approximately one month's nightly applications. The effectiveness of hormone creams is most evident in post-menopause clients, where consistent proliferative effects upon the skin's epithelium improve the skin's softness, fullness and elasticity. Its capacity for absorbing fluid is improved, dehydration of surface layers decreases, and the skin is more able to benefit from moisture preparations applied locally. The response to hormone creams varies with the age of the client, the concentrations of oestrogen, and the duration and method of application. Regular use is necessary, otherwise the skin reverts to its original atrophic condition. It would appear that in clients where the natural oestrogen levels are decreasing, locally applied hormone products satisfy the skin's needs, improve the complexion, and delay wrinkle formation. In younger clients where no malfunction exists, no improvement is evident, and application is unnecessary and may cause unwanted skin effects, such as congestion, open pores and a relaxed texture.

Tissue Extracts

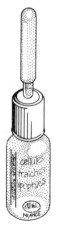

Tissue extracts obtained from the epidermis, ovaries, and placenta of young animals are rich in nutrients including hormones, amino-acids, polysaturates (essential fatty acids), and vitamins. Apart from their success in hydrating an'' nourishing ageing tissue, they can also remedy skin deficiencies such as excessive dryness or oiliness, high colouring and acne. Their action is to increase capillary circulation, and stimulate the metabolism of the skin, they are therefore especially useful in the care of the ageing skin, and on conditions of dehydration.

The method of application may be a 10-day treatment plan, with the serum extracts individually presented in ampoule form, or as a range of products, for all aspects of the home care routine. The treatment is usually most beneficial given in a concentrated form, over 10 days to three weeks, with intervening rest periods between courses.

Moisturizers

The protective and hydrating rôle of the moisturizer on the ageing skin is very necessary to prevent the drying effects of general exposure, causing imperfections of texture and tone. The stratum corneum of the epidermis contains 'natural moisturizing factors' (NMF), which regulate the hydric balance and affect the skin's capacity to retain water. In ageing skin tissue, this ability decreases and moisture must be applied in a cosmetic form as an emulsion or cream. Regular use of moisture products also permits greater absorption of the nutrient creams, extracts etc., applied on a nightly basis, to regenerate the skin.

HOME CARE SUGGESTIONS FOR THE MATURE SKIN

Daily Skin Care

Cleanse

Cleansing should be accomplished gently with an emulsion or cream product, based on hydrating elements, to prevent stripping the skin of its natural oils.

Tone

Tissue-bracing products or mild action tonic may be applied, briskly to the neck and jawline, and gently to the facial area.

Nourish/Protect

A nutrient form of protection should be employed to continue the action of the nightly care, and to prevent further dehydration of surface tissue. Under-makeup concentrates, based on collagen, hormone or tissue extract elements, may be applied to form a thin film over the face and neck.

Makeup

Moisturized semi-liquid, oil-based or cream-textured foundations should be chosen which have fine texture and good covering properties. The tinted foundation is of prime importance in the mature woman for improvement of facial appearance, so it should be advised with care. The texture must be soft and fine to prevent exaggeration of lines, wrinkles etc., the colour should mask imperfections, whilst enhancing the natural colouring. Many of the recent foundation formulations do not require a loose powder application to set them, which avoids the risk of lining and heaviness of texture. If however a powder is required, it should be of a translucent nature, and be sparingly applied and carefully brushed away.

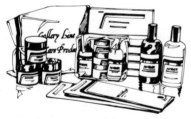

COLLAGEN TREATMENT PRODUCTS

All makeup items for the mature client must be chosen for their softness of texture and subtlety of colour. Powder/cream eye and cheek makeup may be used whilst the skin is still firm, but should be revised to cream textures when a crêpy skin texture is evident. A different attitude to making up the mature woman should be established, which places emphasis on attractive facial coluring and development of individual features and personality. This is preferable to attempting to adapt younger makeup fashions, which would be unsuitable both for the existing skin texture and facial expression, and also for the client's way of life.

Nightly Skin Care

Cleanse

Cream cleansers should be used to remove every trace of tinted preparations and cotton-wool tissues employed for removal. The procedure must be repeated until the skin is thoroughly clean.

Tone

A repeat of the morning sequence.

Nourish

An emulsion or cream nutrient product should be applied according to the firmness of the muscle tone and skin texture. On a firm but finely lined skin, a small quantity of nourishing or hormone cream may be applied with light upward massage strokes until it is completely absorbed by the epidermal layers. On the older skin, with a loss of skin tone, emulsions, concentrates, or moisture/collagen products should be utilized, due to their speed of absorption and elimination of the need for massage and subsequent risk of skin distension.

Treatment routines of hormone creams, collagen, and tissue extracts products can be simply co-ordinated into the daily skin care sequence, and their use explained and demonstrated to the client. The skin care advice to the mature woman should be kept as simple as possible, due both to the time she may feel justified in committing to it and possible confusion that could arise if an elaborate plan is presented. It is preferable to have a simple sequence performed regularly, than a complex one performed spasmodically. As regular cosmetic skin care is of vital importance in treatment of the ageing skin, its value must be stressed to the client, both in terms of prevention of premature ageing and improvement of the existing condition.

WARM OIL MASK TREATMENT
(Using Infrared or Radiant Heat Irradiation)

Warm oil mask therapy functions on the principle of heat penetration, using different forms of heat source to produce a local increase in skin temperature. The therapeutic effects of infrared and radiant heat rays are combined with a cosmetic oil application to produce the oil mask treatment. Natural perspiration is gently induced, and the skin's capacity to absorb cosmetic preparations is increased due to dilation of the superficial vascular network. Respiration of the skin is improved, surface adhesions are freed, and the complexion shows an immediate difference and a sustained reaction in the period following treatment. Increased elasticity, smoothness and softness of texture, and improved colour and skin tone are clearly evident to the client over a course of treatment.

Infrared and Radiant Heat

Infrared rays are electromagnetic waves with lengths of between 4 000 000 and 7 000 Å (400 000 nm and 700 nm approximately). When infrared rays are absorbed by the tissues of the body, warmth is produced at the point where they are absorbed. Various types of heat generators are available, which are usually referred to as non-luminous and luminous generators. Treatment with the luminous generator is known as radiant (visible heat), and infrared is used to describe the radiations from the non-luminous forms. Most heat lamps produce varying proportions of both forms of radiation, and so the terms are rather misleading. The heat emitter is available in:

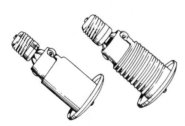

INFRARED AND RADIANT HEAT EMITTERS

1   Non-luminous form, where the heating element is embedded in a fire clay material, and very few visible rays are produced. Infrared rays are produced with wave-lengths between 150 000 and 7 700 Å.

2   A luminous generator, where the element is apparent, and visible rays are produced (radiant heat), in addition to the infra-red rays. The coiled filament surrounds a fire clay emitter, and produces heat, infrared and visible rays of between 40 000 to 6 000 Å when it reaches maximum output. Many of the radiant heat rays have wave-lengths in the region of 10 000 Å.

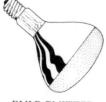

BULB EMITTER

Shorter IR rays penetrate to the deeper parts of the dermis, or to the subcutaneous tissues, while the longer rays are absorbed in the superficial epidermis. (See Chapter 9, Penetration of Rays into the Skin.) Radiant (visible) heat is therefore more penetrating, but has greater irritant properties to the surface tissues, whilst infrared, although less penetrating, is less irritating, and is therefore more frequently chosen for beauty therapy applications.

An irradiation from either heat source produces warmth in the superficial tissues, which is conducted to the deeper tissues by blood circulation.

Effects of Local Application of Infrared Rays

Local irradiation of infrared rays produces a rise in temperature, erythema (an increase in colour due to vasodilation), a calming effect on sensory nerve endings, and increased activity of sweat glands. The sedative effect is enhanced by the general relaxation of the client, due to both the heat application, and the relief of tension brought about by skilful client preparation and handling. All these effects correctly applied can be combined into a cosmetic/therapy routine to produce very satisfactory results.

Indications for Oil Mask Treatment

1 Crêpy, finely-lined, mature skin.

2 Premature ageing of the skin.

3 Dehydration of skin tissue.

4 Preventative treatment on the younger 'dry' skin.

Contra-indications to Oil Mask Treatment

1 Extremely vascular complexions.

2 Hyper-sensitive skins.

3 Very nervous, highly strung clients, due to the need for immobilization during the application.

4 Areas of dilated capillaries must be excluded from the exposure by covering them with damp cotton-wool pads to prevent heat penetration.

Preparations of Oil Mask, and Application

The client is prepared in the normal way, and the skin inspected for areas of sensitivity and imperfections which would affect the infrared exposure and intensity proportions. The infrared irradiation is based on knowledge of the inverse square law, and power of the heat source, and the client's sensitivity to treatment. (See Chapter 9, Inverse Square Law and Lamp Treatments.) As infrared treatments produce an immediate colour change, due to the rise in temperature and evident warmth in the surface tissues, the initial treatment, if applied with caution and attention to these factors, can give valuable information on which future applications can be based.

Preparation of the ray lamp and emitter is completed prior to treatment as 10–15 minutes are required for the IR lamp to reach maximum emission or output. The lamp should be positioned safely and left ready to bring into position, as at all times the safety of the client must be considered. Care of the lamp and reflector will have ensured the equipment to be in good working order, with a polished undented reflector to deflect the rays into the area of treatment. The items required, warm oil, gauze, scissors, bowls, etc. must be prepared with the usual cosmetic commodities, and an efficient sequence established to avoid the necessity to leave the client unattended.

With the approximate distance and timing decided, the client's prepared skin is protected with a gauze mask, cut to shape, which has been saturated in a fine oil (almond), warmed to a comfortable temperature. The face and neck area can be

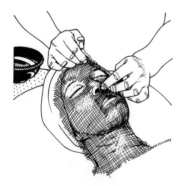

PREPARATION OF GAUZE MASK

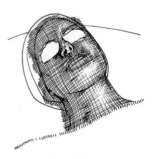

OIL MASK TREATMENT

covered, and the eyes protected, by damp cotton-wool pads if these are to be excluded from treatment, and the mask placed to fit the contours of the face closely. Previously cut lip and nostril holes must be placed in position, and care taken that prominent areas such as the nose tip are not left exposed.

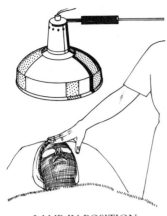

LAMP IN POSITION

With the client comfortably settled, the prepared lamp is placed in position, parallel to the face, at a distance of 18 inches–3 feet, according to the intensity of the lamp, the sensitivity of the skin, and its reaction to the heat if known. The lamp must be placed to ensure stability, with the cross-arm directly over one of the feet, and all adjustable parts firmly clamped. The therapist should stay in close attendance, checking the skin reaction at intervals, until the required result is achieved. Because of individual skin reaction this may vary from 8–20 minutes approximately, and no fixed timing sequence can be indicated. The lamp is removed first, by gently moving its cross-arm away from the client, switched off and left to cool before moving to preserve the life of the IR emitter. Constant attendance during treatment will prevent client interference with the lamp, and minimize the risks of burns, shock etc. occurring.

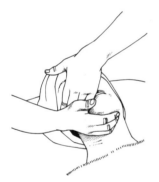

GENTLE MASSAGE TO AID
OIL ABSORPTION

The gauze mask is removed and the excess oil used for further effleurage and light tapotement massage movements, if the skin condition and reaction permits. The superficial skin tissues will absorb as much oil as they require, and the excess can then be removed with soft slightly damp tissues. As the respiration of the skin is increased, oil will continue to be present in the superficial tissues for some time, and the skin will appear unsettled and stimulated for a considerable period. A mild natural-based refreshing lotion may be sprayed over the skin if desired, and moisturizer applied as a final protective step.

Conclusion

The effects and long-term benefits of the oil mask treatment will be seen more clearly by the client the day after treatment. As the routine is classed as a remedial treatment, its application should be promoted as a preventative measure for dehydrated and mature skins, to delay the effects of ageing, and to promote cellular function and biological activity.

REGENERATING TREATMENT FOR THE AGEING SKIN (BRUSH MASSAGE METHOD)

The treatment is designed to stimulate ageing and slackening skin tissues, whilst at the same time removing dead epidermic cells, so that the skin can absorb the regenerating and moisturizing preparations being applied.

Indications for Treatment

1   Mature skin with thickened epidermal layers and areas of discoloration.

2   Dehydrated skin, with fine wrinkling of the surface, but adequate subcutaneous tissue.

3   Slightly atrophied skin, due to neglect, or premature ageing, caused by excessive weight loss or ill health.

Contra-indications to Treatment

1   Hyper-sensitive skin.

2   Loose skin texture, with evident loss of elasticity, and decreased moisture and oil levels. (The treatment should not be applied due to the risks of further skin distension.)

3   Extremely vascular complexions.

4   Areas of dilated capillaries must be excluded from the application.

Preparation and Application

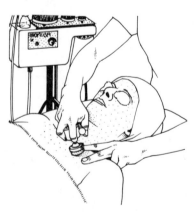

BRUSH MASSAGE ON CREAM

After thorough and intensive cleansing and application of ozone steaming for a limited period, a generous amount of regenerative cream is applied to the skin. Brush massage is applied over the shoulders, neck, and facial areas, with a circular soft-haired applicator for a period of 10–15 minutes, or until the required reaction is achieved. Surplus cream may be removed, and fine tissue oil applied over the treated area. A damp gauze mask is applied and wheat germ gel spread over the porous fabric to form a close contact with the face and neck. Infrared rays may be applied for 5–10 minutes to facilitate absorption if the capillary network is sufficiently covered with subcutaneous tissue.

When the skin appears calm, relaxed and soft, the gauze, containing the oil and wheat germ gel, may be removed and the skin may be refreshed with

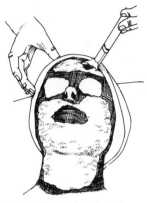

WHEAT GERM GEL ON
GAUZE

spray toning of a camomile dilution. Moisture protection may be used to complete the routine, as facial makeup should not be applied due to the unstable nature of the skin for several hours after treatment.

PASSIVE MUSCLE CONTRACTION TREATMENT (FACIAL FARADIC)

Passive muscle exercise is accomplished by application of a faradic type current to produce contractions of facial muscles without conscious effort on the part of the client. It is of value in the treatment of ageing skin, atrophic and wrinkled conditions and poor muscle tone.

Physiological Effects of Faradic Type Currents

The name 'faradism' was originally applied to the current obtained from a faradic cell. This was an induced alternating current, which produced spasmodic fierce contractions, controlled by the physiotherapist for treatment of damaged or denervated muscle tissues. Modern equipment used for beauty therapy purposes combines various types of currents, which produce similar physiological effects, without discomfort, and these are termed faradic type currents. The current is surged so that the contraction produced closely resembles natural facial exercise and is acceptable to the client. Between each surge there is an interval during which no current flows.

The primary sensation is stimulation of sensory nerves, prickling, slight irritation and resulting erythema in the area. When sufficient intensity of current is applied and the electrode is placed accurately over a motor point, muscle contraction takes place. The surging of the current produce relaxation and prevents muscle fatigue or dis comfort. The working muscles exert a pumping effect on blood and lymphatic vessels in th immediate area, improving cellular function an removal of waste products.

Indications for Passive Muscle Exercise (facial faradism)

1 Ageing skin tissue, with atrophic, withered appearance.

2 Loss of firm facial contours.

3 Evidence of oedema, due to loss of muscle tone, particularly around the eyes. (Medical approval is required to ensure the infiltration is not attributable to any physical systematic condi- tion, i.e. heart complaints etc.)

4 As a preventive measure, to delay the effects of ageing, and promote cellular function, by increasing nutrition to the skin's surface layers.

Contra-indications to Muscle Contractions

1 Hyper-sensitive skins, due to irritation of sen- sory nerves.

2 Highly coloured vascular complexions.

3 High blood pressure.

4 Very highly strung, nervous clients, due to the need for client co-operation.

5 Skin abrasions, due to the discomfort caused.

6 A large quantity of fillings in the teeth, or metal bridge work in dentures, requires adap- tation of contraction positions to avoid dis- comfort.

7 Any area of the face where severe discomfort is experienced within the treatment, such as the frontalis muscle area in some individuals.

8 The muscles should not be worked until the become fatigued. Any sign of fatigue, tremors unwillingness to continue to contract, etc must halt the application.

9 Sinus congestion.

10 Migraine.

SUPERFICIAL NERVES OF THE HEAD AND NECK

The superficial nerves of the head and neck are under the control of the cervical plexus of the nervous system. This plexus lies deep in the neck, opposite the upper four cervical vertebrae.

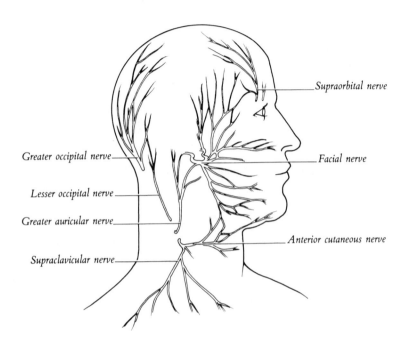

Supraorbital nerve

Greater occipital nerve

Facial nerve

Lesser occipital nerve

Greater auricular nerve

Supraclavicular nerve

Anterior cutaneous nerve

Muscle Contraction. Methods of Application, and Equipment available

There are several methods of producing facial muscle contractions:

(A) Stimulation of Motor Points

With faradic type current applied via an active (cathode) electrode, to the motor point of the muscle, with an indifferent (anode) electrode, completing the circuit placed on the area of good contact (i.e. the spine), or applied in the form of a hand-held electrode.

(B) Facial Electrode Application

Utilizing the same current, the contraction is produced by application of a facial unit, which has built in both the positive (anode) and negative (cathode) electrodes, into the surface of the applicator. Client acceptance due to decreased discomfort has made this a popular method of facial muscle contraction therapy.

(C) Interferential Current Method

Interferential current is the result of crossing two medium frequency stimulating currents, both of which are independently generated in the apparatus, and introduced separately into the area to be treated. The electrodes for each current are placed in diagonally opposite positions and the area of activity is formed where the two currents cross. The main advantage is that a sufficient intensity of current can be used to obtain the desired effect without excessive skin discomfort. The frequency of stimulation (i.e. the difference between the two medium frequencies employed) can be varied easily over a suitable range, usually 0–100 Hz. At the higher end of the range stimulation of tissues occurs but without muscular contractions, unless a very high intensity is used.

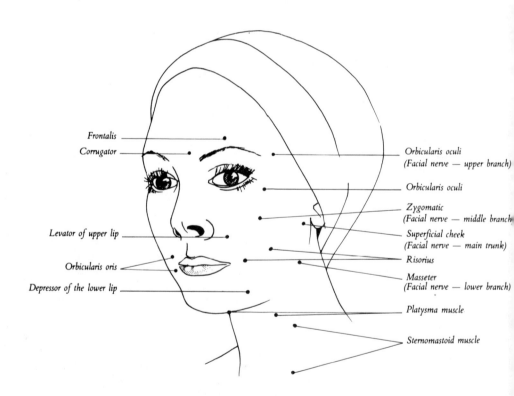

Frontalis

Corrugator

Orbicularis oculi
(Facial nerve — upper branch)

Orbicularis oculi

Zygomatic
(Facial nerve — middle branch)

Levator of upper lip

Superficial cheek
(Facial nerve — main trunk)

Orbicularis oris

Risorius

Depressor of the lower lip

Masseter
(Facial nerve — lower branch)

Platysma muscle

Sternomastoid muscle

MOTOR POINTS OF FACE AND NECK

KNOWLEDGE OF THE EQUIPMENT

As so many forms of specialized muscle contraction equipment are available, with various electrodes and applicators, differing methods of use, and manner of connection, therapists should become really familiar with the apparatus and its controls etc., before embarking on the treatment, to avoid accidents. When concentrating on achieving accurate and comfortable contractions for the client, it is very easy to reach for the wrong control knob and alter the treatment incorrectly, perhaps painfully if not fully acquainted with the equipment.

In professional life any new equipment considered should be investigated fully before purchase, so that complete confidence in the application methods is established before presenting the treatment for clinic purposes. The more elaborate the muscle contraction unit is, the more technical skill will be needed to handle it competently. If skill with a particular piece of equipment has not been obtained during basic training, then it has to be acquired through short courses, from the equipment supplier or from training seminars organized by professional associations. The need for client safety demands that this specific knowledge is acquired.

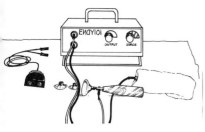

BASIC MUSCLE CONTRACTION UNIT

Electrical therapy requires a therapist to add to her manual and social skills, develop an ability as a technician, competent to handle correctly the equipment to enable the treatment to produce the desired result, whilst maintaining client confidence and comfort. For this reason it is necessary to have basic therapy ability before commencing training in electrical therapy. To gain the technical ability needed it is necessary to use all the professional expertise available and not be afraid to admit a lack of knowledge when faced with new systems of treatment. Electrical therapy treatments can be some of the most popular and profitable in the clinic if applied well and with confidence. The therapist owes it to her clients to see that she has that confidence through thorough training.

Method of Application Facial Faradic

Preparation

The client is prepared in a similar manner for all three methods of facial muscle contraction. The skin is freed from all cosmetic preparations, oils, creams, etc., and the client placed in a semi-reclining or upright position, depending on the area of treatment. The effect of gravity on the facial contours will give guidance as to the condition of the muscle tissue, and the most advantageous electrode position for facilitating muscle contractions. The motor points of facial muscles should be determined in relation to muscle size, position, and bony attachments (if any), and contractions obtained with the minimum of client discomfort. The conductivity of different tissues varies according to the amount of fluid they contain, therefore the epidermis which has a high resistance requires moistened pads, sponges, or gauze coverings over the electrodes to permit a comfortable application without using excessive voltage (intensity control). Fatty tissue acts as an insulator, or buffer, whilst muscle tissue itself is a good conductor, so contractions will be more easily obtained on a thin face than a well-covered one.

All equipment required must be prepared and tested. With the motor point system, the indifferent metal plate must be covered with damp lint and a

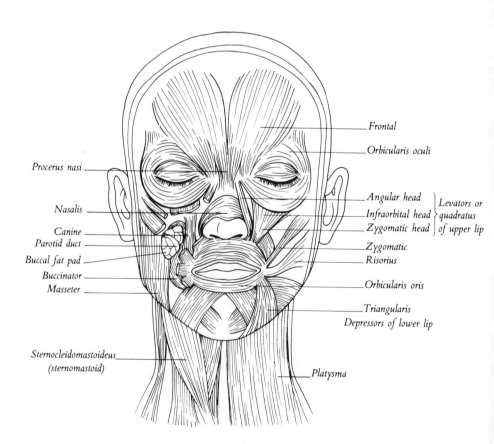

Procerus nasi

Nasalis

Canine
Parotid duct
Buccal fat pad
Buccinator
Masseter

Sternocleidomastoideus
(sternomastoid)

Frontal
Orbicularis oculi

Angular head ⎫ Levators or
Infraorbital head ⎬ quadratus
Zygomatic head ⎭ of upper lip

Zygomatic
Risorius

Orbicularis oris

Triangularis
Depressors of lower lip

Platysma

SUPERFICIAL AND DEEP MUSCLES OF THE FACE

small active button or disc-handled electrode may be selected. The applicator also requires some form of moisture contact over the active areas, either in the form of damp cottonwool or lint, or simply an emulsion cosmetic preparation. The interferential method requires connection via its four leads, and its application also relies on moist viscose sponges, to cover the diagonally placed metal plates.

Application   With Method A (motor points) and Method B (facial electrode), each muscle is worked individually for a limited period, until early signs of fatigue are evident. In a general toning routine each muscle need only be contracted clearly 6–8 times, so that the complete application of the face and neck should not exceed 15 minutes when professional competence is reached. Initially when proficiency is being developed in locating and accurately obtaining clear contractions, the overall period of facial contraction will be much longer. However the muscles will not have received longer periods of contraction, so they should not be fatigued. It is simply that initially muscle contraction is a difficult treatment to become skilled at, and as proficiency grows, the whole procedure becomes more efficient, for both the therapist and her 'client'.

With Method C (interferential system), small electrode pads are used to exercise areas of the face and neck. Each pad has four very small electrodes fitted in it, these electrodes sometimes being called 'points'. Also available are specialized applicators which are applied to a group of muscles, i.e. the neck and jawline, and they remain in place under the control of the therapist for 10–15 minutes. In this way all muscles in the stimulated area, receive identical contraction durations. The treatment is more efficient and less time-consuming.

Motor Point Method

With all preparation complete the application may proceed, with the therapist positioned so that she can both control her apparatus, and watch the effects of the contractions. If using the point system method (A) the covered indifferent plate should be placed between the shoulder blades, and checked to ensure it forms a firm contact, and has no exposed metal areas, or the client may be given the hand roller electrode to hold. The active button electrode may then be firmly placed over the motor point of the selected muscle and the intensity smoothly increased until first the primary reaction, prickling, is felt, and secondly a contraction is obtained. The

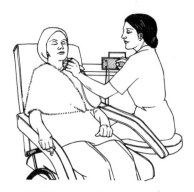

MOTOR POINT METHOD

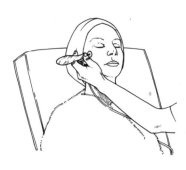

contractions should be visible, but not permitted to distort the face. If a contraction is not evident, the intensity should be reduced, and a slightly different placing or angle attempted until an even movement is formed.

As the effect of the motor point method is so specific and direct if accurately positioned over the nerve connection of the muscles, a long period of treatment is unnecessary. From studying the diagram of the facial nerves it is possible to see how by working closely to the area where the facial nerve enters the cheek area, the whole face can be exercised from one point. This may not always be comfortable because it is so clear a contraction, and so the nerve paths are then followed closer to their muscular connections. This explains why it is possible to obtain contractions of differing degrees of comfort and accuracy, on many different positions on the face. By working on the outer borders of the face, the nerve supply is improved, and this also avoids causing discomfort from excessive filling in the mouth. The mouth and eyes can be worked actively by the motor point method if uncomfortable in treatment, by working on the muscles close to them, which causes a connecting response as the muscles are so interlinked in position. Facial expressions are all controlled naturally via the facial nerve and its branches, so with artificial stimulation the same expressions will occur within the contraction. Because of the intensity of stimulation the nerves receive, the facial expressions can be exaggerated and distort the face. This should be avoided, as it is contrary to the effect trying to be achieved and makes the client embarrassed. Facial stimulation can also produce unnatural movements which the muscles would be unable to achieve naturally, such as pulling down the lower corner of the mouth. Again, as this area cannot benefit from such an action, it should be avoided in treatment. The idea of facial contraction is to tone the muscles in a natural uplifting manner, to minimize the effects of gravity on slack tissues. Any movement that doesn't achieve this end should be excluded from the sequence.

Facial Electrode Method

The facial electrode (Method B) is used in a similar manner to motor points but, due to its increased size, it tends to contract more muscles in the immediate area, due to their interlinking nature and minute size. Positioning to eliminate the unwanted contractions is possible, but for general applications is not really necessary unless the face is being distorted or caused discomfort by the facial movements. Accurate placing of the electrode in relation to the bone structure and muscles of facial expression, will avoid the need for elaborate and annoying repositioning.

When using the facial electrode method therapists should remember that the head of the applicator contains both the active and the indifferent electrodes, both of which must be in contact to obtain a contraction. So as well as ensuring that the electrodes are well protected with moist lint etc. the therapist should also *firmly* but gently hold them against the skin to give the best contact. Care over this matter when initially positioning the electrode or changing its position to improve the contraction will avoid client discomfort or distress caused by making full contact unexpectedly. A low intensity should also be used when moving the applicator head to reposition it, so that it cannot be felt by the client until in the correct place. The process of continual adjustment of the current intensity to bring about successful contractions is an essential element of facial contraction. So the therapist should place herself in such a way that the machine used is like an extension to the actual application. She should be able to see the controls, reach them easily, and thus minutely control the muscular response to the current. Talking to the client to get her response to the treatment provides essential feed-back to the therapist in accurate contraction work. Gently feeling the muscular activity in the area of treatment also provides extra guidance as to the position and the intensity of current needed.

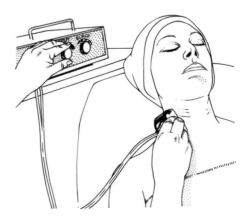

FACIAL ELECTRODE METHOD ON STERNOMASTOID MUSCLE

With all facial muscle contraction it is necessary to realize that a contraction will not be initiated unless a sufficient intensity of current is used, even if the position is accurate. So when correctly placed on a facial muscle, the intensity must be smoothly increased until a contraction comes about. If the intensity needed appears to be excessive, reduce it and check the likely reasons for lack of success. These are nearly always incorrect positioning, poor contact, incorrect control of the equipment, or poor skin preparation.

Routine of Facial Contraction

For a general preventative treatment, the application should commence on the sternomastoid muscles and progress via the platysma, masseter, zygomatic, risorius, orbicularis oris, levators of the lip, to the eye area and the orbicularis oculi sphincter, to conclude on the forehead, with the corrugator and frontalis muscles (if not contraindicated).

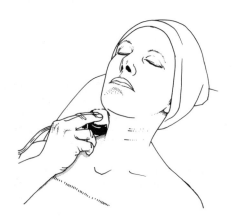 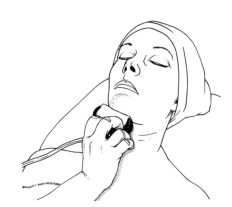

CONTRACTION ON THE PLATYSMA MUSCLE

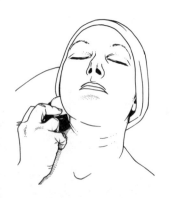 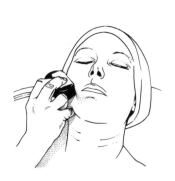 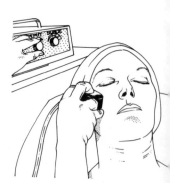

JAWLINE AREA AND
MASSETER MUSCLE

SUPERFICIAL CHEEK
MUSCLES

ORBICULARIS OCULI

Interferential Method of
Facial Exercise

Preparation

The fibre-covered rubber pads should be soaked briefly before the application, then wrung out carefully, and applied moist and warm on to the skin to avoid an uncomfortable treatment. The fibrous covering over the electrodes can be prevented from drying out and preventing a good contraction, by applying a small amount of glycerine over each point just prior to the application. A warm skin can dry out the protective fibrous covering over the points surprisingly quickly, thus spoiling the comfort and effectiveness of the treatment.

With this four-electrode arrangement, it is vital that all four electrodes on the movable pads should be firmly in contact with the skin to obtain a comfortable contraction. This is important with the facial exercise routine, where the pads have to be held moulded around an area, such as the jawline, and where all the electrode points might not be making contact. To avoid a sudden connection of the current, when the circuit is completed, perhaps unpleasantly at a higher level of intensity, the therapist should check for full connection as each new position is applied.

Any apparent need for high-current intensity to achieve muscular activity should also be investigated. Common causes for lack of response in interferential applications include, the electrodes being too dry, poor connections in the electrodes, leads etc. or unsatisfactory skin preparation with creams etc. remaining on the surface. Another common problem is incorrect control or application of the current, through unfamiliarity with the equipment. It is a wise step to check through the applicators, leads, performance of the machine etc. before commencing an interferential treatment, as it is a more involved application. This avoids a really effective and pleasant treatment being marred by poor presentation.

Application

The facial exercise routine commences at the chest, over the upper fibres of the pectoralis major muscles. The current can be applied at a constant frequency for 2–3 minutes, then changed to the 0–100 Hz rhythmically applied for the remainder of the exercise routine. The intensity is increased to a level sufficient to cause increased vascular and biological activity but without any visible spasmodic muscular contractions, and the position held for 30 seconds approximately. The pads are then changed to a diagonal placing which involves different parts of the muscles, and again held for 30 seconds. Actual visible contraction of the superficial facial muscles may be evident even on this frequency if the intensity level is allowed to become sufficiently high to initiate muscular response. Or if the client has a very slim face with little subcutaneous adipose tissue as padding, contractions occur at a very low level of intensity. Adjustments in the intensity control, and by careful positioning will avoid the treatment distorting the features or causing discomfort. For it is not necessary with the interferential method on the face for there to be any actual contraction visible on the surface, and in fact the treatment is *more effective and comfortable* if this does not occur. The client can feel the sensation of muscular activity, and the therapist can discern it through her hands and by conversation with the client, so it is not wrong to talk of contractions when getting guidance from the client on the effects of the application. What is important to avoid is distortion of the features, and discomfort, both of which occur surprisingly easily with any form of artificial stimulation of the facial muscles. This is due to both their minute size and the interlinking nature of their attachments. This is why it is almost impossible (and unnatural) to exercise muscles one at a time, independently, and hope for clear contractions without involvement of adjacent muscles.

With the interferential system (Method C), contractions are obtained using several electrodes mounted in pads (often called exercise pads) or by using specific applicators for different areas, i.e. eye skin applicators, neck and jaw straps, and full face masks.

The interferential system operates on the principle of providing medium frequencies, which increase biological activity within the tissues. If applied in sufficient quantity these are also capable, via *interference* between two slightly different frequencies, of initiating a muscular response.

For facial contractions the intensity or amount of current required to exercise the muscles is very small if the pads are accurately placed. On interferential equipment the level or scale of frequency required for facial work is normally indicated, as the apparatus also provides for full body therapy, and may also include facilities for galvanism. The frequency used for facial work increases the vascular circulation, and improves the general nutrition of the tissues, in addition to exercising the muscles in the area.

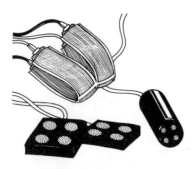

INTERFERENTIAL
METHOD APPLICATORS

The current, whose frequency is shown on a scale with a range covering 0-100 Hz (cycles per second), can be applied at a constant, selected frequency or can be made to vary rhythmically, gradually increasing from zero to 100 and then repeating. To determine the client's tolerance to the treatment, and to adjust her to the sensation, the frequency is applied on a constant (100 Hz) rather than rhythmical basis for the first few minutes of treatment. Getting the client used to the unusual sensation of interferential current takes a little while, as although pleasant it is very unusual, feeling like a running wave passing through the tissues. Whilst the client adjusts to this rippling sensation under the applicators, the therapist is able to use the opportunity to increase the intensity of current to a discernible level, and assess the client's response before progressing in the treatment. This adjustment period on the constant frequency is always necessary when applying the static applicators, such as the neck strap or face mask, but it is not so vital when using the movable pads or eye applicators, as the treatment area is so much smaller. Once clients are used to the treatment their anxiety over the sensation experienced disappears.

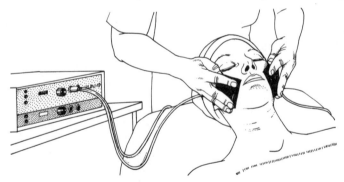

GENERAL FACIAL CONTRACTION

Facial Pads

For a general toning and tightening effect on the facial and neck areas, a pair of flat rubber pads are used, each being fitted with four electrodes arranged in a square. Each diagonally opposite pair of electrodes forms a circuit, this being the correct arrangement when using the interferential method. The main area of activity is directly beneath the pads, being most effective in the area where the current frequencies cross, central to the pads. The close proximity of the electrodes on the facial pads means that the effect of the current is a superficial one affecting only the muscles of facial expression and superficial tissues. So the effect is contained within the area of the facial pads, and does not cause unwanted side effects.

Normally the pads are applied symmetrically in pairs on each side of the neck and face, but they can be used singly to allow easier control of the equipment, if adjustments in current intensity are necessary. This gives the therapist a free hand to regulate the controls of the equipment. If over difficult areas, such as the jawline or forehead only one pad is used, the second pad must be placed safely out of contact (perhaps on the trolley) as it is still active if touched. This is because the pair of pads are attached by a linked set of leads to the apparatus, being designed to be used as a pair.

If the upper breast and sternum areas need particular attention, such as after childbirth and breast-feeding, these positions can be repeated right out to the shoulder areas, and returning on the same path, to link in again with the facial routine at the neck. At the neck the sterno-mastoid and platsyma muscles are treated, with the current intensity reduced if necessary. As the muscles become smaller in bulk, less intensity is required to bring about the correct level of activity. Again two positions are applied, first straight, then diagonal for 30 seconds each. The pads may be positioned in such a way that the face is not distorted due to over involvement of the depressor muscles of the lower lip.

The routine moves on to the jawline in the same manner, taking care to see that all the electrodes are in contact to avoid an unexpected surge of current as contact is made. Initially this area may be best handled by a student using only one pad in contact, placing the other in a safe place, and reducing the current intensity accordingly. This prevents client discomfort or anxiety being caused, whilst the operator gains proficiency in handling two pads in a difficult treatment area.

The treatment progresses to the face, where the current is reduced, and the pads are placed on the superficial cheek muscles so that comfortable levels of activity are achieved. The whole area is activated due to the proximity of the facial nerve, and the pads should be positioned so that the eye is not distorted. The position again changes to the diagonal to bring in all areas of the cheek, eyes and mouth by muscular connection.

The current is again reduced and the treatment concludes on the forehead, taking care over the contact of the electrodes on this bony and sensitive area. The intensity need only be increased to a level that brings about increased vascular activity in the area, to improve the skin circulation and texture. Strong muscular contractions would be particularly pointless and uncomfortable in this area, but circulation improvement is useful to prevent lines, wrinkles etc. forming. The forehead area may be contra-indicated in some individuals due to discomfort, so the therapists should use their own judgement based on the reactions observed, and by talking to the client for guidance.

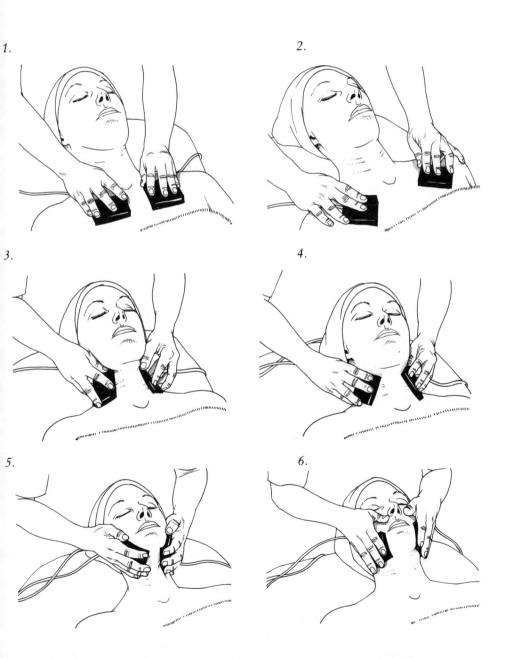

7.

8.

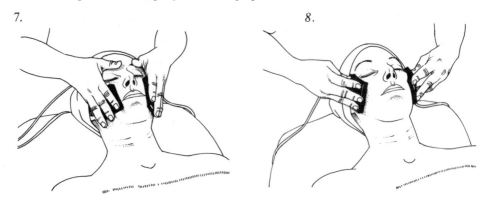

9.

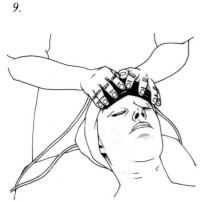

The whole facial exercise routine need not take any longer than a few minutes for all over-toning effects, with each area receiving just a minute or so of activity. If certain areas of the face or neck need more concentrated attention, this can be adjusted within the application, or a static applicator used, such as the jaw strap. Tiny, delicate areas such as the eyes and lips can be treated superficially and in a localized fashion with the small electrode pads designed specifically for the task. These can be used after the general application, or independently, if only these areas need attention. Instances might be bags under the eyes on a young client, or fine lines around the mouth in the slightly older client, from poorly fitting dentures.

FACE LIFTING ELECTRODES

Chin and Jaw Strap

The jaw line applicator is formed of two viscose sponge sleeves of different lengths, which are attached in the middle. The shorter length sleeve is applied around the neck, the longer one around the jawline and cheeks. Firm attachment is made via velcro strips behind the neck and over the head. Accompanying plate electrodes, of metal or flexible conductive rubber, are inserted into the four openings of the moistened sleeves and connected to the terminals of the four conductor cables in such a way that the two conductors of the same colour — red or white — are diagonally opposite. This follows the four-electrode principle already seen 'built into' the facial exercise pads.

The area of treatment lies between the four plate electrodes, and it can be increased or reduced by shifting the position of the plate electrodes. If the orbicularis oculi (eye) and frontalis/temporalis (temples) areas seem to be becoming over-involved in the treatment, which is after all primarily for the jawline improvement, the upper plate can be pushed well down within the sleeves, until they are at lower rather than upper cheek level. Likewise, adjustment can be made with the neck area. These effects may not be noticed until the treatment has progressed sufficiently to be able to see a definite reaction. However, in the initial preparation it is sensible to consider the general position of the active plates, and any effect they are likely to have on any area that lies between the electrodes. Pushing the plates well down within the sleeves provides a smaller treatment area, as nothing that lies beyond the electrodes is specifically involved in the contraction. Any activity then seen is caused by muscular connection, due to the interlinking nature of the facial muscles and their common nervous connection.

So careful positioning of the straps and plates can eliminate areas from the treatment. Excessive fillings in the teeth likely to cause toothache and discomfort in treatment can be adjusted for, so that they do not contra-indicate the routine. The neck strap can be positioned well down the throat, and the jawline straps angled well back, so that they are attached by their velcro strips at the back of the head rather than on the top.

The chin/jaw strap is assembled swiftly after wringing out the sponge sleeve in hot water. The diagonally opposed leads are attached to the electrode plates, which are pushed into the sleeves, making sure they are fully covered by the sponge. The client lifts her head, the strap is attached round the neck fairly tightly to form a good contact, with the velcro strips holding in the leads. The upper sleeve is then attached firmly via its strips, and adjustments made for the position of the plate electrodes. The connecting leads are placed comfortably either side of the client's head, and the contact of the sponge sleeve checked.

Getting the tightness of the chin strap correct takes practice, but if it is not forming a good contact the contractions will not occur comfortably and at a low intensity. When practising the application of this element of treatment in training, it is only necessary to exert a gentle pulling action on the straps at the back of the head and neck, when the treatment is initially in progress, to see what a

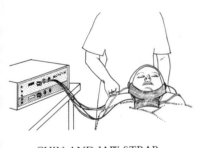

CHIN AND JAW STRAP

difference to the contraction levels firm skin contact can make. Loose connections and the sponge sleeves being insufficiently damp are the main problems encountered in ineffective treatment.

As the entire area within the four electrodes is going to receive an identical duration of treatment, the overall period of treatment need not be prolonged, as the activity produced is so specific. Initially 5–10 minutes overall will be sufficient, progressing to 15–20 minutes treatment over a planned programme of biological activity and stimulating therapy. Improvements in the firmness of the jawline and neck skin are apparent to the client even after one application, especially if the area has been very neglected. Ideally the special neck treatment should be applied 2–3 times a week, either independently or with a half-hour routine including throat packs, masks, brush massage and manual massage with oils or regenerating creams, etc.

The jawline treatment commences on the constant frequencey (100 Hz) for 5 minutes, increasing the intensity gradually until the client becomes adjusted to the sensation. The application is altered to the rhythmical form of the 0–100 frequency, and after a short period of adjustment to the sensation, the intensity may again be increased if necessary, to reach a really active level of muscular contraction in the neck and jawline area. This second stage may be applied for 10–15 minutes.

Any distortion of the features or discomfort experienced can be adjusted for in the initial 5 minute period, but even then there will be instances when the current needs reducing or increasing during the more active period of the treatment. So the therapist must stay in contact with her client and be alert to changes occurring. Gentle reassurance through conversation and the therapist's continuing presence help to make this initially unnerving treatment effective. The therapist is also able in this way, to get guidance from her client regarding discomfort, possible increases in intensity, etc., which will help in the overall effectiveness of the application. For however beneficial the treatment may be, if it has been uncomfortable the client may be frightened off receiving the regular, progressive treatment which is so necessary. In some instances, particularly with a nervous or mature individual, it is worth completing the first treatment at an almost ineffective level, so that she will persevere with the course. Therapists need to use their own discretion about how to progress the treatment to the level required. Extra care is worth the effort.

Facial Mask Electrode

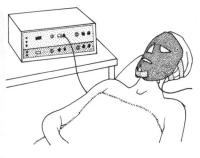

To provide for full facial muscle contraction, a special face mask applicator is available, which has the electrodes built in around the inside borders. This is made of soft rubber, and is applied damp over a very moist sheet of special mask paper to form a good contact. The mask is attached below the chin and behind the head, with firm contact again being necessary. This makes it a difficult treatment to apply in terms of client acceptance, as a feeling of claustrophobia can occur when the mask is working actively. It is a very successful form of muscle contraction, providing continuous, even contractions to the facial muscles, for an identical period of time, but it should only be presented when the client has great trust in her therapist.

The application is very similar to that of the jawline strap, with a need for good connection below the chin, and behind the head. The connection lead in this case is built into the mask, and still operates on the interferential principle, but in this case does not require setting up, making for easier application. The treatment is applied at a frequency of 100 Hz, immediately on to the rhythmical form, with the intensity gradually increased from zero to a comfortable level of activity for the 15–20 minutes of treatment. There is no need for the initial period of adjustment in this case on 100 Hz constant, as the electrodes of the facial mask are arranged in sets of fours, placed so that the areas of treatment are very superficial in effect. The increased vascular activity produced is very effective on slack skin tone, atrophic skin, and post-acne scarring, in addition to the normal benefits of muscular contraction.

Eye Applicator

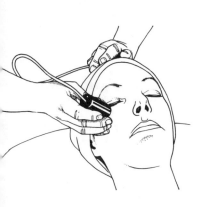

A cylindrical hand held applicator is available for treatment of small localized areas, where only a superficial action is required to achieve results. The four built-in electrodes are so closely placed on the head of this unit, that only a minute area is stimulated at a time. This is ideal for working around the eye on the fibres of the orbicularis oculi muscles, and around the mouth on the orbicularis oris muscle. These muscles are sphincter (circular) muscles which have no bony attachments, but attach into the fascia of other muscles, so being very movable and liable to change. Swelling (oedema), discoloration from poor circulation and tiredness under the eyes, and crêpy skin on the lids can all be helped by interferential treatment. This is accomplished by sending the interferential current superficially through the skin and muscle tissue of the area, the intensity being kept low enough to avoid winking. The eyes feel rested and refreshed, and look clearer after treatment. This is due to the circulation improvement which can help clear blood-shot eyes if caused by simple tiredness. Really blood-shot eyes should be medically checked before treatment, just in case the condition is due to eye strain or is associated with poor physical health.

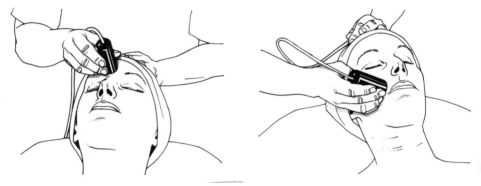

SMALL FOUR-POINT ELECTRODE

Fine downward lines on the upper lip, wrinkles at the sides of the mouth, laughter lines etc., can all be treated in a localized fashion. Frown lines between the brows also respond very well to specific treatment, the etched appearance of the line being eased by the muscular and circulatory response in the tissues.

The applicator is used on the 100 Hz frequency, immediately on the rhymical system, for a few minutes over each area requiring treatment. The fibrous covered electrodes must be well moistened before the application, and must all be in contact with the skin to achieve a contraction. To avoid the tiny electrodes from drying out, the applicator head should be well soaked before the application, and glycerine applied over the covering of the electrodes just prior to treatment. A more delicate approach to using the small applicator is needed, so that small areas can be activated without involving unwanted muscular reactions. Careful positioning makes it possible to eventually exercise all the different parts of the muscles under treatment. The areas of the face that are particularly affected by normal facial expressions causing flexure lines benefit especially from this localized form of treatment.

GENERAL POINTS ON ALL METHODS OF MUSCLE CONTRACTION

The passive exercise operates most efficiently, and with the least client discomfort, if applied around the outer borders of the face. In this way, pain from metal fillings or dentures, and areas of sensitivity on the upper cheeks may be avoided. By following the main facial nerve branches, most areas of the face can be stimulated into action, from outer border positions. If specific treatment is required, on the lip area (for downward lines, caused by weight loss or poorly fitting dentures), the intensity must be carefully regulated to prevent discomfort and subsequent toothache.

Accurate application of all forms of passive muscle contraction is based on the same principles of:

1   knowledge of the position of the muscles of facial expression;

2   the nerve supply, and motor points of the muscles;

3   careful intensity control to facilitate comfortable contractions, and knowledge of the effects of faradic type and interferential currents;

4   skilful client handling and verbal exchange, to determine the sensations experienced, and level of the client's tolerance, and so prevent discomfort and anxiety.

Chapter 11

Treatment of the Arms and Legs (Manicure, Pedicure and Massage)

TREATMENT OF NAILS

Structure and Function of Nails

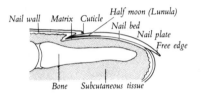

Nail wall   Matrix   Cuticle   Half moon (Lunula) Nail bed Nail plate Free edge

Bone   Subcutaneous tissue

The main rôle of nails is a protective one, safeguarding the sensitive areas of the distal portions of the fingers and toes. They are formed from hard keratinous cells, which are termed onychin, and have a very low moisture content (7–12%), and infinitesimal fat content. The matrix area of the nail is the most important part and is composed of polygonal cells, similar to the Malpighian layer of the skin. The opaque appearance of the nail is due to the presence of keratohyaline, and the white area (lanula) at the base of the nail is thought to be noticeable due to the change of light refraction at this stage or growth, and acts as a dividing level.

Sensitivity and Growth of Nails

The nail rests directly on a layer of prickle cells, overlying an extremely vascular papillary layer containing numerous sensitive nerves, and this explains the pain involved if a nail is injured by pressure, or by being torn below the flesh line. The nail bed and plate grow outwards together, so any injury to the matrix (cell-forming area) may affect both the nail and bed. The rate of growth in nails appears to be fairly constant, at 1 inch in 8 months, with no real difference between the sexes. However, the rate of wear, breakage etc., due to work conditions, health and dirt, varies considerably, and will be the area in which the facial specialist can give the maximum assistance. Eliminating or reducing nail abuse, by sensible guidance, plus a programme of professional treatments, will achieve excellent results.

General good health, a balanced diet, and exposure to sunlight does appear to improve the condition of nails, but some clients will always have frail nails, due to genetic factors, and then control of the condition to prevent further deterioration is the task of the therapist.

Recognition of Nail Diseases, Imperfections and Cosmetic Conditions

Many physical conditions affect the nails, among them psoriasis, rheumatism, eczema, and heart complaints, which may show themselves as transverse ridges, furrows, pitting etc. Any condition of the nails which appears unusual to the beauty specialist should be directed for medical attention, if it is not known to be connected with a systemic state (such as a client who suffers from rheumatism or anaemia).

Primary evidence of a fungus infection may be noticed first within the manicure treatment situation, and may avoid the severe state of decomposition, which can occur if the condition is left unchecked. The fungus may appear at the base of the nail, or at the side, and take the form of a yellow, dull looking patch, in its early stages, whilst in its more active stages the nail may have disintegrated, become messy, inflamed, or decomposed in appearance. Cosmetic treatment of the nails is not permissible, due to the cross-infection risks and interference with the necessary medical care the nails will receive. The manicurist/beautician must safeguard herself and her other clients in this instance, and refrain from treating even the unaffected nails of the hands or feet. Infectious conditions such as athlete's foot, warts, and inflammatory conditions such as onychia, also fall into this category (see Chapter 5, Skin Disorders), and must not be treated on any account.

Minor Imperfections, and Cosmetic Conditions

Fragile nails, brittle or splitting free edges, grooving and white spots, can be controlled and improved by cosmetic treatment and preventative measures.

Injury to the matrix area of the nail causes disturbances which may show as white spots (leukonychia puncta) or irregularities such as grooving. The incidence of both is higher in women than in men, and may be caused by careless use of manicure tools, orange sticks etc., around the base of the cuticle, over the matrix area.

Fragile nails require a preventative and protective programme to minimize de-fatting and de-hydrating elements in their daily care, and to give them additional substance against the wear and tear of daily life. Caustic preparations, washing up liquids, detergents, scouring powders etc., should never be allowed to touch the nails, and rubber gloves (with inner cotton gloves if necessary) should be worn for all abrasive tasks. The professional treatment and home care will be planned to keep the nails supple, replacing lost moisture and fats daily with nail creams, and protecting the nails with specialized adherent enamels, and strengtheners, at all times. A moderate nail length should be aimed at, as, if the nails are over-long, the task will be impossible.

Purpose of the Manicure

Regular and attentive care is necessary if immaculate nails are to be maintained and this point must be stressed to the client. As the nails are so vital to a groomed appearance, the manicure treatment is one of the most popular services that a facial specialist can offer, often in combination with facial applications. The actual procedure frees the cuticle and nail wall from the nail plate, thus avoiding the risk of hangnail formation, caused by the stretched skin splitting away from the nail plate. The outline of the nail is kept smooth, infection is prevented, and only gentle treatment is required to maintain an attractive cosmetic appearance. Regular professional attention will also prevent minor nail damage, splits tears, fragile tips etc., remaining undetected and becoming more serious in nature.

Repairs and remedial home treatment can be introduced immediately to prevent a worsening of the existing condition. The protective rôle of the enamel and adherent strengthening preparations should be exploited to the full, reinforced by an extensive programme of nourishing and emollient creams applied nightly. The addition of massage into the manicure routine increases the skin improvement, delays ageing tendencies such as wrinkled or discoloured skin, and controls areas of senile pigmentation in the mature client, by the addition of bleaching preparations in the massage medium.

The Manicure Treatment: Small Equipment and Preparations Required

The manicure treatment unit should be mobile, attractive in its presentation, and contain all items of small equipment and cosmetic preparations required in the sequence. A small table with an arm rest, bowls for soaking and waste items is the ideal working area, and gives the beauty specialist full control over the hands and arms of her client. Manicure trolleys and baskets are also in common use, due to their convenience of size, but as they lack arm supports, separate provision must be made by utilizing a small cushion. The hand should be raised to the right level for fast efficient work, whilst maintaining client comfort. The manicure unit requires the following items:

Nail and cuticle clippers and cuticle knife.

Emery boards and metal files (everlasting diamond type).

Nail brush, buffer, orange sticks and 2 small bowls for soaking.

Covered cotton-wool containers, waste bowls and container for orange sticks. (All containers should ideally be of stainless steel, but may also be of glass or metal, but not plastic.)

Manicure and hand massage preparations, and nail repair kit.

MANICURE PREPARATIONS REQUIRED AND THEIR USE

Enamel Removers and Solvents

These must be capable of fast, efficient removal, without excessive dehydrating and defatting effects on the nail plate and surrounding skin tissue. Acetone or ethyl acetate is the normal base, with the addition of a small quantity of oil. The natural oil and moisture lost should be replaced by application of a nail cream or oil.

Cuticle Cream

An emollient product designed to soften and nourish the cuticle, and make the nail plate more flexible, by replacing the natural fats lost in daily life through exposure to detergents and drying elements. The nail cream or oil should be used within the manicure sequence, and as a nightly home care treatment, applied to the cuticle area.

Cuticle Remover

The purpose of the cuticle remover is to loosen and release cuticle skin cells, which adhere to the nail plate, without discomfort to the client. The fluid-based alkaline lotion is applied to the previously softened skin with tipped orange sticks, and the procedure accomplishes a swift removal of dead and adhering tissue from the nail plate. Potassium hydroxide is the active ingredient in many cuticle removers, and it also acts as a nail bleach removing nicotine stains effectively.

Paste Polish

Paste polish is used in combination with the buffer application if the nails are ridged, uneven or simply lifeless. If coloured enamel is not required, or if it is a male manicure, paste polish gives a healthy sheen to the nails and does help to minimize evident ridges. Many paste polishes are composed of jeweller's paste formed into a cosmetic preparation for convenience of application. The friction formed during the buffing process increases blood circulation in the nail bed, and the paste polish itself has only a slight abrasive action, with no nourishing elements.

Nail White Pencil

Used to whiten the free edge if clear enamel is preferred, and to give a clean light appearance to discoloured nails. The pencil usually requires wetting before application, and is composed of a soap base with the addition of white pigment. The popularity of white pencils has declined as high-gloss enamels have become increasingly popular. They should always be available for clients who like to appear well groomed but, due to the nature of their work, they are restricted to colourless enamel or simply a buffed sheen, i.e. medical staff, cooks, etc.

Nail Enamels (Polish or Varnish)

The high-gloss cellulose lacquer or enamel so popular at present must have several qualities if its application is to be successful. It must be easy to apply, with an even consistency and colour, and should be fast-drying. It should not be harmful to the nails or stain them with the pigment resins, and it must be long-lasting and highly protective in action. The cosmetic improvement in appearance is well known, and relies on a high lustre and attractive colour choice.

Base Coats

The base coat has a special rôle in the manicure, prolonging the life of the enamel, preventing pigment from the enamel staining the nails, and minimizing irregularities in the nail plate. Its additional effect of increasing the protective element of the enamel application is enhanced by careful choice of the most suitable type of base coat for the existing nail condition.

Nail Strengtheners

Plastic-based nail strengtheners help to prevent the nail becoming fragile or over-brittle. The preparation is used prior to the base coat, or may be incorporated into it for convenience by some manufacturers. Care must be taken to prevent the lotion from touching the cuticle skin, otherwise dryness will result.

Hand Lotions and Creams

The additional exposure to caustic and detergent items that the hands suffer makes regular application of a hand cream an essential item, if the skin is to remain intact and smooth. Within the manicure routine a water-based emulsion type hand cream should be used to permit fast absorption and prevent stickiness. For nightly application and hand/arm massage during the treatment an emollient nourishing cream should be employed, to allow free movement over the area of massage, and to increase the benefit gained from the circulation improvement. The hand lotions are glycerine based, formed into a jelly substance by gum tragacanth, and enhanced by colour and perfume. Hand creams have a similar consistency to a general skin cream, and should have similar quantities of nutrient ingredients, fine texture, and fast absorption to increase circulation and prevent moisture loss.

Nail Repair Kit

The repair kit consists of a liquid nail cement which is used in conjunction with fibrous tissues and solvent, to effect repairs of split and torn nails and reinforcement of fragile tips.

THE MANICURE

Procedure

The manicure position should be prepared with sterile small equipment, cuticle clippers, knives, commodities required etc., and clean towels or disposable paper for preference. The enamel should be the correct consistency, with clean bottle necks, and an adequate choice of cream and pearlized colours available. Regular maintenance of tools and preparations, enamels etc., will avoid cross-infection, and allow fast and efficient work to progress.

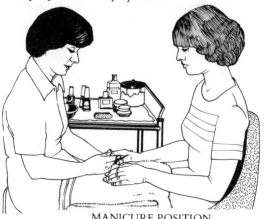

MANICURE POSITION

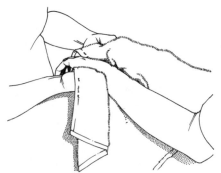

DRYING THE HAND

1   The client's hands should be inspected for nail or skin infections, and then wiped over with a soapy antiseptic solution, and dried thoroughly.

2   All the enamel should be removed in a decisive manner with a pad of cotton-wool soaked in remover. Deep shades or thickly applied enamel require the remover pad to be permitted to soak into the nails for a couple of seconds before it is withdrawn. Final removal should be accomplished with a tipped orange stick, soaked in remover, to clean up the cuticle and free edge.

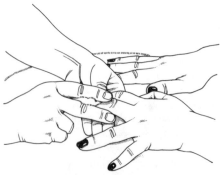

REMOVING ENAMEL

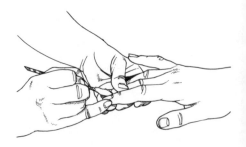

CLEANING AROUND CUTICLES

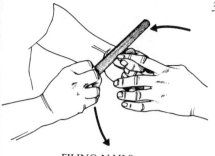

FILING NAILS

3 The nails of the right hand are then filed with an emery board, from side to centre, to form a curve. The sides should not be filed away, but left to give support to the nail. The free edges should then be bevelled to avoid the nail layers splitting apart. Light strokes must be used, with the fine side of the emery board. The free edge should then be checked for smoothness, by running the thumb pad across it to feel for snags, which may need extra attention.

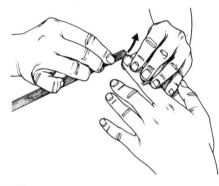

BEVELLING

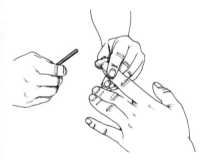

Various corrections can be made at this stage, to improve nail appearance, or flatter the hand shape, the shape created being emphasized by the colour and manner in which the nail enamel is applied later in the sequence.

CHECKING THE EDGES FOR SMOOTHNESS

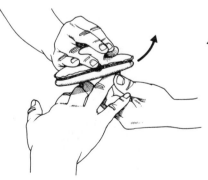

4 Paste polish, if required, is applied at this point by spreading a minute quantity onto each nail, and buffing it off with the chamois covered buffer. The buffer may also be used without the polish for stimulation but, due to the difficulty of sterilizing and cleaning the chamois covering the buffer, this step is often omitted from the sequence.

BUFFING

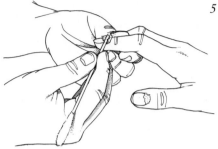

APPLYING CUTICLE CREAM

5   Massage cuticle cream into the nail fold and surrounding skin, with firm rhythmical pressure, covering the first joints and complete nail area. Place the right hand in sufficient warm soapy water to cover the nails and first joints of the fingers only, to prevent accidents occurring if the client moves her hand unconsciously.

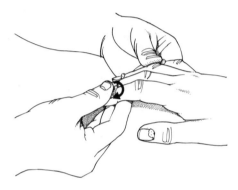

RHYTHMICAL MASSAGE ON CUTICLES

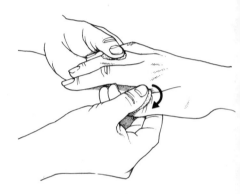

RHYMICAL MASSAGE ON JOINTS

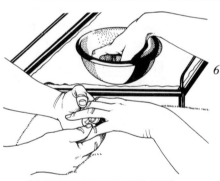

SOAKING THE FINGER TIPS

6   Repeat steps 3–5 on the left hand. If only one bowl is used, the right hand must be removed and dried prior to placing the left hand to soak.

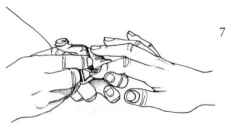

FLOODING THE CUTICLES

7   The right hand is placed in position on the hand rest in preparation for the cuticle work. The cuticles are flooded with cuticle remover, and first a tipped orange stick is used to free the cuticle from its nail plate attachment, and push it gently back to form a smooth nail fold. Keeping the area damp, the cuticle knife may be used for stubborn areas or neglected nails.

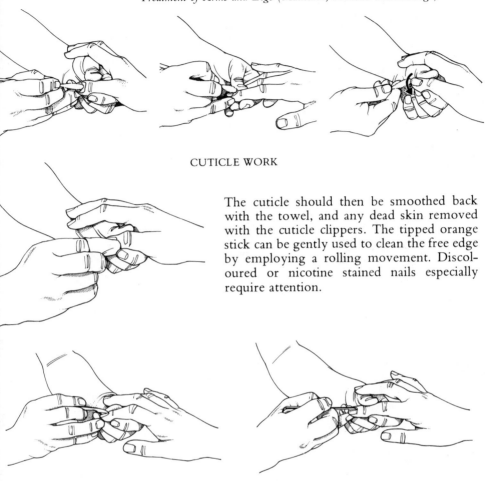

CUTICLE WORK

The cuticle should then be smoothed back with the towel, and any dead skin removed with the cuticle clippers. The tipped orange stick can be gently used to clean the free edge by employing a rolling movement. Discoloured or nicotine stained nails especially require attention.

CUTICLE KNIFE WORK

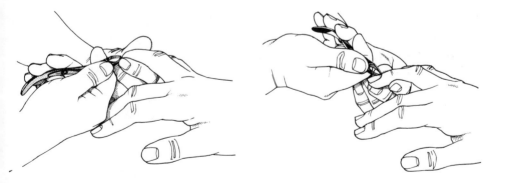

CUTICLE CLIPPERS

8   Remove and dry the left hand and complete step (7).

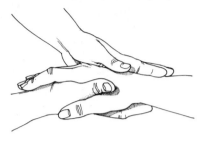

HAND LOTION

9   Apply hand lotion to both hands, smoothing it in with effleurage strokes. The hand massage routine, if required, is applied at this stage of the treatment.

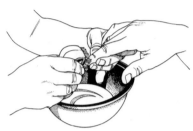

BRUSHING

10   Both hands should have the nails and free edges gently brushed, to release nail layers, loose skin etc., and then the final inspection and tidying up can be completed. Separated nail edges should be bevelled, and any excess dead skin carefully clipped away. The hands may then be thoroughly dried.

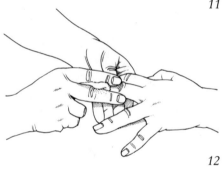

SQUEAKING

11   Enamel remover is then used to remove all soap, oil, cream, etc. from the nails in preparation for the base coat. Long nails should also have the free edge cleaned with a tipped orange stick.

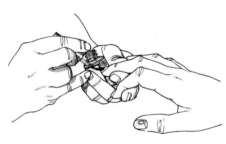

ENAMEL APPLICATION

12   Apply nail strengthener if required, and base coat to both hands, working from left to right to prevent smudging. Light fast strokes should be used to achieve even coverage. The correct base coat should be used for the nail condition, i.e. strong or fragile, and for the enamel chosen previously, i.e. cream or pearlized.

13   Apply the coloured enamel in a similar manner. To achieve sufficient colour density three coats of enamel may be required with pale shades, otherwise two coats of the deeper colours should be sufficient. A top coat may be used on cream enamels only, to add lustre, and is not required on pearl enamel. Four coats,

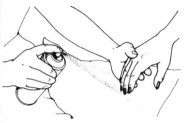

SPRAY APPLICATION

including base, colour, and top coat, is the maximum that should be applied, otherwise the nails will not dry in a reasonable time. Quick-drying spray may be used to set the surface of the nails, taking care to spray away from the client or furniture.

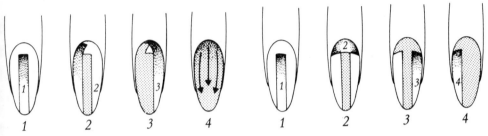

BASE COAT APPLICATION   ENAMEL APPLICATION

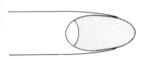

HALF MOON APPLICATION

Some clients prefer to leave the half-moon area of their nails unpainted, and the enamel strokes for this require practise to accomplish an even half-moon area. A slightly different method of application is necessary to prevent flooding of the cuticles. Any enamel which touches the nail wall during the application should be removed before proceeding to the next nail, as once set it is impossible to remove cleanly without leaving a smudgy appearance. Neglected, untidy cuticles also make even enamelling difficult, but excessive clipping should be avoided, and the client encouraged to gradually improve the cuticle appearance by regularly smoothing back the skin, and by nightly application of cuticle cream, to reinforce the regular professional manicure given. Once cuticles have been excessively clipped, they build up an unattractive ridge-like appearance around the nail, and have to continue to be clipped to reduce the hard skin formed. New clients should be encouraged to rely on regular nail attention and professional care to maintain attractive hands, rather than over-zealous treatment applied erratically.

Home Care and Sales of Manicure Preparations

As in facial therapy, nail treatments need to be reinforced by regular care and awareness of elements that will aggravate the nail condition. Fragile nails need the constant protection of strengtheners, base coat, enamel etc., if a reasonable length and appearance is to be maintained, rubber gloves should be worn for all jobs involving detergents etc., and even with all these precautions only a moderate length will be possible. All nails benefit from nightly applications of cuticle cream massaged in, over the enamel, to the nail fold and surrounding skin. Soaking very brittle nails in warm oil is also a very effective treatment, and should prevent the nails being severed at the flesh line.

It is to the manicurist's advantage to see that if her client wishes to change her nail enamel between professional visits, she does so with quality products which will not be detrimental to the nail condition. The client should be encouraged to purchase cuticle cream, strengthener, base coat, enamel and remover from the salon; in this way all her home care needs are fulfilled. If the manicure is performed swiftly, efficiently, and achieves good results, it becomes an essential part of the client's professional grooming needs.

Organization of the Manicure

Care of the Trolley

For the manicurist to be able to accomplish an efficient manicure in the brief time commercially available, it is necessary that her manicure trolley or tray is at all times clean and ready for use. This calls for a neat method of work, replacing items in their correct position, during or at the conclusion of each manicure accomplished. Waste bowls should be emptied after each client, and the tools used, washed, dried thoroughly and sterilized. This may be by cold water methods such as Instrument Dettol, or Savlon, or within a vapour cabinet (formaldehyde) or ultra-violet sterilizer. All these methods rely on the items placed within them being very clean if the sterilization is to be really effective. Then the tools need only be in the sterilization system for 20 minutes, before they may be used again, which is important in a busy salon. Instant sterilization can be achieved by wiping the tools over carefully with surgical spirit, which like the other methods prevents the growth of microorganisms which could cause infection.

Care over sterilization is very important in the manicure routine, as the skin may be open around the walls of the cuticle, and infection could easily result from careless procedures in the cuticle work.

All the items on the trolley should look clean and attractive to the client, who normally has them in view and would notice tatty and dirty preparations.

Client presentation is important in manicure work, as it is a grooming service, and likely to be requested on impulse, if the manicurist and her trolley look appealing. The client is tempted to treat herself, and an extra service is gained, which with luck may become a regular part of her grooming routine.

The manicure products should be ready for immediate use, and items such as enamels, base coats etc. must be of the correct flowing consistency to achieve a fast-setting enamel application. The enamel should flow easily without hesitation back into the bottle from the brush, not form into blobs around the brush. The consistency of new enamels should be noted and if products thicken, they can be brought back to the correct consistency by the addition of a few drops of solvent, applied from an orange stick. Once corrected, the enamel needs to be shaken, and left, ideally for 24 hours, but even 20 minutes can be helpful in improving the flow of the application. For this reason it is a wise step to consult the client about her choice of enamel colour before the manicure commences, so providing an opportunity to check that the item is a good consistency, and if not, making some last minute improvement. Enamels thicken through exposure to air, either caused during the actual application, or through air entering the bottle if tops are left messy. Apart from making it even more difficult to achieve a perfect finish in the enamel application, messy bottle tops spoil the consistency of expensive enamels very quickly. With the need to nave a good selection of cream and pearlized enamels for the clients choice, any additional expense because of poor product care, makes the manicure less able to be operated as a profitable service.

Bottle tops can be cleaned very swiftly using the soiled pads used to remove the client's coloured enamel. The top then forms a good contact with the bottle, and air cannot enter, thus keeping the enamel in perfect working consistency.

The temperature in the clinic can alter the flow of the enamel, making it less easy to apply. Cold temperatures thicken the enamel, whilst high temperatures make the products more fluid and less easy to control. Extremes in climate can make products react strangely, so therapists working in hot areas should try to find a cool storage place for their enamels and base coats.

Manicurists should get into a regular habit of cleaning, stocking up, and checking their trolleys and the preparations and tools required. When the trolley is not in use it can be protected with a polythene cover to prevent dust etc. soiling it. If trolleys are always left ready for use in this way in the commercial clinic, it avoids a scramble to prepare or find all the necessary items when a manicure is requested unexpectedly. Even the tipped orange sticks may be prepared beforehand, an air-tight container should be available to store them so that they do not become soiled. This saves time on the actual routine.

Organization of the Manicure Routine

The main criticism of manicurists being unable to accomplish a good manicure in the time available, 20–30 minutes on average, is mainly due to poor preparation and organization of the routine. With practice it is perfectly possible to accomplish an excellent manicure in 20 minutes, if the client has regular treatment, as the cuticle work will not be protracted. Really neglected hands and nails should be dealt with on a treatment basis, in conjunction with arm massage, paraffin wax applications etc. In this way the treatment remains profitable, and is of more benefit to the client. A simple explanation to the client regarding the state of the nails can help to decide priorities in treatment and is a more professional way to approach the work.

Really neglected nails may benefit from more work on the cuticles to ease them back gradually, and nail enamel would then not be necessary, making the routine possible within the normal time. Fragile nails may need extra protection in the form of nail patches, for which extra time would be allowed if it could not be included in the normal manicure. Discussion with the client about the time needed, and the cost involved, before the manicure commences, avoids client dissatisfaction and places the client in a position where she can decide her priorities.

NAIL REPAIRS

Badly chipped, torn or fragile nails can be improved by three different methods of nail repair: tissue method, nail builder, and artificial nails. None of the methods permits normal heavy daily usage, so the applications are most suitable for clients who do not engage in house work or continuous heavy work. As an instant repair for a special occasion, for career women or professional models, they are all very satisfactory.

Tissue and Nail Cement Repairs

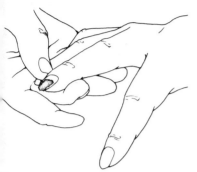

MEASURING A NAIL PATCH

The manicure is completed up to the stage prior to the base coat application. The tear or fragile tip is inspected, and the special tissue torn into a suitable shape to effect the repair. The torn edge permits a stronger repair, and when saturated with nail cement will adhere to the nail plate firmly. The excess tissue protruding over the free edge should be gently smoothed out to fit the nail contour, by pushing it under the free edge with an orange stick. With the client's palm upwards, any rough areas should be smoothed down and extra cement applied if required. When the adhesive has set the manicure can be concluded in the normal way, with a coloured enamel of sufficient depth of tone to allow a good diguise. With care, the repair should last for a considerable time while the nail is growing. A well-applied repair can be reinforced on subsequent manicures by first removing the enamel carefully, and reapplying nail cement over the nail plate and free edge areas, without disturbing the actual repair.

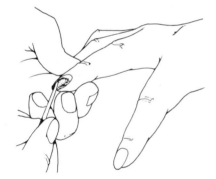

SMOOTHING OUT THE TISSUE

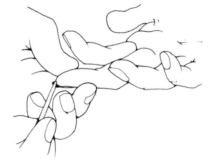

FINISHING THE FREE EDGE

ARTIFICIAL NAILS AND SEMI-PERMANENT NAIL EXTENSIONS

Treatments which improve the look and length of the nails have always been popular with women; hence the consistent sales of artificial nails for home application. Until recent times however, the techniques of nail additions, and nail extension, have seldom provided a sufficiently durable result for it to be a really successful salon application. Now all

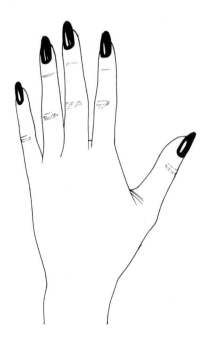

this has changed, due to improvements in the materials used to form the new nails or free edge extensions. These treatments now provide a very popular and profitable area of business for the beauty industry.

Nail additions come in several forms. Artificial nails are made of plastic materials, which can be shaped to fit varying nail shapes. These are designed to be applied for temporary periods, and can be removed and reapplied. Then there are nail extension, which can be used to lengthen the natural nails, either the whole set, or more normally, used as a repair on a broken nail, to match it back to the rest of the nails. These extensions stay in place, until the natural nail has grown sufficiently for the extension to be unnecessary. Durability will depend on the wear and tear the nails receive in daily life. Lastly there are semi-permanent nail additions, where plastic type compounds are applied to cover the clients nails entirely, and extend their natural length. These nails are very tough and durable, and can be shaped with abrasive drills into the desired shape, to suit the clients hand. In-filling is required periodically, around the cuticle area, to keep the nail addition undetectable, making for regular salon attendance and trade in the clinic. The nail additions can be used as a total transformation, or as a nail repair on an individual nail. Like the nail extensions, the nail additions grow out with the natural nail, but because of the toughness of the materials used, and the total coverage of the natural nail, they cannot be removed so readily. So clients need to be advised of the long term nature of their application, and the need for regular maintenance to keep the appearance immaculate.

So the therapist must advise her client regarding the best nail addition for her purpose, by considering its purpose. Temporary nails, perhaps for an evening event, may be satisfactorily fulfilled by plastic 'false' nails, allowing the client to return to her normal length nail the next day. Clients who are able to, and choose to, keep their nails long, may find the nail extensions best for repairing a broken nail. The fact that they are able to retain long nails, being some guidance to the therapist, as to the normal wear they are likely to receive. For the client who is unable to grow her nails long, due to an inherent weakness, but desires this length, nail additions may prove the best solution. A client with weak nails should not however be encouraged to look upon nail additions as a remedy to her weak nails, only as an alternative camouflage of the problem. The only things likely to improve poor nails are better health or a better diet and a reduction in the wear and tear on the nails from daily chores.

Artificial Nails

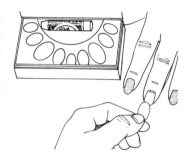

Artificial nails are now available in a wide range of shapes and lengths to suit most hands and so excessive pre-shaping is unnecessary. The chosen nails should be placed to soak while the manicure proceeds to just prior to the base coat stage. The cuticles must be free, the nails clean, and any filing of the false nails completed prior to the adhesive application. Adhesive is then applied to either false or real nails, or both, and the nails placed firmly in position, with the lower edge just beneath the loosened cuticle. The nails can be held in place by small flat rubber straps or bandage if necessary, but modern adhesives effect such a fast bond that this is really unnecessary, and just firm pressure held for a few seconds is sufficient.

The initial shaping of a set of nails should be carefully undertaken, first by making the choice of nails closest to the client's natural nails, although longer, and then by continual checking to determine that the correct curve and shape of nail is being produced by the filing. Once completed, the attachment of a shaped set of nails is an easy task and can be combined quickly into the manicure procedure, adding additional revenue to the sequence. Clients should be advised to wear artificial nails for short periods only, as continual pressure on the matrix area of the nail can cause transverse nail ridging to appear some time after their use.

Nail Extensions

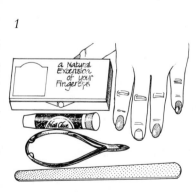

Nail extensions are a new system of false fingernails that rely on a new type of tough fast-acting glue, to bond a plastic shape firmly to the edge of the natural nail. The result both looks and feels like the natural nail, and it files and grows out just the same as the natural nail. The popularity of nail extensions has expanded the clinic's range of manicure services, and it can be a very profitable treatment. Achieving success relies on skill in shaping the extensions to match closely the shape and curve of the natural nails. This, as with the complete false nails, makes the difference between an undetectable result or an obvious one.

Nail extensions take about 10 minutes for repairing an individual nail, and about one hour for the complete set where the client requires extra length, perhaps due to nail weakness when she is unable to grow the nails to the desired length naturally. Charges for the service should be based on the clinic's normal charge-per-hour basis, depending on the member of staff concerned, and the usual rate at which they are costed. With practice it can become a simple addition to the manicuring skills.

Application

1   The nail to be extended is inspected and the nail enamel removed. It needs lengthening to match the length of the other nails. The nail shapes, glue, clippers and file are assembled.

2   The nail shape is selected for size and tested against the natural nail for the correct fit.

3   Nail clippers are used to shape the inner edge of the false nail shape, to achieve an exact fit with the edge of the broken nail.

4   The false nail is held in place against the natural nail—with edges abutting—and adhesives applied at the join. Care should be taken to ensure the nail shape is in line with the natural nail, not angled over, as with the instant bond the new glue makes, it is easy to have it wrongly positioned, and fixed in that position, very quickly.

5   The false nail is trimmed to the required length with nail clippers, and then filed into shape with an emery board.

6   More adhesive is applied to fill in any gaps and ensure the false and natural nails are attached all round the edges.

2

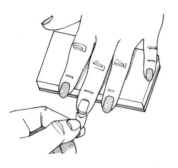

3

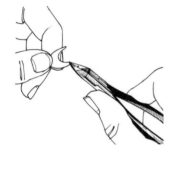

4

5

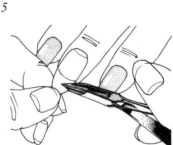

6

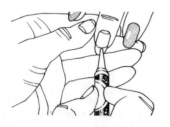

7

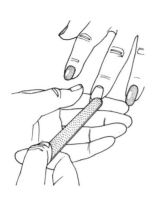

7   The glue dries in a few seconds, and is rock hard in half a minute, when the joint can be filed smooth with the emery board, to make the join indetectable.

8   The treated nail looks natural and feels like a real nail. Because of the differences in colour between a plastic free edge and natural nail, it is more successful in most cases to enamel the nails, so that the extension blends in with the other nails.

9   The final touch of enamel shows off the nails to advantage and makes it impossible to detect the nail extension.

8

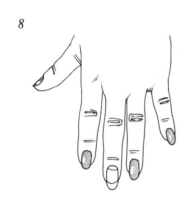

9

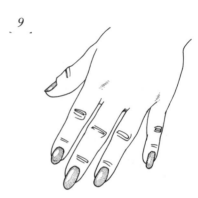

Semi-Permanent Nail Additions/Sculpture

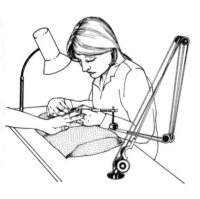

WORKING POSITION

To offer the nail addition service within a clinic requires increased expenditure on equipment and commodities etc. but the popularity of this grooming and fashion-linked service makes the investment well worthwhile. Very little space is needed to offer the nail addition service: simply a working table position to provide a base for the abrasive drill used to shape the nail compound. The entire nail addition system makes a neat and attractive unit, but because of the noise involved when the drill is in use, it should be sited away from the more restful clinic treatments.

Different systems of nail additions vary in their application methods, and the manufacturer's instructions should be followed exactly to achieve good results. Most nail addition treatments are applied to lengthen and transform the client's complete set of nails or to infill the nails around the cuticles, so this is a grooming rather than a repair service. It has to be a comparatively expensive service because of the time taken in applying the semi-permanent nails, from around 1½–2 hours. However, it is proving to be a service that women are willing to pay for to maintain their nail appearance.

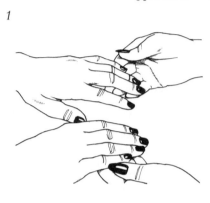

Application

1   Examine the client's nails and discuss the preferred shape and length of semi-permanent nails required. Advise the client about the treatment, its cost, duration, and its need to be maintained by in-filling every three to four weeks. Make sure the client understands the long-term nature of the nail additions, and that they cannot be removed, but must grow out with the natural nails, if the client decides to return to her natural nail length. They can naturally be filed down, if they prove to be too long for the client in her daily life. Many clients unused to long nails will find them hard to get used to, and for that reason it is worth discussing this point with the client in the initial examination. A moderate-length, nicely shaped nail is usually the most successful on clients who have daily chores to cope with. Younger women, with only their appearance to worry about, enjoy really long nails, and have no trouble maintaining them.

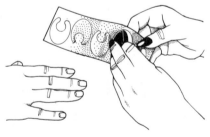

2   A drill with an abrasive head is run lightly over the nail to slightly roughen the surface, and provide a 'key' to which the built on nail will firmly adhere.

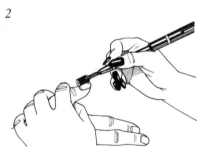

3   A horseshoe shape of adhesive-backed silver foil is fitted around the nail to be treated. This forms a guard on to which the artificial one will be built over the natural nail's tip.

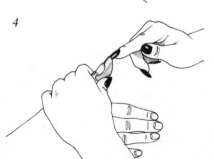

4   Check that the foil is fitting closely under the nail tip and is fixed firmly around the cuticle, without overlapping on to the nail at the sides.

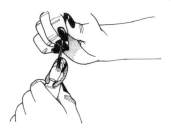

5   The false nail is created with a mixture of powder and liquid, which bonds together to form a clear and strong plastic type compound. It is painted on with a brush which is alternately dipped in the powder and liquid, and applied on to the nail.

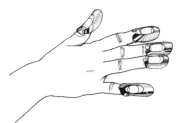

6   The powder and liquid is worked up the nail from the cuticle, over the tip and on to the guard in an approximate nail shape. The other nails are treated in the same way, and the compound is left for a few minutes to set hard. The second hand can be treated in this period, saving time.

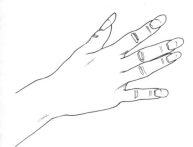

7   When the compound is set, the silver foil is removed from the fingers. The artificial nails will look bulky and uneven because they have been built up considerably to allow for shaping.

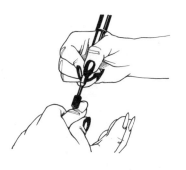

8   Shaping is done with the abrasive headed drill. This is worked lightly over the surface of the artificial nail to flatten and smooth down the compound, to follow the nails natural contours and around the nail tip to provide the required length and shape. Skill in shaping the nails can make the difference between a really natural looking nail, or a very false one, so this stage is worth taking care over.

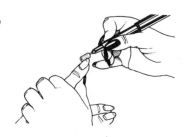

9   Paint the artificial nail with a special vegetable oil before buffing with a smooth textured head fitted on to the drill. Work all over the artificial nail with the buffer to produce a smooth and natural-looking surface.

10

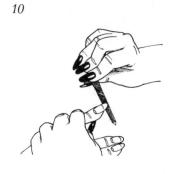

10   Give the finishing touches to each artificial nail with a diamond surface nail file. Emery boards would have no effect on the tough material used to create the nail.

11   Paint the nails in the usual way. The artificial nails respond just like natural ones to nail enamel and remover, though as the nails are so tough, the enamel lasts much longer and does not chip.

12   The new nails are firmly seated on the natural nails and as they grow so a gap will be left at the cuticle. This can be easily filled in by the salon, on an average of every three to four weeks.

11

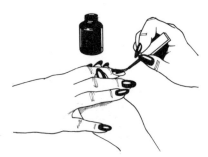

12

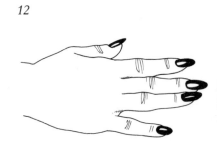

PEDICURE

Pedicure is simply manicure of the feet, but there are slight differences necessary due to the pressures imposed on the feet and their necessity to function in an enclosed space.

The feet should be inspected prior to treatment, for skin or nail infections or conditions requiring chiropody. The purpose of the pedicure should be explained to the client, to prevent misunderstanding as to the scope of the therapist's rôle in foot treatments. Ingrowing nails, corns and excessive callouses should be referred to the chiropodist for attention, and this in turn should develop a reciprocal arrangement for maintenance of foot and nail appearance between those visits.

Implements and Preparations

In addition to the standard manicure preparation and tools, a foot bowl (large enough for both feet), nail clippers, hoof stick, large metal file, hard-skin remover, foot powder, soap solution, and antiseptic are required. Disposable paper is the most hygienic method of drying the feet, and protecting working areas. A foot stool and a low seat are also desirable depending on the location of the treatment. Folded paper tissues may be placed in readiness.

The pedicure treatment may be applied in combination with hair-drying and facial therapy, or given independently, and often includes a foot and leg massage for maximum benefit. The routine may have to be adapted, due to the client's position, but the basic routine remains a guide to the elements required and an efficient sequence.

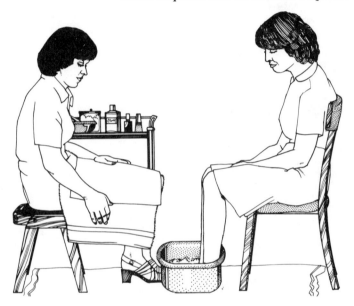

GENERAL PEDICURE POSITION

Contra-indications to Pedicure

The following conditions prohibit pedicure treatment: (1) athlete's foot. (2) nail fungi. (3) onychia (inflammation of the nail fold). (4) eczema. (5) warts (common warts and verrucas). (See Chapter 5, Skin Diseases.)

Pedicure Procedure

1 Prepare all equipment and commodities. Advise client to remove shoes, tights, etc., and provide a gown and a chair if necessary. Place the client in a comfortable position, and put the feet to soak in the foot bowl, half-filled with warm, soapy disinfectant solution. If soaking is not possible, wipe the feet over with a large swab or cotton-wool soaked in antiseptic solution.

2 Remove the right foot from the bowl, dry
thoroughly on disposable paper, remove the
enamel, and cut the nails straight across with
only a gentle curve at the sides to prevent
ingrowing toe nails. File the nails with the metal
file to remove rough edges.

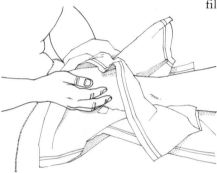

DRYING THE FOOT

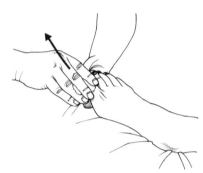

REMOVING ENAMEL

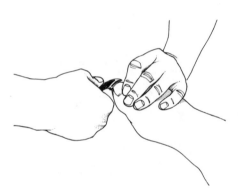

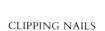

CLIPPING NAILS

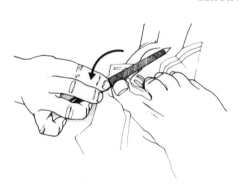

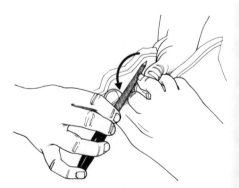

FILING NAILS

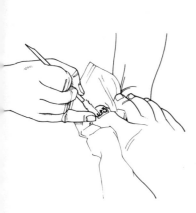

3 Remove the adhering cuticle skin with a combined use of cuticle remover, a tipped orange stick, cuticle knife and rubber hoof stick. Keep the cuticle area moist with cuticle remover to assist the removal of the skin adhering to the nail plate. Alternate the use of the tools as necessary. Smooth back the nail wall to see progress, and if necessary, remove dead and loose skin with cuticle clippers. Thorough work with the cuticle tools and cuticle remover should minimize the need to clip the cuticle skin, thus reducing the risk of infection developing. Any open area of skin, caused by clipping, or overzealous cuticle work, is a possible site for nail fungus to develop, so care should be taken to keep the skin intact wherever possible.

CUTICLE WORK

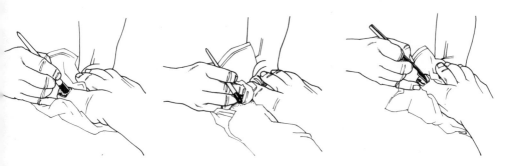

CUTICLE CLIPPERS

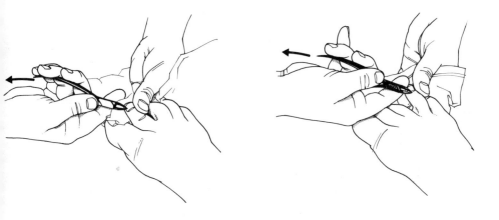

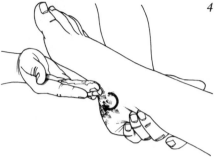

4   Apply hard skin remover if necessary to the heel and toe pad areas, working vigorously to remove callouses, with massage friction movements over the area. This section of the routine should not be prolonged within a normal pedicure treatment. The foot can then be briefly replaced in the bowl and steps 2–4 completed on the left foot.

HARD SKIN REMOVER

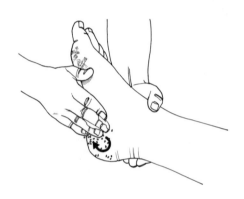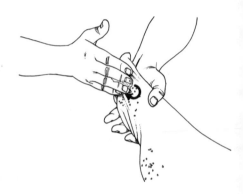

5   Remove first the right foot then the left from the bowl, dry them, push the bowl out of the working area to prevent accidents, and place the feet on either a covered foot stool, or one on the floor (on a clean dry piece of paper) and the other on your lap protected with tissue.

FOOT MASSAGE

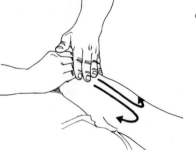

6   Using a suitable foot lotion or powder, massage the feet using effleurage and friction movements. Within the pedicure sequence 2 minutes is adequate, but if foot and leg massage is to be combined into the routine, it is applied at this stage, using a nourishing cream medium. The leg should be well supported to prevent tension occurring in the muscles. Apply powder generously between the toes to help prevent infection.

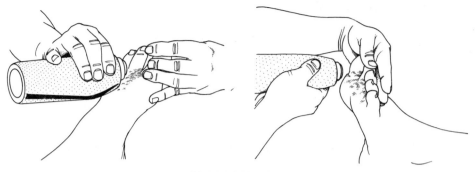

FOOT POWDER

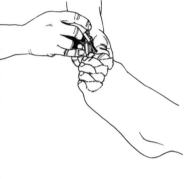

7 Place rolled cotton-wool pieces between the toes of the left foot, clean the nails with remover, and apply base coat, and enamel if desired, in the same manner as in the manicure. Complete steps 6–7 on the right foot.

8 When the enamel is completely dry, remove the cotton-wool, check that the feet are dry and comfortable, and allow the client to replace tights and shoes, offering assistance if required.

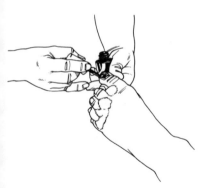

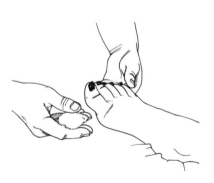

ENAMEL APPLICATION

Complete the treatment by putting equipment and working area in order, sterilize tools, and clean and check all preparations used. Enamels may require attention if they have become too thick and a small quantity of solvent may be added to improve their consistency. Hand-washing completes the routine, to minimize the risk of infection both to other clients and to the therapist.

ANATOMY OF THE
HANDS AND FOREARMS

Anatomically the wrist and hand is a very complex part of the body, containing 29 bones, and a large number of joints and small muscles which permit an enormous range of movements. A knowledge of the superficial muscles only is required, and the antagonistic nature of the flexor and extensor muscles should be understood.

Bones of the Hand

Carpals or Bones of the Wrist

There are 8 bones of irregular size, which fit closely together, held in position by ligaments. The bones articulate with each other, permitting slight movement, and also give attachment to the small muscles of the hand that move the fingers. They are:

Hamate. Triquetrum.
Capitate. Pisiform.
Trapezoid. Lunate.
Trapezium. Scaphoid.

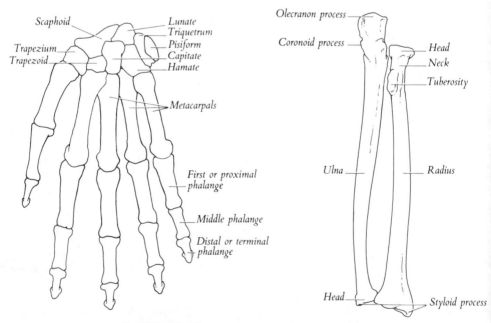

BONES OF THE HAND WRIST AND FOREARM

Metacarpals	The palm of the hand is made up of 5 long bones the proximal ends (those closest to the centre of the body) of which articulate with the wrist bone. The distal ends articulate with the phalanges (finger bones).
Phalanges	The 14 finger bones are also long bones, with 3 to each finger and 2 to the thumb.

Bones of the Forearm

Radius. Ulna.
The ulna bone articulates with the humerus of the upper arm, and only flexion and extension movements are possible.

Muscles of the Forearm

Many of the muscles of the forearm and wrist are termed according to their action, forming two groups, flexors and extensors (flexion and extension actions). Many of the small muscles co-ordinate to form similar actions, so a representative sample of each type of muscle and its action provides sufficient knowledge for the beauty specialist's application of massage in the area.

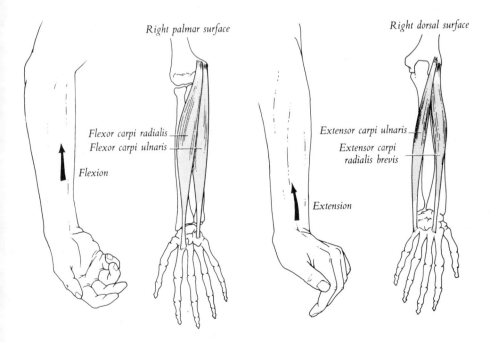

Right palmar surface

Flexor carpi radialis
Flexor carpi ulnaris

Flexion

Right dorsal surface

Extensor carpi ulnaris
Extensor carpi radialis brevis

Extension

LOWER ARM FLEXORS AND EXTENSORS

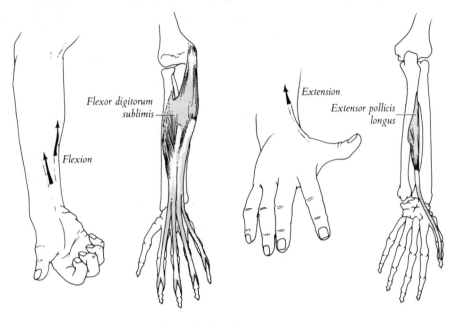

Flexion

Flexor digitorum sublimis

Extension

Extensor pollicis longus

LOWER ARM DIGITAL MUSCLES

Superficial Muscles of the Forearm and Wrist

Muscles	Action
Flexor Muscles	
Flexor carpi radialis	Flexion of wrist and
Flexor carpi ulnaris	elbow joint
Flexor digitorum sublimus	Flexion of fingers, wrist and elbow.
Flexor pollicus longus	Flexion of the thumb.
Extensor Muscles	
Extensor carpi radialis brevis	Extension of wrist and
Extensor carpi ulnaris	elbow joint.
Extensor digitorum communis	Extension of fingers and elbow joint.
Extensor pollicus longus	Extension of the thumb.
Rotation and Flexion Muscles	
Pronator teres	Pronates the forearm (rotation).
Brachioradialis	Flexes the elbow joint.

It can be clearly seen that the flexor and extensor muscles work in opposition to each other, as antagonistics, and that their names relate both to their bone attachments and the action created.

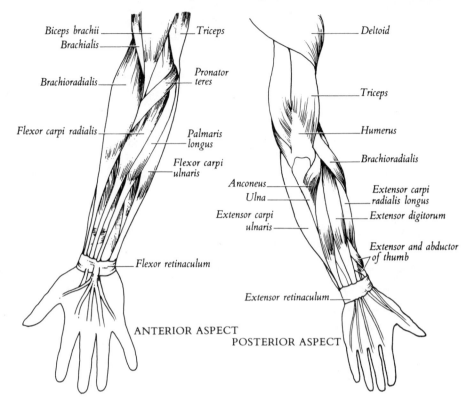

Biceps brachii
Brachialis
Brachioradialis
Flexor carpi radialis
Triceps
Pronator teres
Palmaris longus
Flexor carpi ulnaris
Flexor retinaculum
ANTERIOR ASPECT

Deltoid
Triceps
Humerus
Brachioradialis
Anconeus
Ulna
Extensor carpi ulnaris
Extensor carpi radialis longus
Extensor digitorum
Extensor and abductor of thumb
Extensor retinaculum
POSTERIOR ASPECT

SUPERFICIAL MUSCLES OF THE FOREARM

ANATOMY OF THE FOOT, ANKLE AND LOWER LEG

The foot achieves its function of movement and support by means of a large number of closely articulating small bones formed into arches by their ligament connections to combine strength and flexibility.

Bones of the Foot

There are 26 bones of the foot and consist of:

Tarsal or Ankle Bones   Seven in number: talus and calcaneum, which take the weight of the body, transferred from the tibia bone of the lower leg.
Navicular.
Medial, intermediate, lateral cuneiforms and the cuboid, which form a row of bones.

Metatarsal Bones   Five in number, forming the greater part of the length of the foot.

Phalanges   There are 14 phalanges of the toes and follow the
same pattern as the fingers, with three to the small
toes, and two to the big toe.

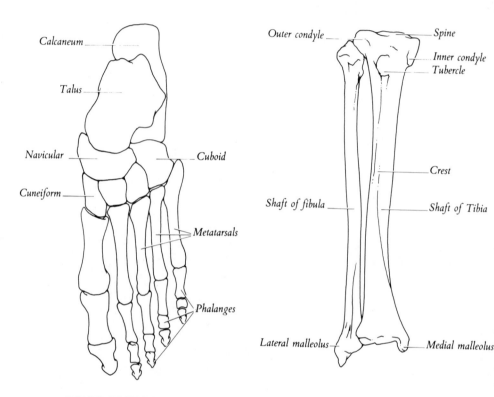

BONES OF THE FOOT

BONES OF THE LOWER LEG

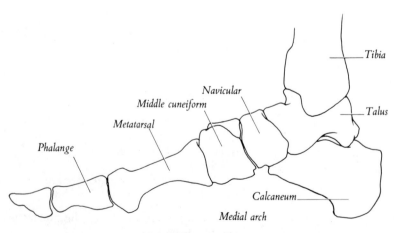

SIDE VIEW OF FOOT

ARCHES OF THE FOOT

There are four arches of the foot; two longitudinal, running down the foot, the lateral and medial, and two transverse arches.

Medial Longitudinal Arch (long main arch of the foot)

The main arch of the foot, placed on the inner aspect, involves the area from the calcaneum bone to the proximal ends of the three inner metatarsal bones; both these bony areas being in contact with the floor, like the ends of a bridge. The suspended area of the arch is formed by the talus, the navicular and the three cuneiform bones, the strength and resilience being gained from the small strong muscles and ligaments which surround the joints.

Lateral Longitudinal Arch (shorter arch)

Situated on the outside (lateral) aspect of the foot, extending from the calcaneum to the cuboid and proximal ends of the outer metatarsal bones.

Transverse Arch

The transverse arch of the foot lies under the metatarsal bones, extending from the outer to the inner aspect of the foot.

BONES OF THE LOWER LEG

The tibia bone bears all the weight and articulates with the femur of the upper leg. The fibula has no connection with the femur. The knee joint permits only limited movement, and is a hinge-type joint. The floating sesamoid-type bone, the patella of the knee joint, is encapsulated within the quadriceps tendon of the thigh muscles, and the patellar ligament, and it supports the action of the thigh muscles.

MUSCLES OF THE LOWER LEG, ANKLE AND FOOT

Many of the flexion and extension muscles produce inversion (inward) and eversion (outwards) movements of the foot, through the tendon attachment to the small bones of the foot and ankle. The longitudinal and transverse arches of the feet, which permit a full range of active movements, are supported by the distal ends of the lower leg muscles, particularly the tibialis posterior muscle.

Muscles of the Lower Leg and Ankle	Action
Gastrocnemius (superficial)	Plantar flexion of foot and flexion of the knee.
Soleus (deep) mainly under the Gastrocnemius	Plantar flexion of the foot.
Peroneus longus (superficial)	Plantar flexion and eversion of the foot.
Peroneus brevis (deep)	Plantar flexion and eversion of the foot.
Tibialis anterior (superficial) Tibialis posterior	Inversion of the foot and support of the long arch of the foot.
Extensor digitorum longus Extensor hallucis longus	Flexion and eversion of the foot and toe extension.
Flexor digitorum longus	Plantar flexion and inversion of the foot.

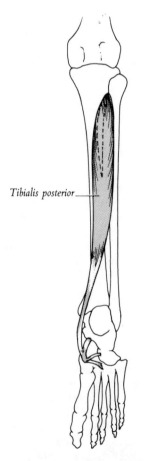

Tibialis posterior

TIBIALIS POSTERIOR

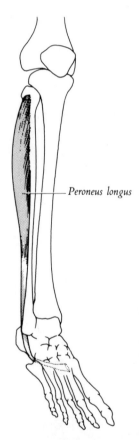

Peroneus longus

PERONEUS LONGUS

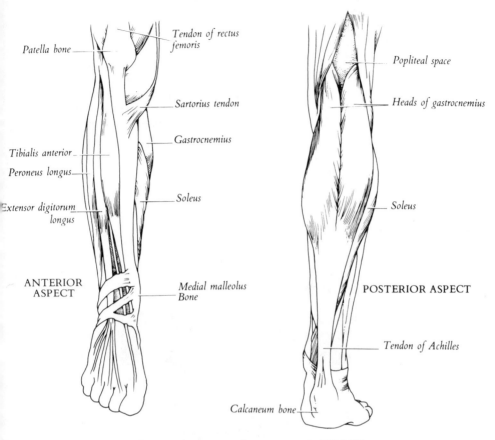

Patella bone

Tendon of rectus femoris

Sartorius tendon

Gastrocnemius

Tibialis anterior

Peroneus longus

Soleus

Extensor digitorum longus

ANTERIOR ASPECT

Medial malleolus Bone

Popliteal space

Heads of gastrocnemius

Soleus

POSTERIOR ASPECT

Tendon of Achilles

Calcaneum bone

SUPERFICIAL MUSCLES OF THE LOWER LEG

Small Muscles of the Foot

The small muscles of the foot are concerned with maintaining and supporting the longitudinal and transverse arches. The muscles include the interossi and lumbricale groups, and together with fatty and fascia connective tissue form the soft-cushioned nature of the sole of the foot.

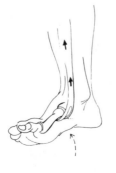

Inversion Movement
Tibialis anterior muscle
Tibia bone (long)
Medial cuneiform bone (short)
Metatarsal bone (short)

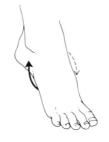

Eversion Movement
Peroneus longus muscle
Fibula bone (long)
Metatarsal bone (short)
Ankle joint (hinge)
Medial cuneiform bone (short)

HAND AND ARM
MASSAGE

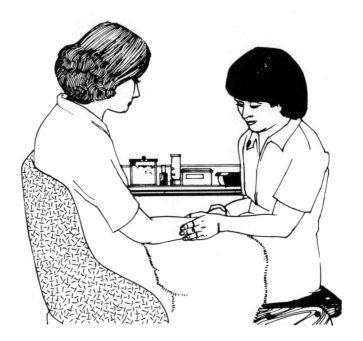

The purpose of the massage is to improve skin texture and appearance by the increase of surface circulation and application of nourishing cosmetic massage preparations. Special bleaching or nourishing and regenerating products may be employed for special effect, or a simple oil or talcum medium may be used. The item chosen must permit massage over an extended area, i.e. 10 minutes per arm, and so should not have a fast absorption rate, unlike the preparations advised for home use, where this is a desirable feature. To gain maximum benefit from the treatment the client's arm should be well supported, either on pillows, or arm rests, to prevent muscle tension and permit full relaxation of the entire arm. The client's clothing must be protected and, if the style of the dress makes disrobing necessary, a gown with loose sleeves or sleeveless should be offered to the client. If the treatment is combined with manicure, preparation for both items must be completed prior to commencement to avoid disturbance.

The manicure routine is completed up to the pre-base coat stage of the sequence, with the cuticle work completed on both hands. The pillow or arm rest may then be used to bring the arm into the correct working position.

SEQUENCE OF THE ARM MASSAGE

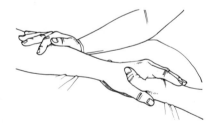

1 The massage preparation is applied with effleurage strokes over the entire arm area. The movement then increases in pressure as a preparation for further petrissage strokes. The elbow, forearm and hand should become relaxed, before progressing to further movements. Repeat 10–15 times approx.

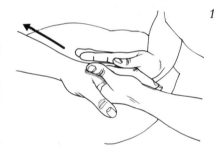

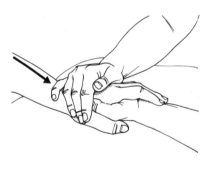

EFFLEURAGE

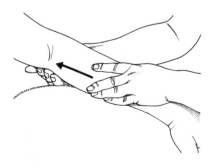

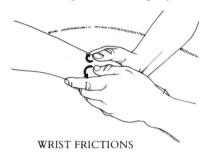

WRIST FRICTIONS

2   Friction movements around the wrist, working with the thumbs in firm rotaries, to increase circulation and prevent stiffness in the area.

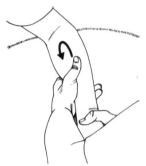

PETRISSAGE ON FOREARM

3   Petrissage movements on the muscles of the lower arm, flexor carpi ulnaris and radialis, brachioradialis and palmaris longus. The pressure should be upwards, and adjusted to the bulk of the muscles under treatment. Effleurage must be used to link the sequence, by returning the hand to the wrist, prior to repetition of the pressure movement.

4   Link effleurage over entire forearm and hand, to re-establish muscle relaxation, repeat 10–15 times.

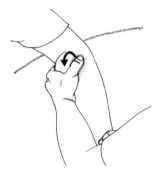

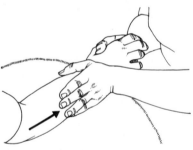

LINK EFFLEURAGE

5   Friction movements around the elbow joint, with the hands either working alternately, one hand supporting the elbow, the other applying massage to the area, or with both hands working together.

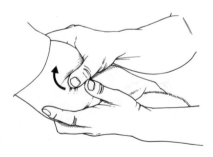

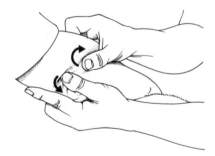

ELBOW FRICTIONS

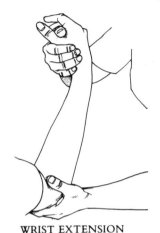

WRIST EXTENSION

6 With the elbow retained in a supporting position, the arm is then lifted into an upright position, and the wrist is rotated into its fullest extension, to stretch the ligaments and muscle attachments of the hand and wrist. The hand should be rotated fully to the left and right, with relaxation in between to prevent discomfort. The interchange of blood and tissue fluids created by the pumping effect of the tendons and ligaments on the joints and surrounding area promotes supple and attractive hands, whilst delaying stiffness and enlargement of joints. 3–4 rotations to the left and right, approx.

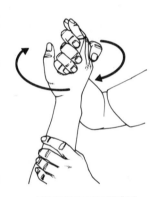 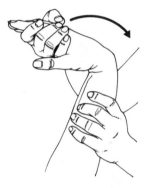 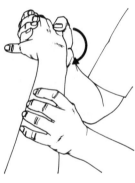

WRIST ROTATION

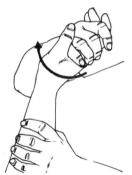 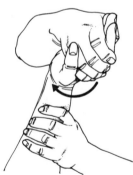

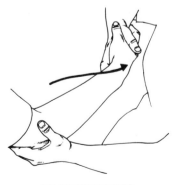

RE-POSITIONING

7 Return the arm to the pillow support, palm upwards, and work with firm rotary kneading petrissage movements over the metacarpal area of the palm. Work with the thumbs from the distal to proximal ends of the bones, returning with effleurage strokes. Repeat 6–10 times, approx.

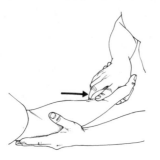

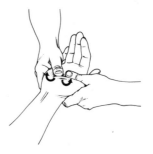

KNEADING ON THE PALM

8   Turn the hand over and apply brisk frictions upwards between the tendons of the fingers and thumb, towards the wrist, returning with effleurage strokes. The thumbs work, and the fingers support the hand to prevent discomfort, and provide a base for the pressure movement to be applied correctly. Repeat 3 times on each set of tendons.

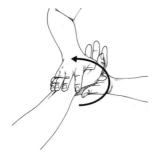

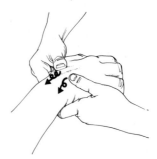

TURNING HAND OVER   FRICTIONS BETWEEN TENDONS

9   The movement progresses to scissor-like frictions, performed by the fingers, under the wrist area. The client's wrist is encompassed by the therapist's hands and the movement is briskly applied, to improve circulation in the joint area.

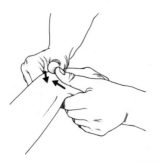

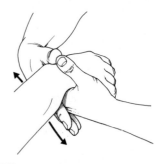

SCISSOR FRICTIONS

10 Link effleurage over the entire arm, alternately applied with right and left hands. Support of the client's arm is maintained throughout. Repeat 10–12 times.

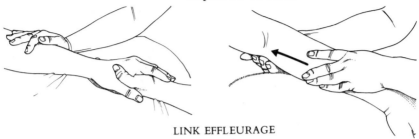

LINK EFFLEURAGE

11 Petrissage movements applied on proximal to distal joints of the phalanges of each finger and thumb, working with even pressure in a rhythmical manner. The hands work alternately, supporting the hand and applying the joint kneading movements.

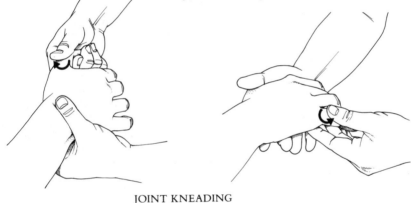

JOINT KNEADING

12 A brisk rolling movement performed with the client's hand held between the therapist's hands, with the thumbs linking through the

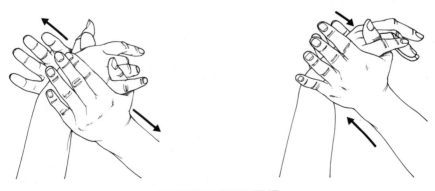

ROLLING MOVEMENT

little finger and thumb, to permit a fast stimulating movement. The circulation stimulation improves skin colour and general functioning, helping to prevent chilblain formation on the fingers in the winter months.

13 Effleurage stroking movements conclude the massage routine, working slowly and evenly over the elbow, forearm, wrist and hand, finishing at the finger tips.

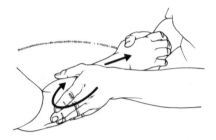

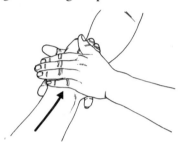

CONCLUDING EFFLEURAGE

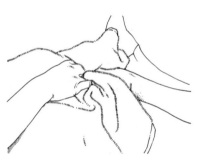

FINAL CREAM REMOVAL

Any remaining oil, cream, etc., should be removed, first with paper tissues or a towel followed by a tonic application to ensure thorough removal. The sequence may be concluded with a dusting of perfumed talcum if desired, to prevent stickiness, particularly in warm weather. The routine is performed on the other arm, and then the remainder of the manicure is completed, if combined, omitting the hand lotion application. A final check should be made to ensure no greasy areas remain at the end of the complete treatment, especially around the elbow area.

FOOT AND LEG MASSAGE

Preparation

The massage may be given independently, or combined with the pedicure, where it is applied on completion of the cuticle work, prior to the enamel application. Ensure that the client is comfortable, with relaxed muscles, regardless of the position in which the massage is to be applied, i.e. prone or in a sitting position. The ideal position for the treatment is with the client in a fairly high armchair and the operator on a lower stool, permitting free movement of the arms and enabling the client's lower limbs to be constantly supported.

The massage may be accomplished with talcum powder or cream, depending on the time of year, and the condition of the feet and legs. In hot weather and for feet that perspire freely, a dusting of powder is refreshing for the client and more agreeable for the therapist. When the temperature is cold or the feet and legs show a dry and scaly skin, oil or cream will be more beneficial.

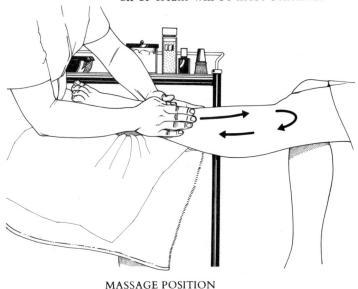

MASSAGE POSITION

Method. Sequence of Movements

1 Superficial stroking (effleurage) over the entire foot and leg area, repeated until the muscles become relaxed.

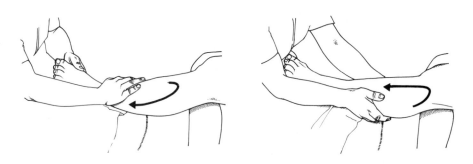

EFFLEURAGE

2   Superficial stroking over the upper surface of the foot, one hand supporting, one working, alternately, from the ankle to the toes.

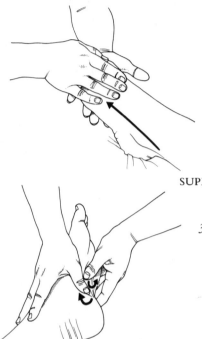

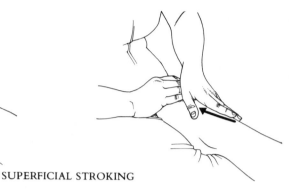

SUPERFICIAL STROKING

3   Thumb kneading (petrissage) over the medial arch of the foot, forming firm rotary movements, progressing from the ankle to the phalanges. The movement returns with a superficial stroke, and the fingers rest lightly on the upper surface of the foot. Repeat 3–4 times.

KNEADING ON THE MEDIAL ARCH

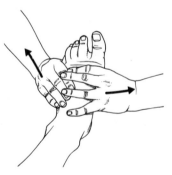

4   Petrissage movement over the phalange joints, with the hands enclosing the area, thumbs in firm contact, fingers overlapping. The movement commences under the metatarsals, with the thumbs exerting firm pressure under the ball of the foot, the toes are pressed firmly but smoothly downwards to their fullest extension, Superficial stroking links and returns the movement, for 4 repeats.

TOE EXTENSION

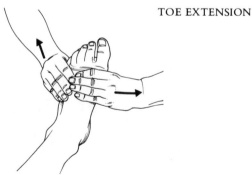

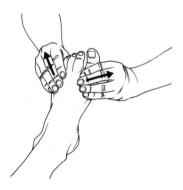

5   Deep kneading over the medial arch of the foot, accomplished with the thumb pad of the therapist's hand, working in firm rotaries, from the heel to the toes. The foot is supported, and so a true petrissage action is achieved.

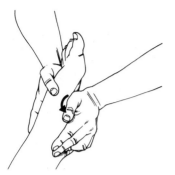

DEEP KNEADING OVER MEDIAL ARCH

6   Digital stroking around the malleolus, commencing at the toes, with index fingers together, and thumbs crossed. The movement progresses with firm pressure to the ankle, the hands divide and return with a superficial stroke to the toes, outside borders of the hands in contact. Repeat 6 times.

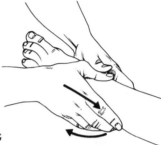

DIGITAL STROKING

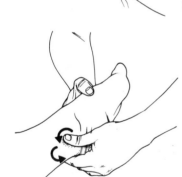

7   Alternate kneading and stroking on the Achilles tendon of the gastrocnemius muscle, with the foot and leg well supported, and both hands working. Firm rotaries are performed with the thumbs either side of the tendon and the fingers link the movement with relaxing effleurage strokes. Repeat 6 times.

KNEADING OF ACHILLES TENDON

8   Superficial stroking over the entire area to re-establish relaxation. Repeat 6–8 times approximately.

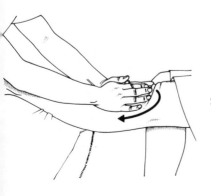

SUPERFICIAL STROKING

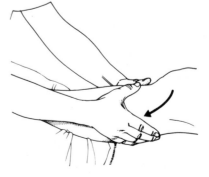

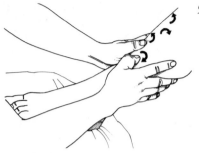

KNEADING ON THE
ANTERIOR TIBIALIS

9   Thumb kneading over the tibialis anterior muscle, working from the attachment on the foot, upwards towards the knee. Thumbs move alternately working with upward, outward pressure, over the entire muscle, returning with effleurage strokes. Repeat 3–6 times.

10   Palmar kneading to calf muscles, working in an upward direction, with the muscles relaxed, and the leg well supported. One hand supports, the other first lifts and exerts outward pressure on the muscles, then relaxes, and moves to a new position. The petrissage movement is applied to the entire calf area, adjusting the pressure, according to the bulk of the muscles. Superficial stroking links the movement, which is repeated with the other hand in a medial direction. Repeat 3 times each side.

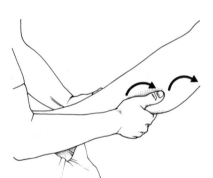
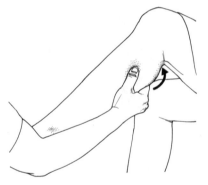

CALF KNEADING

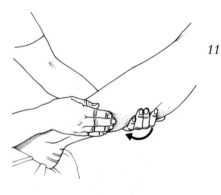

11   Alternate palmar kneading, with both hands working from the knee to the ankle, rolling the muscle in a rhythmical manner. Superficial stroking links the movement, and should be repeated 4 to 6 times.

LEG ROLLING

12   Clapping movement to the calves, performed briskly, with the palmar areas of both hands, formed into a cupped posture. Apply for 20–30 seconds.

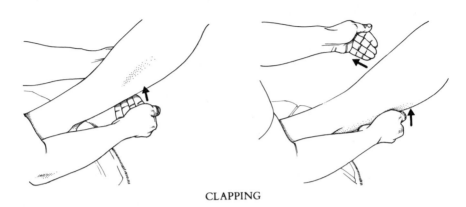

CLAPPING

13   Snatching movement, performed over the toes, with the fingers and thumbs in a light tapotement stroke, rapidly repeated.

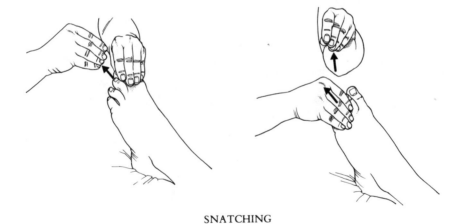

SNATCHING

14   Whipping movement, applied in the same fashion, exerting rapid stimulating strokes, over the toes, to increase local circulation and improve colour. Both snatching and whipping are applied lightly and quickly for 10–20 seconds, and at no time should discomfort be experienced.

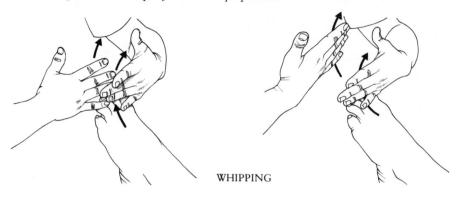

WHIPPING

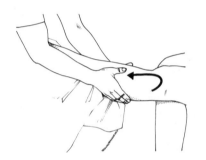

15 Relaxing superficial stroking over the entire foot and leg completes the routine. Repeat 6–8 times slowly, finishing at the toes.

EFFLEURAGE

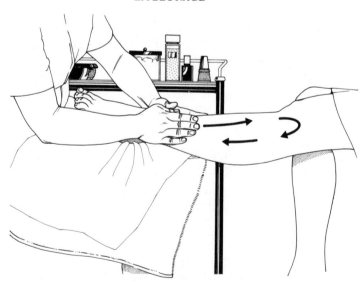

Conclusion

Excess cream or oil may be removed, and the legs toned with mild tonic, and dusted with unperfumed talcum if desired. If applied in combination with pedicure, the routine may then be concluded.

Chapter 12

Waxing Therapy. Heat Applications and Depilatory Treatments

TYPES OF WAX AND THEIR USE

Paraffin Wax

Paraffin wax is used for treatment of stiffness in the joints and improvement of skin texture, colour, and general appearance. It provides a means of generating a steady, high level of heat throughout the tissues, so relieving pain. Paraffin wax is solid and cloudy-white in colour when cold, and has a low melting point. When heated to its working temperature of 120°F (49°C) it becomes clear, completely fluid, and capable of forming a second skin of wax over the treated area on exposure to the air. When sufficient wax encloses the limb, heat is built up, perspiration is induced and relaxation of the tissues results.

Parafango Wax

A mineral-based wax, similar in action to paraffin, but reputed to have additional cleansing, toning, relaxing and invigorating actions on the tissues. Muscular pain is eased, joints are relaxed, and sweating can be induced if a sufficient area is treated. Parafango wax is dark greeny-brown in colour, and requires the same method of application and maintenance as paraffin wax. Its additional effects are credited to the mud-based mineral content of the wax, which is obtainable only from volcanic areas of the world.

Depilatory Wax

Depilatory wax is used for removal of superfluous, unwanted hair. The adhering wax consists of beeswax and resins, plus extra soothing ingredients to minimize skin reaction to the heat, and prevent irritation after hair removal. The wax varies in colour and consistency, according to manufacturer, but normally is pale yellow in colour, forms a solid mass when cold, and has a high melting point and a working temperature of 68°C approximately.

Cool Wax

Cool wax methods of hair removal offer an attractive alternative to normal depilatory wax methods, reducing the preparation and maintenance time associated with traditional hot waxing.

333

Cool wax products are based on a combination of wax, oils and organic substances, and they are water-soluble. They operate at low temperatures of 110°F (43°C) so reducing a fire risk in clinic use. Cool wax is used very sparingly, in conjunction with muslin strips, with both the wax and strips normally being thrown away after use. With practice, cool waxing can be a much quicker procedure for hair removal than the hot wax system. The skin reaction to the waxing is also considerably reduced due to the lower working temperatures needed to accomplish the hair removal.

HOT WAX THERAPY

Contra-indications to Hot Wax Therapy

The arms or legs should be inspected prior to treatment, for conditions which prohibit or limit the wax application.

1 Varicose veins.
2 Defective circulation, i.e. diabetic condition.
3 Skin diseases.
4 Cuts and abrasions.
5 Warts, hairy moles.
6 Stings or sepsis present.
7 Hyper-sensitive skin, from any cause, wind, sun-burn, over-exposure to ultraviolet etc.
8 Any areas of the limbs or body, where extreme discomfort would be involved, due to sensitivity, should be excluded from waxing therapy, i.e. upper inside thigh, breast, and in certain cases of known sensitivity, the under arm.

Any application which places the client at risk, should be avoided, i.e. central eyebrows, due to the close proximity of the eyes, and the danger of liquid wax entering the optic areas.

Safety Precautions

Well-made waxing apparatus which complies with the British Standard of Safety should be employed. The equipment must be earthed or double-insulated, correctly wired, and should have enclosed heating elements to prevent over-heating of the outer casing. The heater should be sited for use on a metal or wood topped mobile trolley, protected with rough paper tissues. Glass trolleys must not be used as the risks of shattering are high, and could result in serious damage to anyone in the vicinity.

The wax should not be left to heat and melt, close to any inflammable materials, plastic goods, curtains etc., due to the risk of fire. Covered containers reduce both the pungent odour of the melting wax, and reduce the fire risk, The wax pans should be free from adhering wax on the rims and bottoms, otherwise they may ignite and cause a serious fire hazard. Regular supervision should be given to the wax, to check its progress, even with thermostatically controlled units, and as modern apparatus is designed with client presentation in mind, it may be prepared within the treatment situation, close to the operator and the client.

The best form of safety precaution in waxing is knowing the best wax for the application, and then becoming proficient in its use and maintenance, thus avoiding areas of danger. The following faults reduce the safety level and proficiency of waxing, and so must be avoided at all times.

1   Overheating the wax.

2   Inadequate protection of the client and working area.

3   Incorrect working consistency, too hot or cool.

4   Neglect in testing the wax heat, in relation to the client's tolerance.

5   Careless application, producing untidy removal and unsatisfactory results.

6   Moving the wax whilst hot.

Wax Hygiene and Maintenance

To maintain efficient performance, ensure a maximum period of usage, and prevent cross-infection, all types of wax must be cleaned and filtered after use. Regular replacement of wax ensures a satisfactory working consistency. The following points will achieve a high standard of waxing technique, and permit fast and profitable treatments to be accomplished with the minimum client discomfort and maximum satisfaction with the results.

1   Strain and clean the wax after use, to remove waste particles, dead skin, perspiration and hairs (in the case of depilatory wax). A fine mesh filter and a moderate heat are employed for the task.

2   Use separate wax containers for application and filtering within the equipment, to avoid altering the heat of the available wax. To prevent slowing down the application, the used wax should be melted and filtered on the fast heat of the equipment, whilst the clean wax is kept at a

moderate working temperature (68°C) by the thermostatic control of the low heat section. A pilot light indicates when the element is actually heating the wax, otherwise its temperature is simply maintained. This prevents a prolonged period of heating, which has a detrimental effect on the adhering properties of the wax and results in unsatisfactory removal.

3   Avoid over-heating the depilatory wax above its correct working temperature, otherwise it will darken and give off a pungent odour. Performance will be less efficient, removal more lengthy due to the brittleness of the wax, and complete hair removal impossible to achieve.

4   Careful choice, and regular cleaning and maintenance of waxing equipment, allows for maximum working efficiency and client safety.

Choice of Equipment

Depilatory Waxing

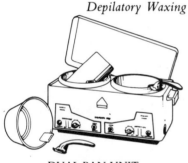

DUAL PAN UNIT

Modern waxing equipment incorporates large capacity containers, fine mesh filters, and is electronically heated. Thermostatically controlled elements heat the wax to its correct pre-set heat (68°C) and maintain the temperature throughout the treatment, thus preventing over-heating and ensuring wax is available throughout the sequence. Portable and clinic models are available, depending on the wax capacity required. Client presentation of equipment demands that the appearance should be immaculate, and rather clinical in design, whilst being easy to keep clean.

Paraffin Waxing

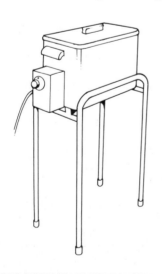

Small quantities of paraffin wax may be prepared in a single unit waxer, but for immersion of limbs a larger bath, with a built-in water jacket and thermostatic controls, is desirable. The wax is pre-heated, and maintained at the correct temperature (48°C) automatically, so minimizing the risks of over-heating or burns. Sufficient time should be allowed for pre-heating the wax prior to treatment, particularly in the case of the larger baths, where 1 hour should be allowed prior to the client's arrival.

PARAFFIN WAX EQUIPMENT

Preparation for Hot Wax Therapy

The working area should be protected with heavy grade polythene sheeting to prevent fragments of wax adhering to the floor coverings, or couch surfaces. Both vinyl and carpet-type floor coverings require protection. The couch should be covered first with polythene, followed by rough paper sheeting, to prevent damage, and speed the clearing procedures after treatment is concluded. Towels, if used, must be protected by disposable paper, as both paraffin and depilatory wax cannot be removed easily from fabric, but form a fast bond. Clients' clothing must be adequately covered and, if a large area is being treated it is preferable for the client to replace her clothing with a salon gown to avoid mishaps. Careful application of technique with the wax at the correct temperature and consistency should avoid unnecessary mess, caused by liquid wax dripping during the application.

PARAFFIN WAX THERAPY

Preparation

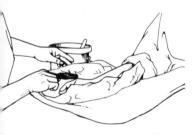

APPLICATION ON THE ARM

Paraffin wax may be applied by (a) painting the wax over the area with a large brush, or (b) dipping the limb into the wax bath. Preparation for both methods involves pre-heating the wax, protecting the working area, and ensuring the necessary commodities are ready for use.

Items required include:
2 sufficiently large foil sheets to enclose the limbs,
2 medium-sized towels,
nourishing cream and spatula,
large brush for application (if used).

The working position should permit safe and efficient wax application, whilst maintaining client comfort. The limb should be washed, or wiped over with a soapy, antiseptic solution, and in the case of hand treatment, all jewellery removed if possible.

Application

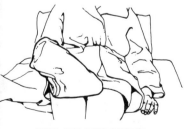

THE ARM WRAPPED

With the client adequately protected, and in a comfortable position, the limbs are covered in a thin film of nourishing cream, and then dipped into the warm wax to form a thin coating. The fingers or toes remain together, and the process is repeated until a fairly thick layer of wax is formed (5–6 times). The limb is then wrapped in foil and towels to maintain the heat. The second limb is treated in a similar manner, and then the client should be allowed a few minutes rest to permit maximum heat build-up to produce a satisfactory circulation improvement.

If a small wax container is employed, the wa
may be brushed on to the prepared limb, whic
rests on a foil sheet, placed over a towel protectin
the operator's lap. When sufficient layers of wa
have been applied, the foil is wrapped firml
around the limb, enclosing the wax, and towel
bind the package to retain the heat. Because of th
fluid nature of the heated wax, care must be take
to protect the garments, towels etc., and the sur
rounding area from drops of wax spilt during th
application.

Removal

Removal is easily accomplished due to th
nourishing cream application. The wax peels off i
one piece, if it has been evenly applied, requirin
the minimum of additional cleaning. The limb wil
be found to be relaxed, warm, with increased circu
lation, improved skin colour and appearance. Th
tissues are in an ideal relaxed condition for manua
massage treatment to reinforce the circulatio
improvement action commenced by the hot wax
If applied, a full 10 minutes massage is desirabl
to release dead skin, ease stiffness and tension in th
joints and muscles, and reinforce the improvemen
in appearance. Senile skin, dehydrated and dr
flaky conditions benefit particularly from paraffi
wax applications, as the action is two-fold, promot
ing internal circulation, whilst achieving a cosmeti
improvement in epidermal cells and skin tissue.

Combined Paraffin Wax and Massage Treatment

If the waxing is combined with manicure o
pedicure and manual massage, the following sequence ensures maximum benefit is gained from the
application. The nails are completed up to the cuticle work, wax is applied to one limb, wrapped and
left. The second arm or leg is waxed, and wrapped
and then the first limb is unwrapped, and massage
is applied. The second limb is then unwrapped
massaged, and the manicure or pedicure completed
in the normal way.

Paraffin Wax Maintenance

Small quantities of used wax may be filtered
through a very fine gauge mesh sieve to remove
waste particles before being replaced for future use.
Larger waxing units incorporate an efficient cleansing system, which functions on the principle o
drawing off the waste elements upon the addition
of water into the wax container. As the wax cools.

it rises to the surface and, when solid, the water debris may be drawn off from a release tap at the side, leaving the wax clean and ready for use.

Paraffin waxing units based on the principle of a container surrounded by a water jacket and heated by an enclosed element are the safest in use, as at no time can the limbs come into contact with an open source of heat during the treatment. The water level must be maintained, by checking before use and by the addition of fluid if necessary, through an opening at the side of the tank.

DEPILATORY TREATMENTS

(for temporary removal of superfluous hair)

The method of removal should be discussed with the client prior to treatment, and advice given regarding the advantages and disadvantages of the various means available. The therapist should have sufficient knowledge of all permanent and temporary methods in order to guide her client. The decision should be based on the quantity of superfluous hair, its location, and rate of growth, facts which may be learnt from the client by conversation and general inspection of the condition.

Depilatory Methods Available (temporary)

Plucking and waxing.
Shaving, cutting, abrasive gloves, and depilatory creams.

Plucking and waxing remove the hair completely from the follicle, leaving an active area of cells which produce a new tapered hair, which appears on the skin's surface after a period of 4–6 weeks. The rate of growth varies amongst individuals but, if rapid regrowth occurs, a more permanent method of superfluous hair removal should be considered.

Shaving, cutting, abrasive gloves and depilatory creams remove the hair only from the surface of the skin, and blunt regrowth is apparent after only a few days. These methods are not employed professionally, but a knowledge of their use and effects is essential, as the client may have applied them as a temporary method prior to and between professional visits. The skin effects of depilatory creams, abrasive gloves and shaving may have caused the skin to be fragile, and more liable to irritation from wax therapy.

Permanent Hair Removal Methods (destruction of the active follicle)

Epilation

Epilation is, removal by short wave diathermy (heat), causing coagulation of the hair root, and surrounding cells, and eventual destruction of the hair-producing properties of the follicle.

Electrolysis

Electrolysis is, removal by galvanic (chemical means), where chemical substances formed at the tip of the needles destroy the hair root and surrounding cells.

Both methods of permanent removal are applied via extremely fine needles, which enter the hair follicles individually. The specialized training for epilation depends largely on a highly developed sense of touch to determine the follicle depth.

Advantages and Disadvantages of Temporary Methods (for client discussion)

Depilatory Treatments (Waxing)

Advantages

1 Large areas of unwanted hair may be removed in one session, giving 'instant results'.

2 Relative low cost and high client satisfaction.

3 Only slight discomfort experienced with correct application technique.

4 Regrowth hair is fine-ended, and feels soft in texture.

Disadvantages

1 Has to be repeated at regular intervals to maintain a groomed appearance.

2 Waxing can occasionally cause regrowth hair to be ingrowing, causing discomfort. Waxing should not be repeated after the condition rectifies itself.

Advantages and Disadvantages of Permanent Methods (for client discussion)

Permanent Epilation and Electrolysis

Advantages

1 Once completed the task never needs repeating.

2 Each regrowth that occurs produces a finer growth. Fine hairs may only require one removal to achieve destruction.

3 The only real solution to excessive hair growth.

Disadvantages

1 Skin reaction may occur in certain cases.

2 Pain may be experienced by some clients.

3 High cost if a large area of superfluous hair growth requires treatment.

Depilatory Hot Waxing Treatment (for superfluous hair removal)

Preparation

Sufficient depilatory wax should be pre-heated to a moderate temperature, whilst the salon preparation is completed and the commodities required assembled. The working area should be protected, and the items for waxing placed close to the waxing area, but not in contact with the heating unit.

Items Required

Surgical spirit, talcum powder, cotton-wool, wooden spatulas or brush for applying the wax, tweezers, and soothing lotion or cream.

When the wax attains the correct working temperature it has the consistency of syrup, and can be tolerated on the inside of the operator's wrist. It must be liquid enough to adhere to the hairs, particularly if they are short, but not too hot to cause discomfort and subsequent grazing of the surface skin.

Client preparation must include inspecting the area for contra-indications, protecting clothing with disposable tissues and ensuring a comfortable position for treatment.

Method of Treatment

When the wax appears to have reached the right temperature and consistency, it should be tested by the operator, and then applied rapidly in strips of 2 inch width, by one of the following methods.

1 Against the growth, smoothing the wax in the opposite direction to the natural hair growth. Shorter hairs are best treated in this way to obtain maximum removal.

2 In the same direction as the growth. The regrowth is reputed to be more natural in appearance, with less risk of breakage during the removal. Hairs must be of moderate length (½ inch minimum) for this method to be fully efficient.

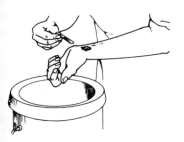

TESTING WAX TEMPERATURE

Good quality wax will remove hairs by both methods, but method (1) is in the most common use, as regular treatment normally permits only a short growth to be evident above the skin's surface, and more satisfactory results are obtained by brushing against the growth than with it.

Application

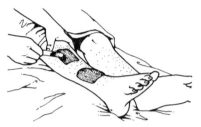

APPLICATION OF STRIPS

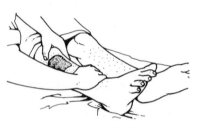

PRESSING DOWN WAX

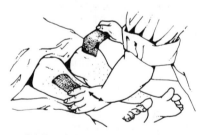

TAKING OFF AND RUBBING

The area should be prepared, after initial inspection, by rubbing surgical spirit vigorously over the skin on a pad of cotton-wool to remove natural oils etc., and make the hairs stand away from the surface. A light dusting of talcum, in the pattern of removal, may then be applied against the growth to make the hairs erect and give guidance as to the application area. Flat hairs which contour to the skin should be given special attention otherwise they will not be removed satisfactorily. A brush or spatula may be used for the application.

During training the wax strips should be 4 inches long by 2 inches wide approximately, to facilitate easy removal and avoid client discomfort. Equal distance should be left between the strips for treatment with a following application. As many strips as possible should be applied at each stage of the treatment, with the ends of the strips covering bare skin whenever possible, in this way reducing discomfort during removal. When application and removal techniques have improved in proficiency, the strips may become 12–14 inches long, by 2 inches wide, so that the length of the leg may be treated in one application, so reducing the time of the removal. Both methods are in general use, and the choice of application will depend on both the client's tolerance to the discomfort of removal and the amount of superfluous hair present.

The strips should be rapidly applied with firm edges, against the growth, to a thickness of ¼ inch. The strips should be evenly applied, with no areas of wax build-up to cause a heat reaction and subsequent grazing to result. When the wax is not sticky to the touch, it should be firmly moulded to the area to increase its adhering properties. It may be removed when it has reached a flexible but semi-set state, by quickly flipping up one end, ripping the strip off with a decisive movement, and following up swiftly with a rubbing movement to alleviate smarting. Removal should follow the contour of the area to avoid wax breakage or stretching of the strip. It should not be permitted to become over-set and brittle, otherwise it will shatter on removal, and the client will experience discomfort, whilst the treatment time will be extended.

Achieving speed and efficiency in waxing can only be gained by practice, and observation and awareness of the correct wax consistency. Preventing the wax over-heating will avoid unnecessary waiting and stirring to reduce the temperature. A half-leg wax (both legs up to the knee) should take ½–1 hour, depending on the degree of hair growth.

Full leg hair removal (including the thighs) may take 1–1½ hours, due to the need for moderately sized pieces on the thighs, because of the sensitivity involved.

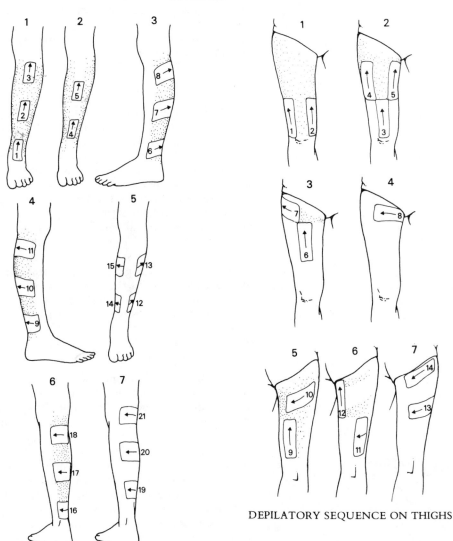

DEPILATORY SEQUENCE ON LEGS

DEPILATORY SEQUENCE ON THIGHS

The fronts of the legs should be completed and the client requested to turn over. The head rest should be dropped and the client made comfortable, and her clothing or gown protected again with tissues. The back of the leg normally requires a different direction of wax application, still against the growth, but around the leg, following its contour. Ths strips should not be made too wide, otherwise removal will be inefficient.

On completion of the waxing sequence, the leg should be inspected, with the client sitting up, and her legs in a pulled-up position, free from the couch. Loose wax fragments should be removed with the rough paper from the couch to improve client comfort and prevent the spread of the wax to the surrounding area. Any adhering wax, loose hairs etc. remaining on the legs may be removed with surgical spirit, and a soothing cream or lotion applied over the area. Stroking movements are used to disperse the heat reaction present. Remove disposable paper, help the client from the couch check for wax pieces, and permit her to replace her own clothing, giving assistance if required.

Red coloration, blotches etc., if evident, will fade within a few hours, a point which must be explained to new clients to prevent distress. It should be suggested that only a moderately warm bath be taken the day of the treatment, to prevent a strong heat reaction being formed. Areas in which the hairs have not been removed satisfactorily may be rewaxed only if the skin does not feel or appear sensitive. The risk of grazing on a mature or sensitive skin would limit the possibility of rewaxing, and so it is a practice which should be avoided if at all possible. Leg hairs regrow over a period of 4–6 weeks, and regular removal should be encouraged. A minimum length of ¼ inch of hair is required to ensure satisfactory results.

Under-arm Waxing

The client should be placed in a semi-reclining or flat position, with clothing and couch surfaces protected with disposable materials. She should be made comfortable, and the wax applied against the growth, either in one piece (in the case of sparse growth), or in two pieces, towards the centre. The upper pieces on both underarms should be applied first, and removed, followed by completion of the lower areas, to produce a complete removal, with the minimum of discomfort.

Regular treatment reduces the amount of hair present at any one time, due to the variation of hair growth. This point should be stressed to the client, as it reduces the discomfort considerably, particularly for young women with a substantial underarm growth.

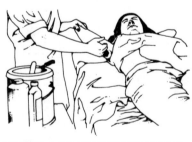

UNDER-ARM WAXING POSITION

The area may be soothed with an antiseptic calming lotion or cream to prevent discomfort and reduce the danger of infection in the exposed follicles. Blood spots (in the case of strong growth) require a light dusting of anti-bacterial powder, after the initial soothing application. No deodorants or anti-perspirant products should be used for 12 hours after waxing to prevent irritation. Results normally last 2–6 weeks, depending on the degree of growth present. The regrowth period is gradually extended with regular removal, as less hairs are available for waxing every time, due to the resting and growing cycle of the hairs.

If after waxing treatment regrowth hairs are evident within a few days, the hairs have been broken off, not removed complete with roots, due to poor technique. Attention should be paid to using the correct method, in both the application and removal of the wax. Regular waxing treatment throughout the year appears to reduce the amount of hair, but this is not in fact the case. The effect is due only to a proportion of the existing hairs being evident at any one time, due to the mass indiscriminate removal caused by waxing. The hairs are all removed at different stages of their growth, and subsequently grow back, at different rates. Regular waxing becomes part of the client's basic grooming habits, and is a very successful salon treatment.

COOL WAXING

Advances in product efficiency have made cool waxing a very popular and effective method of temporary hair removal. The reduced maintenance involved also makes them a popular system with the busy therapist.

Cool wax systems include a thermal heating unit, clinic size for body applications, and facial unit for lip wax etc. plus the semi-liquid wax, muslin strips, and after care lotion. A 32oz capacity heating unit is suitable for body work, and an 8oz for facial work, because of the small amounts of wax required. The cool wax is heated in the thermostatically controlled heating unit, till it becomes clear and warm, (110°F, 43°C) and will spread over the skin and hairs easily. The thermal unit takes only 10–15 minutes to warm the wax to a working consistency, which is a useful point for unexpected waxing clients. The wax may also stay at this temperature all day, without causing odours, making it possible to offer waxing therapy at very short notice.

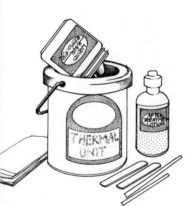

Application

A small quantity of wax is applied to the area of treatment, using the edge of the spatula, at an angle of 90° to the skin. The wax is *pushed* along the skin *with the direction of hair growth*, to form a *thin* film. A muslin strip is then placed over the wax, so that its edges are free, and pressed down firmly, to make a good bond. The strip is then removed with a quick

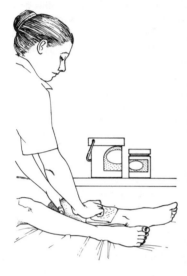

action of the wrist, *against* the hair growth direction, contouring to the shape of the treated area. The strips should not be lifted upwards on removal, otherwise poor removal will result. Rather, they should be almost folded back on themselves, to give maximum leverage to the wax-covered strips.

Even though a rigid pattern of application is unnecessary, a methodical approach to the hair removal should be adopted, to achieve a fast and effective result. A large area of wax can be applied, as it does not set, but remains fluid at body temperature, and the muslin strip re-used until it will not pick up any more hairs. Depending on the clients hair growth, its density and pattern of growth, only 2–4 muslin strips may be needed for a half-leg wax.

On women where the leg hair growth is dense and vigorous, the normal method of cool wax application is used, to reduce discomfort. The wax is applied in strips 1½–2 ins wide by 6–8 ins long, to match the shape of the muslin strips which actually remove the hairs. The hair growth direction is followed closely, and the muslin strips discarded as soon as they fail to remove the hairs effectively. The strips of wax can be reapplied over a previously treated area, as there is very little heat reaction to cause problems. However the less overlapping the sequence contains, the faster the entire sequence will be, which makes it more comfortable for the client, and more profitable for the clinic. Also the actual trauma to the skin, associated with any form of waxing, when the hairs are actually ripped out, should not be applied more than is absolutely necessary, otherwise dilated capillaries or skin grazes can form.

Sparse hair growth, where the muslin strips are not going to be so quickly loaded with hairs, can be treated more generally. Here the wax can be applied to an area, for example the front of the leg, or a forearm, and the muslin strip applied, removed, and reapplied till the hairs are all removed in the area. Care should still be taken to follow the direction of the hair growth during the wax application, and to work against it during the removal.

No special preparation of the skin is necessary with cool waxing, only on the upper lip, or under arm areas need the skin be cleansed with water to free it from perspiration etc. This is because the wax is formulated to cling to the hairs rather than the skin, and less skin shedding occurs. This also makes it more suitable for sensitive or mature skins that would be contra-indicated to hot wax therapy for their hair removal.

After the removal of the hairs in the area is completed, any wax remaining on the skin is simply washed off with a sponge, being water-soluble. Then a soothing after treatment lotion or cream is applied.

A half-leg wax can take 10–15 minutes for sparse growth, up to ½ hour for difficult and heavy growth. Therapists will find once they have mastered the rather different application methods of cool waxing, that it is a faster system of waxing, as less time is spent waiting for wax to heat or cool as with hot waxing. The reduced preparation and maintenance time however, probably produce the greatest time saving overall.

Cool waxing can be applied on all areas of the body and face, apart from those contra-indicated for reasons of extreme sensitivity. There must always be enough hair present to provide some traction for the wax to grip, otherwise results will be patchy. Lip and chin hairs, unwanted eyebrow hairs, and side burns can all be removed with care, as long as the normal precautions for working in these areas is followed. As the cool wax is so controllable, there is less risk of it getting into the eyes, nose or mouth, but the therapist should still be aware of the risks, and work carefully. Special applicators are supplied for tiny areas of treatment, likewise removal strips, shaped to fit the contour of the lip or eyebrow area. If these are not available, they can be easily made by the therapist, so that she has the right tools for the job.

Application on the Thighs

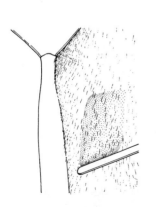

Normally forming part of a complete leg wax, application on the thighs should follow closely the direction of hair growth, to gain satisfactory removal results. Apply the wax thinly, using the edge of the spatula, following a strip pattern. Position the muslin strip over the coated area, keeping the edges free of the liquid. Bond the strip to the area with several firm strokes of the hand, working again with the direction of the hair growth. Grip the bottom of the muslin strip, and peel back *sharply* against the direction of hair growth, contouring the hand closely to the skin whilst ripping off the strip. The hairs should be removed completely, with hair bulbs intact. Repeat the same treatment for the entire front thighs area, altering the wax application direction according to the hair direction. Bend the knee to wax the knee cap.

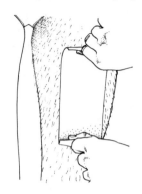

Complete the entire front legs if complete leg waxing is intended, then sponge off the remaining wax, and soothe the skin with after-care lotion. Complete the back of the legs in the same manner, taking special care over swirling patterns of hair growth on the back of the thighs, using smaller areas of wax application in this instance. Avoid the popliteal cavity at the back of the knee during the application.

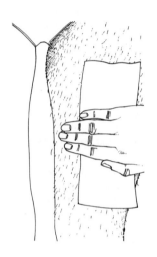

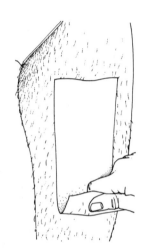

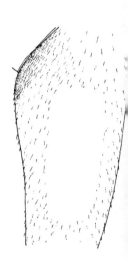

Application on the Lower Legs

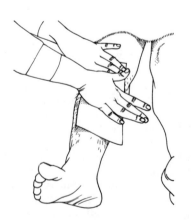

The lower leg is a simpler area of treatment than the thigh, normally having more straightforward hair growth directions. Again the hair growth direction is followed, as seen rather than assumed. Hairs may grow towards the ankle on the front of the leg, and inwards or downwards on the calf. Special positioning may be necessary around the ankles if hair is present. The application and after-care methods used on the lower leg are identical to those on the thigh. As it is often possible to wax the entire lower legs from the front, by repositioning the client, rather than getting her to turn over, the final sponging off and after-care lotion can be left till both legs are complete.

For large clients, or those with difficult hair growth patterns, the front and the backs of the lower legs should be treated separately, like the thighs. This allows greater access to the hairs and is

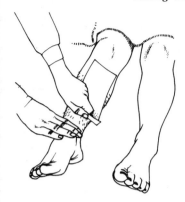

more comfortable for the client. When the fronts of the legs are completed, the client turns over, is repositioned comfortably, and the back is treated. If at any stage the treatment seems to be making the client uncomfortable, or tense, because of the position she is placed in to complete the wax, she should be repositioned if at all possible. This is not only to improve her acceptance of the routine, but also to prevent any unnecessary tension being present, to add to the overall uncomfortable sensation inherent in any procedure, however efficiently applied.

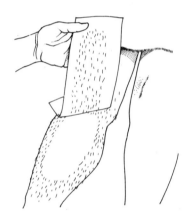

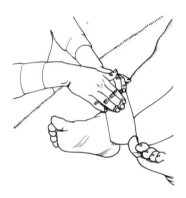

Bikini—Inside Thigh Area

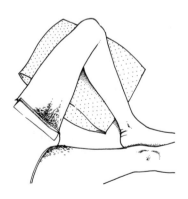

The client is placed in a comfortable semi-reclining position, with the leg to be treated first, bent at the knee and supported by a small protected cushion. This allows the client to relax her knee against the support, and prevents tension in the inner thigh muscles, which would add to the discomfort experienced. The clients clothing and the surrounding treatment area are protected with paper tissues. Avoid over-exposing the client unnecessarily, but make sure the area to be waxed is in accord with the client's requirements. If the waxing is in preparation for wearing a particularly scanty bikini, the areas that need clearing should be discussed briefly before commencing the waxing.

New clients should be advised of the sensitivity of waxing in this area, and the waxing approached progressively, so that clients can decide when they are satisfied with the result, or wish to conclude the treatment. If the hair growth is particularly dense or strongly rooted in nature, then much smaller areas may be waxed at a time, still keeping to the basic application pattern, to reduce client discomfort. If clients are to persevere with inside thigh waxing, as a regular part of their grooming, this is an important point in client handling and treatment adaptation.

On normal hair growth, the direction of the hair is followed, and the application made in three main sections, altering the application direction to match the growth direction of the hairs. Again, apply *with* the growth, and after pressing down well, remove *against* the growth, contouring to the area. Hold the skin taut with the other hand whilst quickly ripping off the strips, and immediately press firmly on the waxed area to alleviate any smarting of the skin.

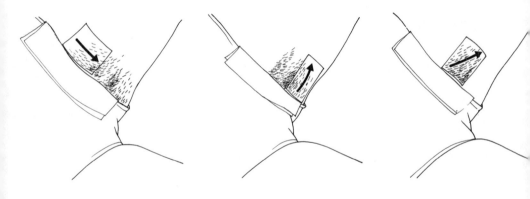

Complete one inside thigh at a time to avoid re-positioning the client unnecessarily, and apply soothing after-care lotion to settle and protect the skin. On an initial wax on a heavy growth, minute blood spots may appear where deep hairs have been removed. This normally only occurs on exceptionally strong growth, and will not continue to occur if the client gets into a regular pattern of waxing. This is because less hairs will be present for waxing on subsequent occasions, due to the disruption in the natural growth cycle of the hairs. If blood spotting does occur it indicates a need for extra after-care attention, and advice to the client, to avoid irritation or infection occurring. It may also be advisable to reduce the application area of each section of wax, perhaps dividing each section into two. This will not only help to reduce the spotting, but will reduce the damage to the skin, and discomfort for the client.

With both inside thighs complete, the area is sponged down with tepid water, and soothed with after-care lotion. The protective tissues may then be removed, and if the abdominal area does not require waxing, the treatment is complete. Advice should be given about avoiding tight underclothes initially, which would tend to rub on the area, adding to skin irritation. Also very hot baths, or use of vaginal sprays should be avoided for the first 6–12 hours after the wax, as these could irritate the skin whilst it is still a little sensitive. So certain clinical treatments should not be booked together, such as sauna and waxing, as both stimulate the skin, and the combined effects could cause soreness. If the client prefers to combine heating treatments with waxing, the routine must be arranged so that the skin is back to its normal temperature, before the wax is applied. So the waxing would come last in the sequence, rather than first which would probably mean further aggravation to the skin from subsequent applications. Even with cool wax, where the heat reaction is greatly reduced, it is necessary to use common-sense in treatment planning, to avoid client discomfort, and to ensure a good result.

Abdominal Area

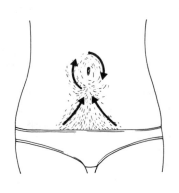

If the abdominal area requires waxing, this may be completed in combination with the inside thigh area, or independently, depending on the hair growth present. The wax is applied in an identical manner to normal cool waxing, but very careful attention to the hair direction is necessary to achieve good results. Small areas should be treated, following the hair growth direction meticulously, whether it grows upwards from the groin, or in a circular pattern on the abdominal area. The softness of the skin in this area presents a problem in certain cases, such as in post-pregnancy skin softening, or in the older client. Position the client so that her abdominal area is as taut as possible, which will improve the removal. The best position is often perfectly flat on a couch, rather than semi-reclining which tends to bunch the soft abdominal tissues, even on a slim person.

When the muslin strips are removed, the skin should be held firmly to reduce skin trauma and discomfort, and the waxed area immediately covered with the free hand to reduce the sensation experienced. Any hairs which are not removed successfully on the initial wax application, because their direction is different from the bulk of the hairs in the area, can be rewaxed. This should be kept to a minimum however, as even with less heat reaction to the waxing procedure, the skin is still undergoing considerable traction and discomfort through the removal process, and could become sore.

Normal after-care lotion application completes the procedure, after sponging the skin of any remaining wax fragments.

The Under-arm Area

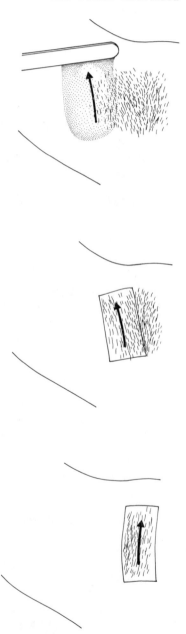

The under-arm area is very responsive to waxing therapy. This is particularly so for dark-haired clients, who will always experience an under-arm shadow after normal depilatory methods, e.g. chemical depilatory methods, shaving etc. This is because the dark root of the hair is still visible through the pale under-arm skin, and stubble is soon present above the surface, as the hairs are simply cut or dissolved away at the surface of the skin. So waxing is a great improvement, both in appearance, and freedom from hairs for a longer period, 3–4 weeks being an average regrowth period.

Sensible positioning of the client is important to ensure a successful result, and to maintain client comfort. The client is placed semi-reclining, with one hand placed behind the head, and the elbow bent. The arm may need positioning until the under-arm area is flat, rather than concaved when more difficult to wax efficiently. Tissues are placed to protect the clients underclothes and the working area. Both under-arm areas can be waxed simultaneously if preferred, but as the treatment is so fast, with no waiting for the wax to set, that there is no real advantage in this method of work. Also if one arm is completed at a time, it does save aching arms for the client.

The direction of the hairs is studied closely while the area is wiped with tepid water. This removes perspiration from the skin, and prepares it for the wax. The skin is dried, and the wax applied to a small area, pressing firmly with the spatula in the hair growth direction. The muslin strip is applied and removed swiftly, holding the skin firmly to reduce discomfort. The process is repeated until the entire area is clear. If the hair growth is in a spiral pattern, divide up the application and follow the direction closely. This avoids unnecessary rewaxing of hairs which have been left behind after the general application. The shorter the visible hairs are, the more care must be taken over the direction of the wax application, if a successful result is to be achieved.

Again, as with the bikini area, coarse deep-rooted hairs may present blood spots initially, until the growth is thinned out by regular waxing. So the wax should be applied in really small sections, and meticulous attention given to after-care and home advice for the client. This would involve advising the client to avoid the use of anti-perspirants, deodorants, highly scented talcs etc. in the area for several hours after treatment. A certain amount of pre-advice on under-arm waxing, when the client books the treatment is also valuable. It is desirable to avoid booking the wax to coincide with some special event in the client's social life, where the use of a chemical deodorant or anti-perspirant would be imperative. Also to suggest that clothing is worn that is not tight in the arm-hole, when coming for the waxing application. Any friction in the area may well cause soreness and is better avoided.

Naturally, many clients who wax regularly have sparse growth, and find only minimal after-care is necessary. But for clients with very dense growth, or who are on their initial waxing treatment, a few points of advice can make all the difference. It can make the treatment more comfortable and bearable, and produce a satisfied client, who will become a waxing devotee, rather than one who never returns for any treatment, and is lost to the business.

After each under-arm area is completed, the remaining wax fragments may be sponged off and after-care lotion applied.

Arms

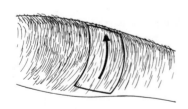

The arms are extremely easy to treat, as the skin is firm and the hairs grow in the same general direction around the arm. The wax is applied, and removed systematically in the normal way, until the desired result is achieved. The wax may be applied over a larger area, and the muslin strip applied, removed, and re-applied until all the hairs are removed. The muslin strips are discarded when they become loaded with hairs, and unable to remove the hairs satisfactorily. According to the density of the hair growth, the use of one muslin strip per arm is normally adequate.

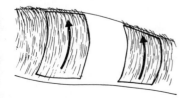

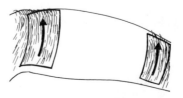

After completion of the hair removal, the arms are sponged down, and soothing lotion applied.

Lip Waxing

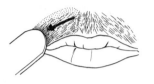

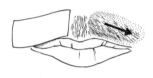

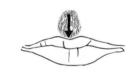

The lip area is cleansed gently and any makeup etc. removed thoroughly. The skin is then wiped over with tepid water, and dried carefully. The wax is applied *with* the growth, in one area at a time, in three sections, using a spatula and taking care not to get wax in the mouth or up the nose. First the hair on one side of the lip is cleared, using specially shaped removal strips, and ripping off swiftly against the growth. Next the other side of the lip is cleared, and lastly the sensitive area under the nose is treated. Care should be taken not to wax a larger area than is necessary, otherwise fine vellus facial hairs will be removed, giving the face an unnatural appearance. Also the wax should be applied to include the fine hairs right on the lip line, and the longer hairs sometimes present at the sides of the mouth. This can be accomplished simply, by taking care to apply the wax right down to the actual lip skin, and elongating the side lip sections. Any hairs left will be visible and spoil the overall effect, both in terms of client satisfaction, and achieving a perfect result.

The lip area, when complete, is wiped free of remaining wax and soothed with after-care lotion. Makeup ideally should not be applied for a couple of hours until the skin is settled, but if it is requested should be of a covering and medicated type to avoid infection.

Eyebrows

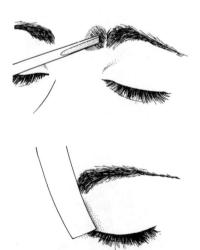

Cool wax can be used effectively to shape the brows, as its less runny consistency and low temperature make it more controllable and therefore safer to use in the eye area. Makeup is removed from the area, and the shape of the proposed brow considered and discussed with the client, using a mirror if necessary. A tiny quantity of wax is applied, using an orange stick or small stiff brush, and the unwanted hairs are parted from the main brow shape. The hairs are removed following the *natural* direction of the hair growth, not the direction in which the hairs have been placed by the wax. Using a narrow specially shaped removal strip, the wax is pressed down onto, and the strip removed with a quick ripping movement, against the direction of natural growth. Small areas may be cleared

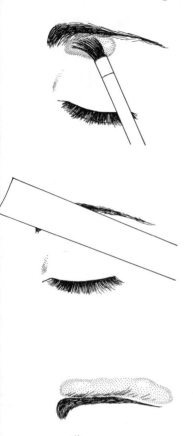

at a time, first under the brows and then over the brows if necessary; also, in some cases, up to the natural hair line in the temple areas.

If at any stage it is desirable to consult with the client as to the shape or thickness of the brow, the proposed shape can be shown to the client and modified if necessary. It need only be shaped by parting the unwanted hairs with the wax, and if this does not meet the client's requirements, can be washed off, and a new shape re-applied. In this way full client satisfaction is assured, in the most efficient manner. As with traditional eyebrow shaping, the client consultation to achieve the correct shape for individual taste is the most important factor. Even if the shape does not appear ideal to the therapist, she must be guided by her client if she wants to retain her custom. Women have stronger views about the shape they prefer their eyebrows than any other element of their facial appearance. So be prepared to guide rather than dictate to the client how her eyebrows should look. With a little tact and diplomacy, clients will normally come around to a more fashionable eyebrow shape.

Cool wax permits fast shaping of the brow, and can help promote this area of business as a profitable service within the clinic. For strong hairs or very heavy overgrown brows, it does cut down the client's discomfort and skin irritation if applied skilfully.

When the brows are completely shaped to the client's satisfaction, they can be wiped over with after-care lotion, and the treatment concluded with camouflaging medicated cream if desired.

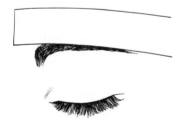

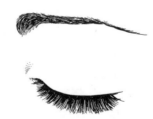

Chapter 13

Business Organization, Salon Procedure and Equipment Choice

METHODS OF WORK

There are many different work possibilities for the qualified beauty specialist or therapist, depending on her experience, mobility and main fields of interest. Information regarding the potential and demands of varied situations is useful in deciding which application best suits individual needs and personal circumstances. The main area of primary work is normally general salon work, which permits techniques to become established and confidence to grow in client handling and treatment sales ability.

General Salon Work, Beauty Clinic

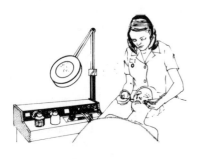

All aspects of facial and body treatments are normally available to the client, from cosmetic and remedial facial therapy, through the full range of figure improvement services, and including grooming aspects such as depilatory and epilation applications. In a large clinic a facial specialist is able to apply all aspects of her training and, if she holds additional body therapy and epilation qualifications, all areas of treatment may be undertaken, giving a varied and interesting work range.

Store Salon

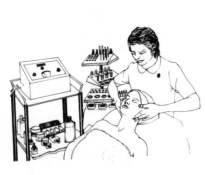

A beauty unit within a store situation is an increasingly popular position for a facial specialist. The work is normally confined by space and facilities, to cosmetic facial treatments, and may be offered in combination with electrology. A growing method of work is for the facial cubicles to be operated on a franchise basis, with the therapist working for a large company, and having the advantage of national advertising and bulk supplies of cosmetics. A trend towards increasing the electrical facial treatments improves the specialist's work range, and produces more satisfactory results. Skin care advice, cosmetic sales, and artistic makeup applications make this an ideal field of work for the facial specialist or therapist most interested in facial therapy and cosmetic applications. Epilation qualification increases the range of work, and is highly desirable both for client satisfaction and convenience, and as a means of additional revenue.

Home Visiting Practice

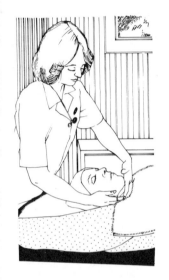

The flexible hours of a mobile practice make it a suitable means of work for any therapist governed by restricted hours of work due to family commitments. It can also be particularly suitable applied on a full or part-time basis for an area with a widely spread population, i.e. a rural location. Facial, body, depilatory and epilation applications may be offered on a visiting basis, providing sufficient organizational ability is used, to avoid time wastage, both on travel and preparation on arrival. Booking of treatments to co-ordinate areas of work for certain days or periods of the week is essential, and of course a reliable means of transport is a necessity.

The varied income of a visiting practice makes it more advantageous for a highly experienced therapist used to promoting treatments, who is limited by circumstances only from fulfilling normal salon hours. A newly qualified woman might find it difficult to be suitably adaptable and organized in order to secure a regular income from it. Clients may prefer evening appointments on occasions, or weekend treatments, and a visiting therapist must be prepared to sacrifice part of her normal leisure time, in booking and completing treatments, if she is to fill her working week. The rewards however for a skilled operator, both in freedom and income, can be extremely good, as long as the necessary time required is spent on organization of the business. An account must be kept of incomings and outgoings, car expenses, special insurance, stock etc., and provision made for tax deductions, as these will be demanded on a yearly not weekly basis, as with P.A.Y.E. contributions.

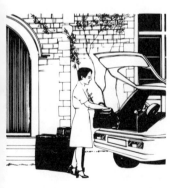

The Health Hydro

The health hydro work situation is normally divided into facial therapy and body work aspects, and therapists have to decide to concentrate on one aspect of their training. This practice is changing as the standard of general therapy training is improving, and the therapists are better able to work in close liaison with nutritional, health, and

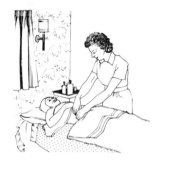

homeopathic experts, and can fulfil their wishe
regarding the therapy treatment, under their gen
eral guidance.

Because of the total supervision and controllec
and restricted diets of the hydro guests, a more
remedial programme of health, face and figure
improvement is normally attempted. This sort o
total approach will appeal to therapists interested ir
body treatments, based on diet, exercise, manua
massage, and electrical muscle-toning applications
Facial specialists often apply a wide range of facia
treatments for relaxation and skin improvemen
purposes, and may also be involved with depilatory
and grooming treatments. Treatment and makeur
advice, linked with cosmetic sales, is also an important area of business within the hydro beauty clinic
and makes up a proportion of the specialist's
income, through sales commission. Residence is
normally required whilst working within the
hydro situation, due to the slightly varied work
hours, compared to a salon and, in some cases, the
isolated position of the hydro. These points are
compensated by longer periods of time off, anc
personal use of some of the hydro's facilities during
free time.

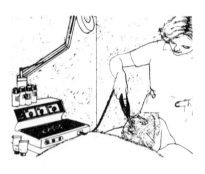

Television Makeup Artist (trainee)

Entry into the field of television work is gradually becoming less restricted, and opportunities for
an interesting and exciting field of work are available for suitable applicants when vacancies arise.
Competition for acceptance on a full-time training
course is fierce, and interviews function on a selective basis, the choice being made from suitably
trained or experienced women. The background
requirements are of an 'A' level academic record,
with an interest in art and history particularly, and a
minimum age restriction of 20½–21 years, with
preference being given to mature and adaptable
personalities. Throughout the paid training period,
experience is gained in all aspects of makeup artist's
work. The varied work hours and involvement of
the programme production demand that the job is a
major interest in the life of the trainee, and it cannot
be compared with the normal salon situation. For
artistically inclined facial specialists of the correct
age, background and general experience, it can be a
fascinating field of work, with high rewards of job
satisfaction and income.

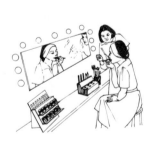

TREATMENT PLANNING
AND PROMOTION

The treatments offered will be based on the following factors: first the type of work situation, whether an independent clinic, linked with hairdressing or health facilities, or a home visiting practice, and, secondly, the area in which it is intended to trade. A highly populated urban area requires a different approach from a mainly residential location, but may support similar levels of turn-over by simply promoting a slightly different range of treatments for the client's needs.

The age range and general inclinations of potential clients gives guidance as to the amount of time and money that they are likely to spend, and should help in deciding the range of treatments and their charge. A professional or commercially involved clientèle will require fast efficient grooming treatments to maintain appearance, but may have little time to spare for relaxation sequences, however much they might benefit from them. Retired or wealthy clients with less demands on their time will enjoy soothing routines and will appreciate the manual aspects of therapy, and the personal attention given to them. Younger clients desire results, and so expect highly efficient treatment sequences, requiring that the salon is equipped with remedial electrical apparatus of a more specialized nature, i.e. ozone steaming or a galvanic unit.

Most therapy practices have a mixture of elements, and it is wise when setting up the business initially to allow a fair measure of flexibility until a clear pattern of client needs emerges. Skilful promotion can sell almost any beneficial treatment to a client, if a good measure of confidence in knowledge and techniques has been achieved, and a sense of trust established. Advertising promotions linked with the time of year or any new apparatus the salon has acquired, are normally very successful, if all resulting enquiries are dealt with sympathetically by a knowledgeable receptionist who is capable of converting them into treatment bookings. As the beauty therapist business appears fairly complicated to the average person, advertising, stressing the qualified status of the staff, is a sensible step.

Staff membership of professional organizations including those which operate in conjunction with the major examination boards, denotes a high standard of skill and illustrates to the potential client the value placed on her receiving a safe and successful treatment.

**Factors which Influence
Charges for Therapy
Treatment**

The location of the salon and the overall cost
its overheads, business loans, rent, rates, equipme
and staff costs must be considered when decidi
the scale of charges that will operate. The high
cost is usually that of the skilled staff involved, a
where personal attention is required througho
the duration of the treatment; this fact must
reflected in a high cost per hour. Treatments requ
ing more general supervision, or not demandi
such a high level of skill, i.e. manicure, make
applications etc., can be costed on a lower basis, d
to the reduced staff costs involved. Remedial fac
therapy, where skill and experience are
paramount importance, in the choice of electri
and cosmetic applications, will be the most expe
sive aspect of the clinic's treatments, due both
staff costs and the additional equipment expenc
ture involved.

Many salons operate on a charge per hour bas
with the main bulk of the treatment carried out
the therapist, formulated at a figure which return
certain percentage of profit, related to the over
costs, and capital investment involved. The level
this price per hour must be set according to t
location of the salon, its competitors' prices, a
the type of clientèle it attracts. This meth
demands good facilities, a wide equipment choi
and skilled staff, experienced in treatment prom
tion, to achieve success. Bookings of treatme
courses have benefits for the client and the busine
as the forward planning enables the appointmen
to be placed at convenient times in the week, a
forms a solid base for other bookings. T
arrangement also permits a discount to be given
the client, usually a bonus treatment, on advan
course payment of the 8 or 12 treatment booking

Specialized treatments such as epilation, ve
treatment, facial muscle toning, bio-peeling etc
will naturally be costed at a higher rate, due to t
additional skill involved. Specialist qualificatio
training, and experience are required in order
promote these treatments, and these factors may
reflected in advertising in order to build this aspe
of work. The clients for the specialist services w
be drawn from a wider area, particularly if simil
facilities are not available within a reasonable pro
imity, and this will enlarge the reputation a
status of the business.

Equipment Choice

When a facial cubicle is set up, basic items should be given priority, leaving more remedial specialized equipment for addition at a later stage, if immediate purchase is impossible. Application of basic facial techniques will reveal where additions need to be made, preventing unnecessary, expensive mistakes. However, the more skilled in promotion of treatment the therapist is, the greater will be her initial needs, and greater, subsequently, her income.

Basic Facial Cubicle Layout and Equipment

A sound basic facial treatment module would include:

1 A flexible treatment couch, ideally capable of multi-position action, to permit a full range of facial treatment, plus arm/leg applications, depilatory treatment, and electrology. As it is a major item of expenditure, consideration should be given to the different facets of treatment which may be offered eventually, and limitations of use avoided. A couch which provides client and operator comfort, makes for relaxation and efficient application of techniques, whilst preventing operator strain.

2 A trolley or vanitory unit, large enough to support a range of small equipment, as well as towels, cosmetic preparations and small implements. A shallow drawer provides a useful site for small sterilized tools, brushes, tweezers etc., and is a safe home for delicate items such as epilation needles, holders and forceps, if this service is offered.

3 A wall-mounted or mobile magnifier, for skin inspection, and magnification purpose. A cool light is essential, to prevent client discomfort and avoid eye strain, particularly for epilation purposes.

4 Storage cupboards incorporating a wash basin, or a vanitory unit, to provide washing facilities and storage for towels, bulk cosmetic containers, equipment etc. The storage space should be close to hand, to prevent unnecessary noise and movement during the treatment.

5 Facial steamer or ozone steamer, for skin cleansing and balancing, and antiseptic effects (ozone steaming).

6 Vibratory massage unit, for facial stimulato
purposes, and relaxation of tense muscle fib
in the shoulder area.

7 Facial vacuum massage unit for deep sk
cleansing, toning, and treatment of fine lir
and blocked pores.

8 Spray toner, for pressure toning and ma
removal.

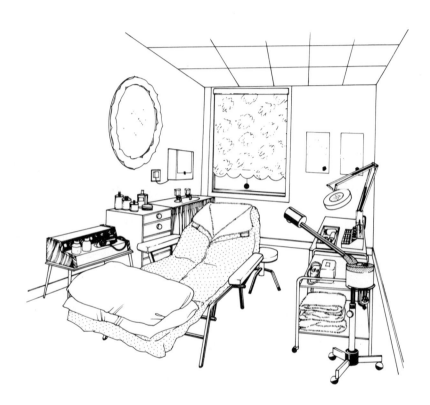

9 Brush massage unit, for thorough cleansing ar
electrical massage, as an alternative to manu
methods.

   Treatment elements such as vacuum, vap
orizers, and brush massage, can be obtained a
combined treatment units, being mounted on
pedestal base. This saves space and improve
the ease of application for the beauty specialis
However it does mean that the equipment car
not be shared between working therapist
operating in the same clinic. So choice woul
depend on personal circumstances, and th
amount of use the equipment was likely t
receive.

10 A small sterilizing cabinet, for the maintenance of sterile tools, brushes, sponges etc., after washing and wet sterilization routines. Regular use of sterilization routines is essential to prevent cross-infection within the salon, and gives the client confidence in the hygienic nature of her personal treatments.

11 Facial waxing unit, for superfluous hair removal by depilatory means.

12 Small equipment, and basic commodities, including cotton-wool containers and waste bin, manicure and pedicure tools, tweezers, brushes, lash and brow tinting preparations, and mixing palette, orange sticks, spatulas, cosmetic sponges, cotton-wool and gauze, fine oil and talcum powder, soothing lotion, and mask preparations.

13 Makeup and treatment preparations. Small quantities of creams, lotions etc. may be kept on the trolley, ready for use and client discussion, with bulk quantities remaining with all the other basic ingredients, not required for immediate use, in an adjacent storage area. A range of treatment preparations would normally include:
Cleansing milk for dry skin (nutrient emulsion).
Cleansing milk for greasy skin (cucumber, lemon etc.)
Cleansing cream for mature complexions or delicate skin, or where a heavier foundation has to be removed.
Tonic for skin refining and bracing on the normal skin.
Tonic for a delicate skin.
Astringent lotion for an oily but not blemished skin.
Corrective lotion for disturbed, blemished, seborrhoea conditions.
Massage cream for normal to dry conditions, dehydration etc.
Light rich emollient massage cream for mature complexions.
Medicated cream for greasy, blemished conditions, to provide a drying and healing action.
Moisturizing lotion, jelly or emulsion for the younger dry skin.
Moisture emulsion for the slightly greasy skin.
Moisture cream or under makeup nutrient base for mature complexions.
Mask ingredients, basic clay types, including calomine, magnesium carbonate, kaolin, fuller's earth.

Mask mixing lotions, including rose water, orange flower water, witch hazel.

Prepared masks for varied skin conditions.

Drying medicated mask for blemished or discoloured skins.

Biological, non-setting masks for delicate, dehydrated, and mature complexions.

Lash extension kit.

Makeup Items

Testers of foundation colours, powders, lipsticks, eye makeup and cheek blushers or shaders should provide an adequate range of makeup for normal day purposes. Additional items for special effects should be available, but need not be kept on the trolley for general use. The range of shades used within the makeup application will depend on the proprietary brand of cosmetics sold by the salon. Some of the treatment houses have only a limited range of makeup items, which can be restricting to the artistic abilities of the beauty specialist. Choice of a range of preparations should be based on a need for a full range of treatment items, with an exclusive image, which will fit the price levels charged by the salon for treatment. As the finished makeup demonstrates the skill of the therapist, it is important that the shades available are subtle, and the textures fine, in order that she may do justice to her therapeutic applications by applying the finishing touch of a flattering makeup.

Cubicle

This basic facial cubicle would provide for a wide range of manual and cosmetically biased facial treatments, and a selection of electrically based treatments. It would be a useful service linked with hairdressing facilities, or within a store situation. The range of treatment offered would include cleanse and makeup, a makeup lesson, cosmetic facial therapy, (including massage, mask, and makeup applications), eyelash and brow tinting, eyebrow shaping, lash extension, and lip and chin waxing.

Treatments based on electrical therapy would include vibratory and deep skin cleansing facials, combining brush massage, steaming, and vacuum methods into the cosmetic and manual applications. Although not remedial in nature, the treatments could be combined in a wide range of different ways to suit varying age groups. The basic cubicle would also act as a base for more remedial, advanced or specialized applications when required, for which additional apparatus and skill would be needed. The most obvious addition to extend the treatment possibilities, being an epilation unit. Many basic treatment cubicles would in fact have this aspect of treatment as a standard requirement because of the popularity and need for electrology. Additional qualification is needed however to provide this valuable treatment addition.

Additional Apparatus to Permit Remedial and Specialized Applications

High-frequency unit, for direct and indirect high-frequency applications.
Galvanic unit, for deep skin cleansing, toning and stimulation, through desincrustation and iontophoresis.
Pulsed air massage unit, for lymphatic drainage, and skin stimulation purposes.
Facial muscle toning equipment, for mature skin treatment, and improvement of facial contours.
Ray treatment equipment, for application of ultraviolet tanning and skin improvement, and infrared for oil mask applications.
Waxing equipment, for paraffin waxing of face and limbs, and depilatory treatments for superfluous hair removal.
Epilation unit, for permanent removal of superfluous hair, and treatment of thread veins etc. (if qualified).

A facial unit equipped to this level would permit a very full range of treatments, both manual and electrical. The facial aspects would be extended and developed to include the maximum amount of body work possible within the facilities available. Remedial and specialized aspects could then be increased, and the clinic could then offer, in addition to the basic routines the following sequences:
Continental facial treatment,
Pore treatment (electrical aspects to include ozone steaming, HF or UV).
Facial faradism, either linked with facial therapy or applied independently.
Bio-peeling,
Viennese facial, with indirect HF,
Brush massage facial,
Oil mask treatment,
Paraffin wax mask treatment,
Heat therapy, for stiffness in the upper back and shoulders,
Facial tanning and skin improvement treatment, with UV,
Epilation, and related minor cosmetic treatments, removal of milia, etc.

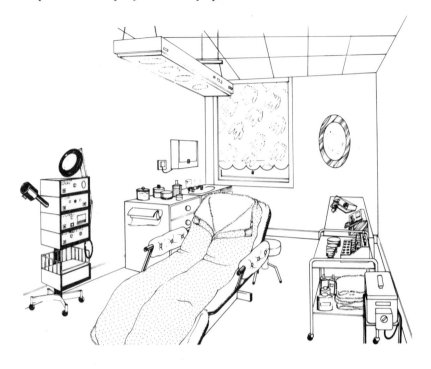

HOME VISITING
PRACTICE EQUIPMENT

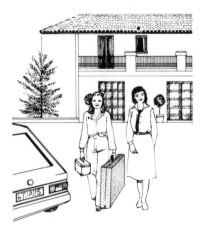

Equipment for a mobile visiting practice must be neat in design, sturdy in construction, and should ideally be in a combined multi-purpose unit. If purely manual and cosmetic treatments are to be offered, these present no real problem, apart from finding a suitable position for treatment within the client's own home. Electrical applications require more forethought and planning to avoid time-wasting. Electrical connections should be checked to ensure the correct fittings are available to apply the treatment. Multi-purpose facial units, enclosed in a carrying case, present the maximum convenience, time and space saving, and are efficient in use. A cosmetic treatment case, either purpose-built or adapted from another use, i.e. a baby box, can carry small quantities of creams, lotions etc., in unbreakable containers. Bulk quantities of treatment preparation may be stored at home in a cool place and used to refill the treatment containers when necessary.

Carrying electrical apparatus in a mobile practice presents particular problems, due to the delicate nature of the equipment, and damage which could result in transit. Special containers built to contain the small equipment reduce the likelihood of intermittent performance but a heavier toll on maintenance is unavoidable and should be allowed for in overall costings. Foam-lined containers lessen the effects of transporting the apparatus, but the choice of equipment should reflect the rôle it has to fulfil. A combination portable unit, providing vacuum (suction) vaporization, galvanic, and high-frequency current permits a wide range of treatment, and is ideal for a mobile practice or a small facial unit where space is limited. Depilatory and epilation applications are also popular areas of treatment, due to the privacy ensured for the client, and can be applied with ease, if attention is given to the working position. A mobile couch may be desirable for leg waxing, and does of course extend the range of possible treatments, as it provides the necessary support for more extensive therapy.

BEAUTY THERAPY QUALIFICATIONS AND METHODS OF TRAINING AVAILABLE

Beauty therapy qualifications may be obtained in a variety of ways, either within an educational situation (Further Education or Technical College, or Adult Education Centre) or by commercial means through a training school or private college.

Internationally recognized qualifications are offered by the International Health and Beauty Council (IHBC), Le Comité Internationale D' Esthétiques et de Cosmetology (CIDESCO), the International Therapy Examination Council (ITEC), and the City and Guilds of London Institute, and the Confederation of Beauty Therapy and Cosmetology. All these organizations act as examination boards for beauty qualification, some on an international basis through approved associations in individual countries. These operate on a national level to provide training to the international standard. Some provide qualification only in the United Kingdom (City and Guilds of London Institute, and the Confederation of Beauty Therapy and Cosmetology), though the training standard is recognized internationally.

The difficulty of obtaining truly worldwide recognized qualifications, is slowly being overcome, as the work of these examination boards in setting an international level of competence, is being increasingly accepted. This will mean that eventually a minimum period of training and skill will entitle a qualified therapist to work anywhere in the world without restriction. It is because of the differences that exist on minimum age of training, duration of course, and its content, and educational entry requirements, that until now qualified therapists have found employment restricted, outside of their country of training.

So it is to the profession's advantage to have international organizations which promote the industry, and have the strength to obtain world wide recognition of the therapists professional status. Therapists can support these organizations by joining the national associations which are affiliated to the international organization. In the United Kingdom, the IHBC is supported by the National Health and Beauty Council (NHBC), whilst CIDESCO has chosen the British Association of Beauty Therapy and Cosmetology to represent them as the British section, and provide an international qualification to students who first pass the Confederation examination at the required level.

So when considering training, look at the opportunities provided by the major associations, and realize that the standard that they have set worldwide has had to be earned. So if the possibility of an internationally recognized qualification is desirable, expect to be required to meet entry requirements on age, academic achievements, etc. and to train for a specified period, according to the level of course chosen. The therapist's work is to a professional level, so the training must be also to safeguard client interest.

Course Content

Depending on the level of the training undertaken, the facial specialist will be required to have a sound knowledge of physical science, cosmetic chemistry, and anatomy, to support the practical skills obtained. The information will all relate to the application of the practical techniques, and is necessary to protect the clients wellbeing. As the apparatus and cosmetic applications become more sophisticated, the facial specialist has to extend her knowledge of the systems of treatment available.

So the training is a blend of technical expertise, manual skills and artistic ability, and it should be of sufficient duration to allow confidence to develop in client handling.

Very often facial therapy is studied in conjunction with body therapy and electrology, to provide the therapist with a wide range of employment opportunities, and to give variety in the work itself. Full therapy training is normally of one year's duration in a private training school, and two years in an educational establishment, due to the educational vacation periods. In the longer educational courses, more time is also spent on related topics to round out the student's experience and build confidence and social skills. Art, drama, social studies etc. all play their part in developing individual confidence and personality, which is so vital in the therapist's professional work.

PROFESSIONAL BODIES AND AWARDS

City and Guilds of London Institute

City and Guilds Beauty Therapist's Certificate 761 (2 year full time Further Education Course, United Kingdom)

This certificate covers all aspects of facial and body treatments, and is provided on a two-year basis at selected colleges throughout the British Isles. Students must be at least 18 years old, and have a minimum academic qualification of three 'O' level GCE subjects. Due to the competition for places, colleges can be very selective in their choice of applicant, and may demand a higher level of GCE passes than the minimum requirement. Tuition is divided between theoretical and practical aspects of therapy, permitting confidence to develop in client handling and practical techniques. The longer period of training makes this an ideal course for the younger woman, and allows skills to become established under the guidance of an experienced lecturer.

City and Guilds Certificate in Electrical Epilation. 761–3

Run in conjunction with the Beauty Therapist's Certificate, the training covers both theoretical and practical aspects of permanent hair removal by electrical methods. Students have the opportunity of clinical practice and can build up knowledge of individual case histories of clients during the training period. A minimum of 200 hours of practical epilation application is the requirement specified by the examination board, before students may enter for the final examinations. So this qualification denotes a very high standard of electrology skill and knowledge.

International Health and Beauty Council

*National Health and Beauty Council
(United Kingdom)
The International Beauty
Therapist's Diploma*

This course is more widely available, on a one or two-year basis, at Further Education Colleges, private schools, and training establishments. The course covers all aspects of salon work, facial and body treatments, figure improvement, and cosmetic applications, plus background theory relating to the practical subjects.

Some colleges in the United Kingdom combine the International Beauty Therapists course and the City and Guilds Beauty Therapist's Certificate, over a two-year period. In this way benefiting from the wide range of subjects covered, whilst establishing practical skills through salon sessions and client handling. Students are encouraged to undertake training in related subjects such as electrology, and remedial camouflage, during the two-year training period, to enhance their career prospects and extend their experience of remedial aspects.

More frequently the course is run independently over a one-year period and attracts a proportion of more mature applicants, who may have previous experience in nursing, commerce or cosmetic work.

The International Beauty Therapist's Diploma is one of the best known and respected of therapy qualifications available around the world.

*The Beauty Specialist's
Diploma*

The Beauty Specialist's Diploma covers all aspects of facial therapy, grooming treatments and arm and leg applications. It is often a forerunner to full therapy training, as the demand is increasingly to offer a full service requiring all-round qualifications. The beauty specialist's course is available on a one-year basis in the college situation, often followed by a further period of body work training. It is available in commercial schools, private training establishments etc., on a full or part-time basis, and provides full facial qualification, which is nationally recognized. The course covers practical and theoretical aspects of facial therapy, cosmetic and physical science, and business organization.

The Certificate in Epilation

Normally taught in conjunction with full-time therapy courses, to provide additional basic qualifications in electrology, and depilatory treatments.

*The Diploma in Advanced
Electrology*

The course covers advanced techniques of electrology, and is a progression from the Certificate in Epilation. Students must possess the certificate level of qualification, or be exempted by reason of alternative professional qualification, before they can commence training at the advanced level. The course covers specialized aspects of permanent hair removal, and minor cosmetic electrology, treatment of dilated capillaries, skin tags etc. A very high standard of practical and theoretical knowledge is required for successful completion of the course. Qualification is by examination only, covering both practical work and theoretical knowledge of anatomy, electro–physics, and the functions of the endocrine system.

Remedial Camouflage Diploma

This qualification covers all the techniques used to camouflage by cosmetic means, severe skin blemishes, scars, and pigmentation abnormalities. Also included is the cosmetic post-operative treatment of plastic surgery patients. Entry to training is restricted to those who already possess a basic beauty qualification in facial therapy, or who have considerable clinical experience or are concurrently training for a IHBC qualification. (Beauty Specialist's Diploma, or International Beauty Therapist's Diploma).

The Confederation of Beauty Therapy and Cosmetology

Esthéticienne Diploma Course

The Esthéticienne Diploma course covers facial and body therapy and electrology, and is organized by the British Association of Beauty Therapy and Cosmetology. It is examined by the Confederation of Beauty Therapy and Cosmetology, which is the British board recognized by CIDESCO and permitted to offer qualification to the international CIDESCO level, to students able to meet the necessary requirements.

On successful completion of the Esthéticienne Diploma course, having gained a pass rate of a minimum of 65% or over, in all sections of the exams, students at selected schools can take further studies to reach the CIDESCO standard of qualification. Approval to offer the CIDESCO course is only granted to a small number of schools and educational establishments in the United Kingdom at present. Normally available as a one-year full-time course in private schools, and two years in Further Education Colleges.

The Esthéticienne Diploma course taken independently has a minimum training period specified by the Confederation, and would normally be of 7–8 months in a private school, and a year in the Further Education College (due to educational vacations).

Beautician Diploma Course

This qualification covers all subjects relevant to a beauty operator, practising facials, manicures, makeup, waxing, eyelash tinting etc. The course duration is for 300 hours of training.

Electrolysis Diploma Course

Covering practical electrology and theoretical studies of anatomy, and electrical science. The course requirement is for 240 hours of study.

Le Comité Internationale D'Esthétiques et de Cosmetology (CIDESCO)

The international CIDESCO Diploma has been recognized for over 30 years and held in esteem in more than 27 countries around the world. The CIDESCO training is uniform in all countries, being of at least one year's duration, plus a probationary period of six months, before the full Diploma is granted. Training *must* be of at least 1200 hours duration, for practical and theoretical work, and covers facial and body therapy, cosmetic applications, treatment of the hands and feet, and waxing therapy. Study options are also offered, to extend the student's range of experience, and these can be tailored to the student's natural interests, and area of chosen work. The study options include electrical epilation, care of the breasts, scalp treatments, specialized massage, care of the body and rhythmical movement.

Students must be a minimum of 18 years old before they sit their final examinations, though many CIDESCO students are older than this minimum, as maturity of outlook is a very desirable asset for a therapist. Students are also expected to have a sound educational background, so that they may benefit from the training undertaken. With the courses offered in the United Kingdom, and examined by the Confederation of Beauty Therapy and Cosmetology, the entry requirements are for a minimum of 3 subjects at GCE 'O' level (or the equivalent, at the discretion of the college). Good oral and written ability in the language of the country, plus a sound background to the science studies are necessary. Anatomy, cosmetic science, and physics are all taught as related theory on the course, to support the understanding of the practical work.

Exacting conditions for recognition at a CIDESCO training school, as regards facilities, qualification and experience of staff, etc. ensure that a high standard of tuition is received, which will meet the international standard. After successful completion of the course, students must work in a first-class beauty centre for a further six months, after which they can apply for the full CIDESCO Diploma. This does ensure that only serious career-minded therapists are recognized by CIDESCO.

All these factors work towards enhancing, and maintaining the professional status of beauty therapists/aestheticiennes, wherever they work in the world. Through national and international conferences they are also able to keep up-to-date with their fast-changing profession, and get first-rate information on techniques, medical advances and the latest procedures in manual and electrical therapy.

International Therapy Examination Council (ITEC)

ITEC provides an independent examination system, which is widely recognized around the English speaking world. Qualifications are offered through registered training establishments, for all levels of facial and body therapy.

Beauty Therapy Diploma

The course covers both facial and body therapy, and the related theory of anatomy, electrical science, and cosmetic chemistry. Students are able to work in a practical situation, to gain clinical experience, at the same time as studying for the theory examinations.

Esthéticienne Diploma

Training covers the beauty aspects only of facial therapy, and is designed to concentrate on manual and electrical therapy, with related background theory.

Institute of Electrolysis Courses

The Institute offers associate or full membership to its potential students, depending on their age and general background. The associate member will normally attempt full membership when age and circumstances are acceptable to the Institute's Council. The main qualification, the Diploma in Remedial Epilation (DRE), is normally taught on a personal basis by a registered tutor within a clinic situation. The diploma course covers all aspects of skin and hair histology and demands an extremely high standard of operating technique in practical epilation. Training is normally full-time, available on a private basis, through tutors, and entry to the Institute's membership is by examination only.

PROFESSIONAL MEMBERSHIP

Beauty Education International

'Beauty Club'

An international organization whose aim is to raise the standards of beauty therapy by means of training, education, equipment information and supply, and management consultancy. The aim is to motivate, communicate within the beauty industry through membership, news letters, instructional material (books, tapes, etc.), and supply information about basic and post-graduate training.

Beauty Club acts as a reference point for all those involved in the beauty therapy industry, and keeps them informed of the latest developments in the field around the world. Membership is open to all those who work within the beauty industry or related fields—all are welcome to join and learn.

BENEFITS OF PROFESSIONAL MEMBERSHIP OF THERAPY AND ELECTROLOGY ORGANIZATIONS

Professional membership provides a means of keeping up to date with new techniques, equipment, and information, through periodic meetings, news bulletins, and social gatherings of members. It maintains a professional status for the members and serves to promote a high standard of practical and theoretical knowledge. It builds a good relationship with the medical profession and other well-known organizations, which creates a good working atmosphere based on mutual trust and respect.

Insurance for professional work is available either linked with annual membership, or is offered at preferential rates due to the level of skill acknowledged by the insurance companies.

Most beauty therapy organizations have a membership list or a national register of qualified operators, listing their qualifications, and range of treatments. These lists are available to the general public, either from private or press enquiries, or through public libraries, etc. This practice of joining the larger organizations is growing as younger operators see the advantages of gaining a professional status, which it is hoped will eventually lead to government recognition of the need for full registration to safeguard the public from untrained therapists.

USEFUL ADDRESSES

Professional Organizations and Examination Boards

Further information on courses available from the following Examination Boards and professional organizations:

Aestheticians' International Association Inc
5206 McKinney, Dallas, Texas, USA

American Electrolysis Association
710 Tennent Road, Englishtown, NJ07726, USA

Beauty Therapy Club

Ellison, Brindley Road South, Exhall Trading Estate, Exhall, Coventry, UK (Tel 0203 362505)

Esthetic and Beauty Supply, 180 Bentley Street, Markham, Ontario, Canada L3R 3L2
(Tel 479 2929)

The Association of Suntanning Operators
32 Grayshott Road, London, SW11, UK

Australian Federation of Aestheticians and Beauty Therapists
PO Box 2078, Brisbane, Queensland 4001, Australia

British Association of Beauty Therapy and Cosmetology
Sec. Mrs D. Parkes,
Suite 5, Wolesley House, Oriel Road, Cheltenham GL50 1TH, UK

British Association of Electrolysists
Sec. Hilary Peacock, 16 Quakers Mead,
Haddenham, Bucks HP17 8EB, UK

British Biosthetic Society
2 Birkdale Drive, Bury, Greater Manchester, BL8 2SG, UK

City and Guild of London Institute (Exam board for Beauty Therapy/Electrology)
46 Britannia Street, London, WC1 9RG, UK

CIDESCO—Le Comité International D'Esthétiques et de Cosmetology (International Exam Organization)

CIDESCO Secretariat, PO Box 9, A 1095, Vienna, Austria

Confederation of Beauty Therapy
and Cosmetology
Ed. Sec., Mrs B. Longhurst, 3 The Retreat,
Lidwells Lane, Goudhurst, Kent, UK

International Aestheticiennes (Independent
Examining Body for Beauty Industry)
First Floor, Regent House, Heaton Lane,
Stockport, UK

International Therapy Examination Council
(ITEC)
3 The Planes, Bridge Road, Chertsey, Surrey,
KT16 8LE, UK

Institute of Electrologists (Diploma in Remedial
Epilation—DRE)
Sec. Mrs E. Derbyshire, Lansdowne House,
251 Seymour Grove, Manchester, MI6 0DS, UK

National Federation of Health & Beauty
Therapists
PO Box 36, Arundel, West Sussex, BN18 0SW,
UK

The Northern Institute of Massage
100 Waterloo Road, Blackpool, FY4 1AW, UK

Skin Care Association of America
16 West 57 Street, New York, NY USA

South African Institute of Health
and Beauty Therapists
PO Box 56318, Pinegowrie 2123, J. Berg,
Republic of South Africa

MAGAZINES AND TRADE PUBLICATIONS

Beauty Therapy Club by Ann Gallant
(International Club for all those involved in the
Beauty Industry—publications/fact sheets/
guides/books/video tapes, etc)
details from Ellison, Brindley Road South,
Exhall Trading Estate, Exhall, Coventry, UK
(Tel 0203 362505)

Esthetic and Beauty Supply, 180 Bentley Street,
Markham, Ontario, Canada L3R 3L2
(Tel 479 2929)

Health & Beauty Salon Magazine
Hair & Beauty Magazine
Hairdressers Journal
Trade publications for the Hair and Beauty
Industries, details from Reed Business
Publishing, Quadrant House, The Quadrant,
Sutton, Surrey, UK
(Beauty Salon Magazine Editor—Ms Marion
Mathews) (Tel 01 661 3500)

Skin Care Magazine
The National Journal of Esthetics
140 Main Street, El Segundo, California 90245,
USA

Cosmetics Magazine
Specialists magazine for those involved with the
sales of cosmetics, toiletries, makeup, skin care
etc.
The Gooderham 'Flat Iron' Building,
49 Wellington Street East, Fourth Floor,
Toronto, Ontario, Canada M5E 1C9

International Beauty & Hair Route
Specialist magazine for electrologists, skin care
and esthetics, beauty therapists
Editor: Mr D. Copperthwaite
PO Box 313, Port Credit Postal Station,
Mississauga, Ontario, Canada

EQUIPMENT DESIGN AND DEVELOPMENT

Ann Gallant Clinic Design, and Equipment
Development through Ellison, Brindley Road
South, Exhall Trading Estate, Exhall, Coventry,
UK (Tel 0203 362505)

Esthetic and Beauty Supply, 180 Bentley Street,
Markham, Ontario, Canada L3R 3L2
(Tel 479 2929)

?MENT MANUFACTURERS

Ann Gallant Beauté Therapy Equipment
Esthetic and Beauty Supply, 180 Bentley Street,
Markham, Ontario, Canada L3R 3L2

Beauty Gallery Equipment by Ann Gallant,
manufactured by Ellison, Brindley Road South,
Exhall Trading Estate, Exhall, Coventry, UK
(Tel 0203 362505)

Cristal (Equipment)
86 Rue Pixérécourt, 75020 Paris, France

Depilex Ltd and Slimaster Beauty Equipment Ltd
Regent House, Dock Road, Birkenhead,
Merseyside, L41 1DG, UK

George Solly Organization Ltd
50A Queen Street, Henley-on-Thames, Oxon,
RG9 2DF, UK

Soltron Solarium and Sun Beds
Josef Kratz, Vertriebsgesellschaft mbH, Rottbize
Straße 69–5340, Bad Honnef 6, W. Germany

Silhouette International Beauty Equipment
Kenwood Road, Reddish, Stockport, Cheshire,
SK5 6PH, UK

Taylor Reeson Ltd
96–98 Dominion Road, Worthing, Sussex, UK

Nemectron Belmont Inc
17 West 56th Street, New York, NY 10019, USA

Simplex Spas
42b High Street, Cuckfield, Sussex, UK

HOF, House of Famuir
Beeston Grange, Sandy, Bedfordshire, SG19 1PG
UK

TREATMENT PRODUCT SUPPLIERS

Gallery Line—by Ann Gallant, Professional Clinic
and Resale Treatment Products/Ampoules, from
Ellison and Co Ltd, Brindley Road South, Exhall
Trading Estate, Exhall, Coventry, UK

Ann Gallant Beauté Therapy Products,
Professional Clinic and Resale Treatment
Products/Ampoules, from Esthetic and Beauty
Supply, 180 Bentley Street, Markham, Ontario,
Canada L3R 3L2

Arnould-Taylor Para-medical Products
Essential Oils, Specialized Masks, etc.
James House, Oakelbrook Mill, Newent, GL18
1HD, Glos, UK

Ella Baché
8 West 36th Street, New York, NY 10018, USA
and from Zena Cosmetics (UK) Ltd
5 Harrington Road, South Kensington, London,
SW7 3ES, UK

Eve Taylor Essential Oils
Blended Oils for Aromatherapy
Institute of Clinical Aromatherapy
22 Bromley Road, Catford, London, SE6 2TP,
UK

Clarins UK Ltd
150 High Street, Stratford, London, E15 2NE,
UK
Specialist skin care from France—oils, creams,
lotions of natural origin

Germaine de Capuccini, Professional Cosmetics
Mallorca, 81-08029 Barcelona, Spain
Advanced treatment and resale product line for all
aspects of facial and body care

Payot Ltd
139a New Bond Street, London, W1Y 9FB, UK
Specialist skin care preparations for professional
therapy and resale

Thalgo Cosmetic/Importex
5 Tristan Square, Blackheath, London, SE3 9UB,
UK
Sea-based natural skin care and body health
products.

Robertier Collection (Perfume)
Townsend Chambers, Amherst Hill, Sevenoaks,
Kent, TN13 3EL, UK

Lady Esther Cosmetics
L E Marketing Ltd, PO Box B143,
10–12 Westgate, Huddersfield, West Yorkshire,
UK
Makeup and nail product range

Robert Tisserand Aroma Cosmetics
Professional treatment oils for aromatherapy
from Hairdressing and Beauty Equipment Centre
262 Holloway Road, London, N7, UK

Elisabeth of Schwarzenberg/Andora Products
13 Windsor Street, Chertsey, Surrey,
KT16 8AY, UK
Specialized masks, creams, ampoules, skin care,
etc. for professional therapy

Pier Auge Cosmetics
from Harbourne Marketing Associates, Oak
House, 271 Kingston Road, Leatherhead, Surrey,
KT22 7PJ, UK

Yin Yang Beauty Care
45 Charlton Street, London, NW1 1HT, UK

Queen Cosmetics Ltd
Dept BS/D, 130 Wigmore Street, London,
W1H 0AT, UK
Hypoallergenic range of skin care and makeup for
professional use and resale

French Complexion
Symot House, 22a Reading Road, Henley-on-
Thames, Oxon, RG9 1AG, UK
Agents for French makeup and skin care range,
Jean Pierre Flurimon

Jean d'Aveze Cosmetics
Professional skin care
Information from Marie Odile, 1346B High
Road, London, N20, UK

Babor Treatment Products
from Malcolm James Ltd, 131 Clarence Gate
Gdns, London, NW1 6AN, UK

Cleor UK Ltd
Morle Consultancies, 176 Kensington High
Street, London, W8, UK
Specialized treatment products and oils for
professional beauty clinics

EQUIPMENT AND PRODUCT SUPPLIERS

Beauty Wholesalers to the Industry

Many of the larger wholesalers will act as agents for the equipment and products previously mentioned. They offer a comprehensive and convenient service to the beauty professional and offer most of the best names in the equipment and product business. Some also manufacture their own equipment and products or make it under licence to the international standard of the parent equipment or product company. Most wholesalers offer both cash and carry facilities (where good cash savings are made) and mail order services to help the busy professional. Technical help is usually available in the form of expert guidance about the equipment and products from an experienced therapist/sales person, and in the form of information sheets, catalogues, treatment guidance notes, or a mailing list offering the best buys currently available to help the therapist. The range of services now offered by the wholesalers is very comprehensive, and full clinic planning services are normally available if planning a new clinic or redesigning one. Most wholesalers can supply a full range of body, and skin care equipment, related treatment products, exercise equipment, saunas, sun beds, and spas, supplying the industry's every need on a national and international basis.

— E. A. Ellisons and Co Ltd, Brindley Road South, Exhall Trading Estate, Exhall, Coventry, UK (Tel 0203 362505)

Full range of equipment and products for the beauty industry, including the Beauty Gallery Range by Ann Gallant, the Gallery Line Clinic Product Line, and Beauty Club, information and technical advice to the industry—clinic planning, training, design and product devlopment. Technical advice from a trained therapist, training and demonstration clinic for full range of equipment, including Sterex, Duelli waxing systems, Sterex disposable epilation needles, Beauty Gallery equipment, Gallery Line products, plus full range of basic product lines for the hair and beauty industries.

Offers a most comprehensive and efficient service to the beauty professional with cash and carry, mail order, technical advice, planning assistance. Supplies everything needed for the therapist to achieve success in her business: equipment, products, knowledge, and friendly support.

— Esthetics and Beauty Supply, 16 Coldwater Road, Don Mills, Ontario M313 1Y7, Canada

Extensive range of equipment, supplies and services to the beauty therapist and esthetician, including the 'Ann Gallant' Beauté Therapy Equipment, skin and body care products, makeup and nail ranges, plus 'Beauty Club' for Canada and U.S.A. Able to supply a total service—from a complete package for a new business, to basic supplies for the beauty professional. Offers technical advice clinic planning, training, a wide choice of equipment, installation and service of equipment, plus a selection of products, makeup and nail lines for business success. A skilled and supportive service from trained therapists, with training and demonstation clinics, and in association with 'Ann Gallant' post graduate training and access to the latest international advances.

— Hairdressing and Beauty Equipment Centre, 262 Holloway Road, London, N7, UK

Comprehensive range of hairdressing and beauty equipment, agents for the Italian 'Dale' beauty equipment, for the aroma mist steamer, and for most leading makes of equipment, sun beds, spas, sauna, exercise and health related equipment. Not a manufacturer, but a stockist of a very comprehensive range of equipment. Not a supplier of products. Technical advice available from a trained therapist on the use of the equipment. Small training clinic.

— House of Famuir, Beeston Grange, Sandy, Bedfordshire, SG19 1PG, UK

Equipment and product supplier, and manufacturer of own range. Comprehensive range of salon supplies, wax, basic and specialized products fo professional therapy. Small training clinic an technical therapy advice available to aid the ther apist.

— Oritree Ltd, 3 Moxon Street, London, W1, U]

Full range of equipment and products, makeup wax supplies, nail products and many small resa] items to increase retail sales in the salon. Trainin clinic and technical advice available.

— Ashton and Fincher Ltd, 8 Holyhead Road Birmingham, B21 0LY, UK

Large group of wholesale/cash and carry supplie for the hairdressing and beauty industry, wit] bulk supplies, wax, towels, small range of beaut equipment. No training clinic or therapist fo technical advice. No information sheets/trainin guidance available, but help with choice of equip ment from experienced staff. An efficient an friendly service to therapists.

— Taylor Reeson Ltd, 96–98 Dominion Road Worthing, Sussex, UK

Comprehensive range of equipment, including that of their own manufacture, plus bulk prepara tions for salon use. Agents for GTE Italian equip ment. Suppliers of the Epitherm 'Hot bead ster ilizer', able to give advice on clinic layout. Nc trained therapist on the staff, but experienced staf able and willing to help with choice of equipment.

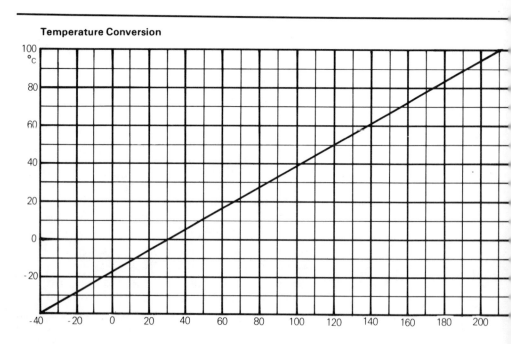

Temperature Conversion

Height Conversion

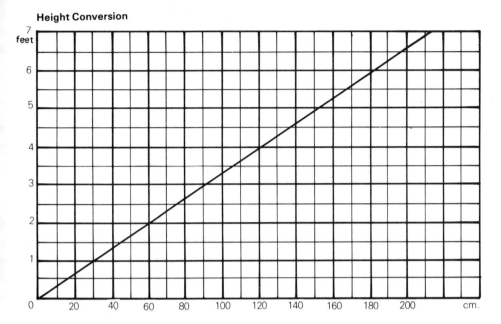

Measurements Conversion (inches/cm)

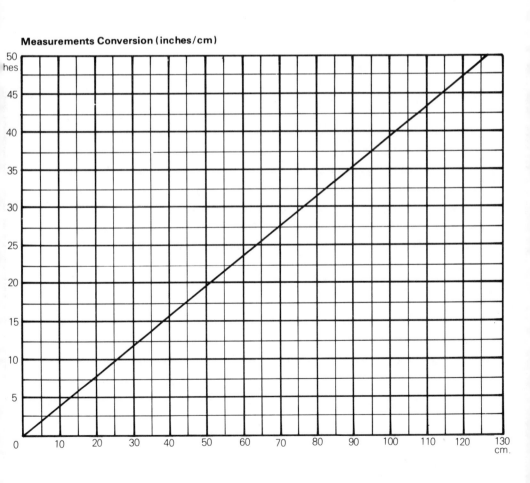

Volume Conversion

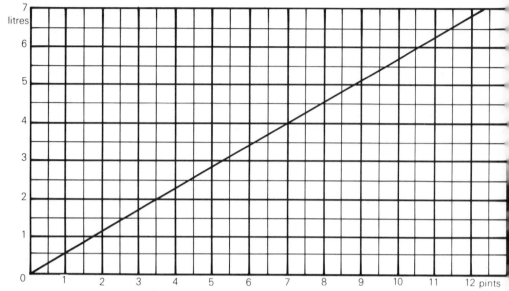

Weight Conversion

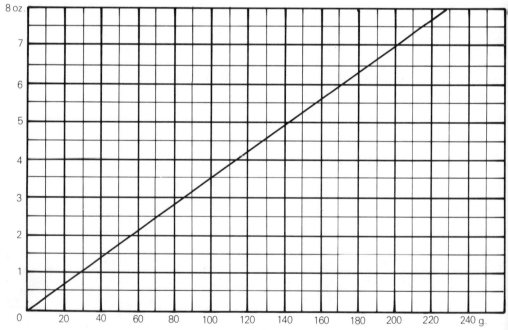